"CHEST PAIN" →

Edited by

J. Willis Hurst, MD
Consultant to the Division of Cardiology
Emory University School of Medicine
Former Professor and Chairman
Department of Medicine 1957–1986
Atlanta, Georgia

and

Douglas C. Morris, MD
Director, Emory Heart Center
J. Willis Hurst Professor and Vice Chair
Department of Medicine
Emory University
Atlanta, Georgia

Futura Publishing Co., Inc.
Armonk, NY

Library of Congress Cataloging-in-Publication Data

"Chest pain" / editors, J. Willis Hurst, Douglas C. Morris.
    p. ; cm.
Title presented in quotation marks, followed by right arrow symbol.
Includes bibliographical references and index.
ISBN 0-87993-482-4 (alk. paper)
    1. Chest pain. I. Chest Pain—etiology. 2. Angina Pectoris—diagnosis. 3.
Chest Pain—diagnosis. 4. Diagnosis, Differential. WF 970 C5255 2001]
RC941 . C569 2001
616.1—dc21   2001018961

Copyright © 2001

Futura Publishing Company, Inc.

Published by
Futura Publishing Company, Inc.
135 Bedford Road
Armonk, New York 10504
www.futuraco.com

LC #: 2001018961

ISBN #: 0-87993-482-4

Printed in the United States of America on acid-free paper.

Dedication

This book is dedicated to William Heberden, whose classic description of angina pectoris in 1768 is considered to be one of the great masterpieces of clinical observation.*

*The first description of angina pectoris was made by William Heberden at a meeting of the Royal College of Physicians in London in 1768. His discussion, entitled Some Account of a Disorder of the Breast, was published in 1786 in their Medical Transactions (II 59).

Preface

The purpose of this book and the explanation of its nonconventional title are discussed in detail in Chapter 1. Here, however, is a brief explanation for publishing yet another book.

We physicians have become sloppy in our assessment of "chest pain" at a time in history when we should be becoming more knowledgeable about the subject. We hear words such as "atypical chest pain" and "noncardiac chest pain" as the final diagnosis of patients who may have been subjected to several high-tech procedures. Patients know that those words are not diagnoses, as do referring physicians who send their patients for the high-tech procedures. These designations reflect the fact that the consulting physician has been unable or unwilling to resolve the problem and the lack of resolution renders appropriate therapy impossible. Accordingly, the patient's problem remains incompletely addressed, unresolved, and unrelieved, and both the patient and referring physician are poorly served.

The format used in each chapter was designed to emphasize the approach physicians should use in their effort to identify the cause of "chest pain." We obviously have not listed and discussed all causes of "chest pain" in this book. As time passes other conditions will be added, but we believe the list of conditions we have included in this little book is a fair beginning.

I appreciate the help of the authors who were willing to use the format designed for each chapter. I thank Patsy Bryan for converting the crude diagrams made by the authors into interesting illustrations. I thank Carol Miller for her tireless effort in preparing the manuscript. I thank Mr. Steven Korn, Chairman of the Board of Futura Publishing Company, who immediately grasped the need for such a book and discussed its development with me on numerous occasions. I also thank the very talented Kirstin Bellhouse, also at Futura, who shepherded the book through the publishing process.

Finally, as always, I thank my wife, Nelie, who wonders when I will put my pen down. No Nelie—no book.

J. Willis Hurst, MD

I thank Dr. Hurst for allowing me to accompany him in this project. The project was the result of an idea of Dr. Hurst's which arose from our early morning sessions with the medical house staff at Emory University Hospital.

I hope the book hearkens us back to a time when the history of the patient's illness was diligently and earnestly elicited, carefully recorded, and studiously pondered. Weren't we all taught that the patient's history was the most valuable part of the data base? Yet, today the tendency is to hurriedly dismiss the history as inaccurate, uninterpretable, or irrelevant in a rush to accept some high-tech approach as the purveyor of the "truth." We toss it aside in favor of some high-tech approach.

I also thank my wife, Terry, for allowing me to intrude on "family time" to join Dr. Hurst in this endeavor.

Douglas C. Morris, MD

Contributors

Rabih R. Azar, MD, MSc
Assistant Clinical Professor of
  Medicine
University of California, San
  Francisco
Division of Cardiology
San Francisco General Hospital
San Francisco, California

S. Wright Caughman, MD
Professor and Chairman
Department of Dermatology
Emory University School of
  Medicine
Atlanta, Georgia

Richard O. Cannon III, MD
Acting Chief, Cardiology Branch,
  NHLBI
National Institutes of Health
Bethesda, Maryland

Stephen D. Clements, Jr., MD
Professor of Medicine (Cardiology)
Emory University School of
  Medicine
Atlanta, Georgia

Karen Drexler, MD
Assistant Professor
Department of Psychiatry and
  Behavioral Sciences
Emory University School of
  Medicine
Atlanta, Georgia

Marc D. Feldman, MD
Medical Director, Center for
  Psychiatric Medicine
Vice Chair, Clinical Services
Director, Division of Adult
  Psychiatry
Professor, Department of Psychia-
  try & Behavioral Neurobiology
University of Alabama at
  Birmingham
Birmingham, Alabama

Bernard L. Frankel, MD
Professor; Director, Consultant
  Liaison Psychiatry
Department of Psychiatry
Emory University School of
  Medicine
Atlanta, Georgia

Michelle M. Freemer, MD
Pulmonary and Critical Care
  Fellow
University of California, San
  Francisco
San Francisco, California

Steve Goldschmid, MD
Section Head, Gastroenterology
Associate Professor of Medicine
University of Arizona
Tucson, Arizona

Andrew P. Gutow, MD
Assistant Professor
Department of Orthopaedic
  Surgery
Emory University School of
  Medicine
Chief of Orthopaedic Surgery
Atlanta Veterans Affairs Medical
  Center
Atlanta, Georgia

Jessica Haberer, MD
Medical Resident, 2nd Year
University of California, San
  Francisco
Department of Medicine
San Francisco, California

James C. Hamilton, Ph.D.
Assistant Professor of Psychology
Department of Psychology
University of Alabama
Tuscaloosa, Alabama

David J. Hewitt, MD
Assistant Professor of Neurology
Emory University School of
  Medicine
Atlanta, Georgia

J. Willis Hurst, MD
Consultant to the Division of Car-
  diology
Emory University School of
  Medicine
Former Professor and Chairman
Department of Medicine 1957–1986
Atlanta, Georgia

Talmadge E. King, Jr., MD
Constance B. Wofsy Distinguished
  Professor of Medicine and Vice
  Chairman, Department of
  Medicine
University of California, San
  Francisco
San Francisco, California

Joseph Lindsay, Jr., MD
Director of the Section of
  Cardiology
Washington Hospital Center
Washington, D.C.

Calvin O. McCall, MD
Assistant Professor of Dermatology
Emory University School of
  Medicine
Atlanta, Georgia

Joseph I. Miller, Jr., MD
Professor of Surgery
Division of Cardiothoracic Surgery
and Chief of General Thoracic
  Surgery
Department of Surgery
Emory University School of
  Medicine
Atlanta, Georgia

Stephen B. Miller, MD
Professor of Medicine
Emory University School of
  Medicine
Atlanta, Georgia

Douglas C. Morris, MD
Director, Emory Heart Center
J. Willis Hurst Professor and Vice
  Chair
Department of Medicine
Emory University
Atlanta, Georgia

Joseph K. Perloff, MD
Streisand/American Heart
  Association
Professor of Medicine and
  Pediatrics
Director, Ahmanson/UCLA Adult
Congenital Heart Disease Center
Los Angeles, California

Robert C. Schlant, MD
Professor of Medicine (Cardiology)
Emory University School of
  Medicine
Atlanta, Georgia

Mark E. Silverman, MD
Professor of Medicine (Cardiology)
Emory University School of
  Medicine
Chief of Cardiology, The Fuqua
  Heart Center of Atlanta
Piedmont Hospital
Atlanta, Georgia

David H. Spodick, MD, D.Sc
Director, Cardiovascular
  Fellowship Training
Saint Vincent Hospital at
  Worcester Medical Center
Professor of Medicine
University of Massachusetts
  Medical School
Worcester, Massachusetts

Vinod H. Thourani, MD
Senior Resident in General Surgery
Thoracic Surgery
Department of Surgery
Emory University School of
  Medicine
Atlanta, Georgia

Paul F. Walter, MD
Professor of Medicine
Cardiologist—Electrophysiologist
Emory University School of
  Medicine
Atlanta, Georgia

J. Patrick Waring, MD
Professor of Medicine
Emory University School of
  Medicine
Atlanta, Georgia

David Waters, MD
Chief of Cardiology
San Francisco General Hospital
Professor of Medicine
University of California, San
  Francisco
San Francisco, California

Nanette K. Wenger, MD
Professor of Medicine
Emory University School of
  Medicine
Division of Cardiology
Consultant, Emory Heart and
  Vascular Center
Chief of Cardiology
Grady Memorial Hospital
Atlanta, Georgia

Byron R. Williams, MD
Linton Bishop Professor of
  Medicine
Emory University School of
  Medicine
Chief of Cardiology
Crawford W. Long Hospital
Atlanta, Georgia

Contents

PART VII
Diseases of the Gastrointestinal Tract as a Cause for "Chest Pain"

PART VIII
Diseases of the Gallbladder as a Cause of "Chest Pain"

PART XI
"Chest Pain" Caused by Diseases of the Aorta

PART XII
"Chest Pain" Related to Emotional or Psychiatric Conditions

PART XIII
"Chest Pain" of Controversial Origin

PART XIV
Final Comments

An Explanation of the Title and General Comments

J. Willis Hurst, MD

An Explanation of the Title

The unusual title of this book is "Chest Pain" →. The uniqueness of this title lies in the fact that there are quotation marks around the words *"chest pain"* and an arrow follows them. The reason for these markings is described in the following sentences.

The word *"chest"* is enclosed in quotation marks to indicate that patients sometimes have an odd view as to anatomic landmarks that identify the location of the chest. Accordingly, the word *"chest,"* as used in this book, is defined as being located from the waist up. The physician should ask the patient to demonstrate where the unpleasant sensation is located. The patient should respond to the request by using one of his or her fingers to *circumscribe the area of "pain."* The patient's response will immediately disclose useful information to the physician regarding the *location* and *size* of the area of discomfort. The use of a diagram of the anterior and posterior view of the *"chest"* to illustrate the location of the patient's *"chest pain"* in the subsequent chapters of this book emphasizes the importance we place on these features (see Figures 1–1 and 1–2).

William Heberden used the words *angina pectoris*—or *"strangling in the chest"*—to describe the symptom we now recognize as being due to myocardial ischemia.[1] He did not know the cause of the *"chest"* discomfort, but realized that it was serious because some of the patients who were afflicted with it subsequently died.

Heberden also wrote that one of his patients had an *"uneasy sensation in his left arm"* while walking. This account documented that Heberden re-

From: Hurst JW, Morris DC (eds): *"Chest Pain"* →. © Futura Publishing Co., Inc., Armonk, NY, 2001.

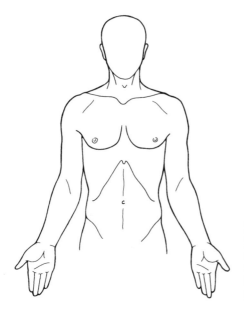

Figure 1–1. Frontal view of the upper portion of the human body. The size and location of the "chest pain" described in this book will be illustrated on diagrams that are similar to this one.

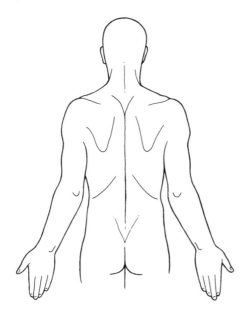

Figure 1–2. The upper portion of the human body as viewed from the back. The size and location of the "chest pain" described in this book will be illustrated on diagrams that are similar to this one.

alized that the pain of angina pectoris was not always limited to the *pectoral* region. We now know that the *"pain"* of angina pectoris may radiate to non-chest locations and may be located solely in the jaw, neck, left or right arm, elbow, wrist, back, etc.

Therefore, because the *"chest"* is thought by patients to be located from the waist up, and because the discomfort may be felt in areas others than the actual chest, the word *"chest"* is enclosed within quotations marks.

The word *"pain"* is enclosed in quotation marks for the following reason. As mentioned above, Heberden, in his early classic description of the condition, used the words angina pectoris which means *strangling* in the chest.[1,2] Every word imaginable has been used by patients, including physicians who are patients, to describe the unpleasant feeling in the *"chest"* that is labeled angina pectoris. The adjectives used by patients to describe the discomfort range from "terrible pain" to "a sternal whisper." The physician must try to find the word a patient uses and, having found it, use it whenever he or she talks with the patient about the *"chest pain."* For example, I always asked one of my patients who felt a *shoe box* in his chest when he walked, "How is your shoe box, Mr. Smith?"

The *arrow* following the words *"chest pain"* has a specific purpose. It indicates that the doctor does not know the cause of the patient's *"chest pain"* and that a differential diagnosis must be listed. To further explain—Larry Weed created the *problem-oriented record* in 1967.[3] It has four components: The *Defined Data Base,* the *Problem List,* the *Initial Plans,* and *Progress Notes.* By adhering to this organizational structure, the physician will proceed in an orderly, stepwise fashion from the accumulation and recording of data, to the cataloguing of the problems, to formulating plans for further resolution and management of these problems, and finally to charting the progression of the patient through this management scheme. When the information available is sufficient to allow the physician to resolve the problem to a specific diagnosis, this diagnosis should be numbered, titled, and stated on the *Problem List.* When the doctor identifies symptoms, physical findings, or abnormalities in the "routine" laboratory examination, but lacks sufficient data to make a specific diagnosis, he or she should state what is known with certainty on the *Problem List.* Such a poorly resolved statement should be followed with an *arrow* (→). The arrow signals that the doctor does not know, at that point in time, what the cause of the abnormality is. Undiagnosed *"chest pain"* falls in that category. An arrow after such a designation implies that the physician must create a differential diagnosis based on the data he or she has collected. The list of possibilities composing the differential diagnosis should be included in the *Initial Plans* of the problem. It is never acceptable to write "rule out angina" on the *Problem List* or the *Initial Plans* because to do so avoids the thought-process needed to create a differential diagnosis. When such an entry is placed on the *Problem*

List or *Initial Plans,* one wonders if the doctor knows the characteristics of conditions other than angina or if he or she is only interested in angina. Also, it is never acceptable to write "probably angina" on the *Problem List.* Here again, the problem should be stated as *"chest pain"*→ and a differential diagnosis should be developed and listed in the *Initial Plans.*

General Comments

"Chest pain" is a common complaint and may be caused by a myriad of conditions. The complaint may signal the presence of a serious and potentially lethal disease, or a worrisome but benign problem. The reaction of the patients with the complaint varies considerably; they may belittle or ignore the complaint when it is caused by a serious disease, or be disabled from the discomfort when it is due to an innocuous condition. Surprisingly, such responses by the patient may occur irrespective of the patient's knowledge of the cause of the discomfort. The most peculiar aspect of the problem is that the severity of the *"chest pain"* does not always parallel the seriousness of the disease that causes it. For example, the patient with life-threatening unstable angina pectoris may experience only mild "chest" discomfort while the patient with brachial plexus neuropathy may have *excruciating pain* although life is not threatened. The patient may confuse the physician by having two or more different causes of "chest pain." This, of course, challenges the diagnostic ability of the most skilled physicians.

The Approach to the Patient

The acquisition of information and its interpretation are the most important parts of the examination of the patient. The nascent physician may not believe that a peculiar type of *"chest pain"* is really due to coronary atherosclerotic heart disease. He or she may label the complaint as atypical chest pain. With more experience, however, he or she may refer to the same complaint, as "another patient with angina pectoris in whom the discomfort is located in what I formerly thought was a strange and atypical location."

At times, the abnormalities found on the physical examination identify a clinical setting in which a certain etiology of *"chest pain"* is likely to be present, but this does not eliminate the possibility that some other condition is responsible for the "pain." For example, a patient with the physical findings associated with thoracic outlet syndrome may also have angina pectoris due to coronary atherosclerotic heart disease.

The physician must remember also that the discovery of an abnormality that could cause the *"chest pain"* using a high-tech procedure does not guarantee that the patient's complaint is caused by the condition that has been discovered. Great skill is often needed to determine that the "chest pain" is actually caused by the abnormality found using high-tech procedures.

The characteristics of the patient's *"chest pain"* are so important that this aspect of the examination of the patient is emphasized in this book. *The time-honored statement is still true today—it takes a lifetime for physicians to learn how to take a history.* This difficulty occurs because the patient must be able to relate how he or she feels and the physician must be an excellent listener and highly skilled at the interpretation of the patient's statements. Generally speaking, nascent physicians can't do that—it takes years of diligent work to learn how to elicit an accurate history from a patient. Also, physicians who are the most skilled realize that it takes various lengths of time to elicit the history of individual patients. A system of health care delivery that does not allow the physician sufficient time to elicit an accurate account of the patient's symptoms will be responsible for erroneous diagnoses and the misuse of expensive high technology.

We agree with the brilliant Paul Wood[4] who in 1956 wrote the following page about history taking. (The passage is reproduced here with the permission of the publisher.[4])

> To take an accurate and relevant history is one of the most difficult and important arts in medicine. Sometimes, a complete diagnosis can be made from the history alone, and not infrequently the possibilities can be whittled down to two or three. A good history should at least indicate the system involved, or it should point unerringly to some group or groups of diseases. A common mistake is the failure to analyse any given symptom sufficiently; in cardiovascular work this applies especially to pain, breathlessness, palpitations, and syncope. The student is usually taught to encourage the patient to tell his story in his own words, and to record them more or less verbatim. Yet such an account may be verbose, irrelevant, inaccurate, and misleading. It is an axiom that the leading question must be avoided at all cost; yet again, an experienced physician must know that the ability to put the appropriate leading question at the right moment, and the intelligent interpretation of its reply, are invaluable. It is not pretended that leading questions may not lead to false information, if the power of their suggestion is not appreciated by the questioner; and it is agreed that much may be lost by failure to allow the patient freedom and time to express his complaints in his own way; but the average patient will not mention half the available information until he is pressed, and the data freely given must be checked as at the bar. For example, in the differential diagnosis between a neural and non-neural somatic lesion, an accurate description of the quality of the pain may determine the issue immediately; yet the majority of patients will volunteer no information concerning the quality of pain, and if asked to describe it will do so inadequately. They may say it is aching or sharp, but fail to enlarge on this, even when urged to do so. In answer to the leading question, "Does it tingle?", however, they may reply at once in the affirmative.

It is essential to realize that the matter does not end there: that such a positive reply to a leading question demands the most penetrating cross-examination, until the questioner is satisfied that the pain really does tingle, and that the patient is not merely saying so because it seems the easier answer. It is scarcely too much to say that the best history-taker is he who can best interpret the answer to a leading question. Appropriate leading questions can only be asked, however, when the proffered history has provided sufficient data upon which to work, and if the physician has sufficient knowledge of the possibilities then entailed. It is this latter factor which makes it easier for the expert than for the student.[4]

The famous Sam Levine knew how to ask a leading question that was not misleading. He would ask a patient, "I suppose your chest discomfort is worse walking down hill and is relieved walking up hill?[5] If the patient replied, "Absolutely not, the reverse is true," then from such a response, Dr. Levine knew he had not misled the patient by his leading question because the response of the patient was counter to the insinuation expressed in the question. With such a reply from the patient, he diagnosed angina pectoris with considerable confidence.

I cannot close this introductory chapter without emphasizing two additional facets of the problem.

It is not uncommon for patients to make their own diagnosis as to the etiology of their chest pain. Advertisements on television hawking the value of certain drugs that are said to relieve indigestion due to gastroesophageal reflux reinforces the erroneous view that the patient can diagnose their own *"chest pain."* Such advertising does a great disservice because, we must always remember, years ago sudden death, undoubtedly due to coronary atherosclerotic heart disease, was thought to be caused by "indigestion."

Doctors may fall into the same trap of self-diagnosis. One of my physician patients diagnosed his chest discomfort as tracheitis even though it only occurred when he mowed the lawn. He actually took antibiotics for the complaint. He finally realized that he might have "coronary pain" when he developed prolonged, severe, retrosternal "pain" which signaled, even to him, that he was having a "heart attack."

One could believe that the physician mentioned above had little knowledge of the "chest pain" due to myocardial ischemia. To contradict that view it is worth recalling the events associated with the "chest pain" experienced by Dr. Paul Wood himself. Paul Wood was, without argument, the leading cardiovascular clinician of the fifties and sixties. He was a master diagnostician. He wrote in the 1956 edition of his book, *Diseases of the Heart and Circulation,* the following sentences which are reproduced with the permission of the publisher.[6]

A second point of general interest is that patients rarely appreciate what is a heart symptom and what is not. The most classical example of this is the well-known paradox that patients with angina pectoris (including doctors) often complain of indigestion, whereas those with dyspepsia or left inframammary pain may be convinced that their hearts are at fault.[6]

Note he realized that doctors also misdiagnosed angina pectoris as indigestion and by inferences suggests that the psychological trick of *denying* the presence of a serious disease occurs in physicians as well as in members of the public at large.

Now let us look at Paul Wood's reaction to his own "chest pain." According to the classic historic account by Mark Silverman, MD and Walter Somerville, MD, Paul Wood himself fell into the common trap of misdiagnosing himself. The passage is reproduced here with permission from Excerpta Medica, Inc.[7] They wrote:

> . . . That weekend, while wrestling with weeds in his garden pool, he experienced "indigestion." Two days later, while seeing patients in his private consulting room at 44 Wimpole Street, Wood again complained of indigestion and took several antacid tablets that did not relieve his discomfort. An electrocardiogram, taken by his secretary, displayed ST-segment elevation in the inferolateral leads.[7]

A final comment is added here to emphasize that physicians must know their patients as persons in order to elicit an accurate history. A hasty inquiry will often mislead the doctor and an intense interrogation of the patient, as performed by lawyers, is not the way to obtain accurate information. By this I do not mean that the physician must have known the patient as a person for a considerable period of time—I simply mean that the physician must develop the skill required to understand the patient's personality and how it influences his or her responses to questions. Doctors must be aware of the emotional makeup of patients because it may influence the symptoms themselves or alter the ability of patients to describe their symptoms to others, including their physicians.

References

1. Heberden W. Some account of a disorder of the breast. *Med Trans Coll of Physns London*, 1772;Vol II:59–67.
2. Heberden W. Commentaries on the History and Cure of Diseases. In *Angina Pectoris*. Printed for T. Tayne, News-Gate, London, 1802, pp. 366.
3. Weed LL. Medical Records, Medical Education, and Patient Care. Chicago, IL, The Press of Case Western Reserve University, 1969, pp 1–273.
4. Wood P. Diseases of The Heart and Circulation, 2nd ed. Philadelphia, PA, JB Lippincott Company, 1956, p 1.
5. Levine S. Personal communication.
6. Wood P. Diseases of The Heart and Circulation, 2nd ed. Philadelphia, PA, JB Lippincott Company, 1956, p 2.
7. Silverman ME, Somerville W. To die in one's prime: The story of Paul Wood. *Am J Cardiol* 2000;85:75–88.

Part I

Skin Disease as a Cause for "Chest Pain"

Although the definition of "chest pain"→ is discussed in Chapter 1, the definition is repeated here so that communication is clear.

The quotation marks around "chest" imply that different patients have different definitions of the word "chest." Here we use the word to indicate pain located above the waist. Then, too, *angina pectoris* is not always located in the pectoral region—it may be felt only in the jaw, neck, shoulder, elbow, or wrist. Therefore, the word "chest" implies that other parts of the upper body may also be involved with painful syndromes.

The quotation marks around "pain" imply that patients may assign other terms to their discomfort, such as indigestion, burning, ache, etc.

The arrow after "chest pain" implies that the physician initially may not know the cause of the symptom, so a differential diagnosis must be established that fits the available information.

2

"Chest Pain" in Patients with Herpes Zoster (Shingles)

Calvin O. McCall, MD and S. Wright Caughman, MD

General Considerations

Herpes zoster (shingles) is the reactivation of a latent varicella-zoster virus infection of sensory nerves. It typically produces a painful, unilateral, vesicular eruption in a dermatomal pattern, often involving the chest. Atypical presentations can occur in which the classic eruption is absent. Such presentations cause diagnostic confusion because the pain of herpes zoster can mimic visceral pain, including the pain due to myocardial ischemia.

Clinical Setting

Varicella (chickenpox), the precursor of herpes zoster, is a disease of childhood. Herpes zoster can occur at any time after varicella, but it is uncommon in childhood. The incidence of herpes zoster increases with age. The majority of patients are affected after the age of 50 years. It equally affects both sexes[1] and all races.[2] Although many patients have only one episode, recurrent episodes of herpes zoster are possible, especially in immunocompromised patients.

Characteristics of the "Pain"

Patient's characterization of the "chest pain"

The course of herpes zoster and the accompanying pain can be divided into the prodrome, the eruption, and postherpetic neuralgia. In all

From: Hurst JW, Morris DC (eds): *"Chest Pain"* →. © Futura Publishing Co., Inc., Armonk, NY, 2001.

stages the patient typically reports unilateral pain, but with variable characteristics.

Prodromal pain is of most significance in the differential diagnosis of "chest pain" because it may occur several days prior to the appearance of any cutaneous signs. At this stage of the disease some patients perceive the pain as intense and localized, while others find it vague and difficult to localize. It may be described as sharp, stabbing, shooting, or boring. It may also be described as a deep aching, burning, or itching. Generally the pain is most intense in a single dermatome, but it is not unusual for it to involve one or more adjacent dermatomes. The pain may be constant or intermittent, and it may radiate. Radiation may involve any contiguous part of the body including the patient's arm, lateral neck, or jaw.

The character of herpes zoster pain may change and the origin of the pain becomes apparent once the cutaneous eruption appears. The presence of erythema and vesicles may be accompanied by an increased sensation of itching and burning. This itching and burning may replace or be superimposed on preexisting painful sensations. The vesicles persist for 2 to 3 weeks before they dry, become crusted, and resolve.

After the eruption fades, some patients (especially the elderly) continue to have pain known as post herpetic neuralgia. This pain remains most intense in the affected dermatome(s), may be constant or intermittent, and may radiate. Patients describe this pain similarly to that of the prodrome, but it may be more easily triggered by tactile stimulation. If the disease has followed a characteristic course and the patient is an adequate historian, the etiology of post herpetic neuralgia is obvious and does not present diagnostic confusion. However, in cases with minimal cutaneous findings or a poor history, the origin of post herpetic neuralgia may be difficult to determine, presenting the same diagnostic confusion as with prodromal pain.

Common location of the "chest pain"

The pain associated with herpes zoster is typically unilateral and concentrated in one to three dermatomes, most often in the thoracic region.[1,3] As shown in Figures 2–1 through 2–4, herpes zoster can cause retrosternal, left or right sided chest pain, often accompanied by left or right flank and left back pain. The pain may also radiate to the left side of the neck, shoulder and arm. This left or right thoracic presentation is further illustrated in Figure 2–5. The pain associated with such a presentation can easily be confused with the pain of angina pectoris or myocardial infarction, but, when present, the cutaneous signs allow the correct diagnosis to be made.

Additionally, herpes zoster is common in the distribution of the trigeminal nerve. Although not likely to cause pain in the thorax, involvement of the trigeminal nerve may be associated with unilateral pain in the neck and jaw that can be confused with the pain of myocardial ischemia or infarction.

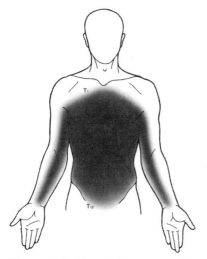

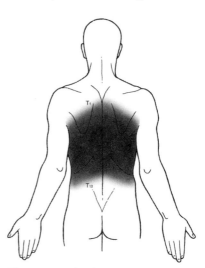

Figure 2–1. The dark area on the frontal view of the chest indicates where the pain of herpes zoster may be located. The pain itself does not occupy the entire black area; it is limited to a dermatome(s) within the area.

Figure 2–2. The dark area on the back of the chest indicates where the pain of herpes zoster may be located. The pain itself does not occupy the entire black area; it is limited to a dermatome(s) within the area.

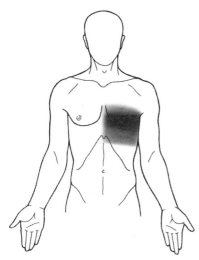

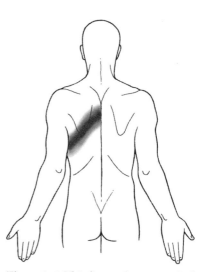

Figure 2–3. This figure shows a typical frontal distribution of the pain of herpes zoster. The black area indicates the location of severe pain in the dermatome. The gray area indicates the spread of less severe pain to adjacent tissue.

Figure 2–4. This figure shows a typical distribution of the pain of herpes zoster on the back. The black area indicates the location of severe pain in the dermatome. The gray area indicates the spread of less severe "pain" to adjacent tissue.

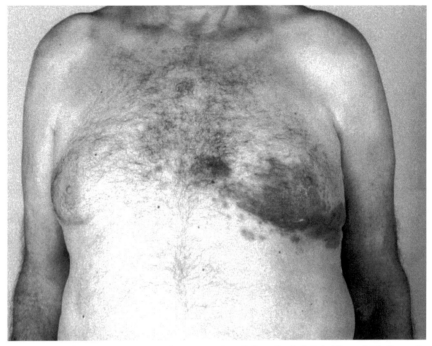

Figure 2–5. Herpes zoster, eruptive stage, involving the left 3rd, 4th, and 5th thoracic dermatomes.

Uncommon location of the "chest pain"

The pain of herpes zoster is less easily localized than is the associated cutaneous eruption; thus, it is more likely to be perceived as crossing the midline. Some patients report symmetric, bilateral pain but this is unusual. Also unusual is pain localized to the entire trunk, or only in the midline of the chest or abdomen.

Size of the "painful" area

The pain of zoster can involve an area as small as several centimeters, or it may involve one entire half of the trunk. More typically the pain involves all or most of a unilateral dermatome and its adjacent dermatomes.

Duration of the "chest pain"

The pain of classic zoster must be divided into three stages. The pro-dromal pain typically lasts 1–3 days. Pain associated with the eruptive stage may last 1–3 weeks. As the eruptive phase clears the pain may sub-side, or persist as post herpetic neuralgia. Unfortunately, post herpetic neuralgia may persist for months to years and cause considerable mor-bidity and even debilitation.

Tenderness of the chest wall

Tenderness to palpation and hyperesthesia in the affected area may occur during all stages of the disease.

Precipitating causes of the "chest pain"

Movement of the affected region and tactile stimulation of the over-lying skin are often reported to aggravate the pain.

Relief of the "chest pain"

Rest, narcotic and non-narcotic analgesics will usually relieve the pain during the prodromal and eruptive stages. Post-herpetic neuralgia may require additional measures (see "Treatment"). However, more valuable than any active intervention, the passage of time improves the pain of herpes zoster.

Associated Symptoms

In a minority of patients, cutaneous sensory deficits will occur in re-gions affected by herpes zoster. The patient may report numbness or tin-gling in the affected region. In less than 5% of patients, motor paralysis, in-cluding motor dysfunction of the limbs, diaphragm, and bladder will occur in areas served by motor nerves that are contiguous with the in-volved sensory nerves.[2] These dysfunctions may occur with typical herpes zoster or with zoster sine herpete (see below). Complete recovery of sen-sory and motor function occurs in most cases.

Associated Signs

Physical examination

Although the patient may present with pain, early in the course of her-pes zoster there may be no signs of cutaneous disease. Patients in severe pain may appear agitated, splint the affected area, appear tachypnic—

breathing rapid, shallow breaths—but diaphoresis is uncommon. Erythema is usually the first cutaneous sign and the patient may report burning or itching in the erythematous area. Initially the erythema is faint without induration. In time, the affected area may become indurated and clearly dermatomal, but in many cases the erythema is patchy and only roughly confined to a given dermatome. In most cases palpable, pinpoint vesicles develop in the erythematous region. Initially, the vesicles may be too small for the clinician to appreciate that they are fluid-filled and they may be mistaken for papules. When the lesions are large enough for adequate visualization, their vesicular quality becomes clear. The vesicles concentrate in one dermatome and its adjacent dermatomes. Scattered distant vesicles are not uncommon but there should be less than twenty-five outside the main area of involvement.[2] Late in the disease process the vesicles may become cloudy and may be characterized as pustules. Erosions and shallow ulcerations eventually develop in severe cases or those cases complicated by bacterial infection. The erosions and ulcerations are also usually dermatomal and often result in segmental scarring or pigmentary changes that may persist for months to years after resolution of active disease.

"Routine" laboratory tests

Routine laboratory tests reveal no specific abnormality.

Exceptions to the Usual Manifestations

Generally, patients present in mild to moderate distress regardless of the stage of their disease. It is unusual for a patient to complain of marked systemic symptoms; however, occasionally malaise, headache, and fever are significant enough for the patient to seek medical attention. Infrequently, patients present in acute distress with extreme pain, nausea and vomiting, shortness of breath, or diaphoresis.

Though most often diagnosed by its dermatomal distribution, herpes zoster and its associated pain can persist for days to weeks with no cutaneous signs. This is known as zoster sine herpete.[4] The exact frequency of this presentation is unknown, but it is assumed to be infrequent. It is also uncommon for lesions to significantly involve more than one dermatome and its adjacent dermatomes. Blisters spanning four or more dermatomes, numerous distant lesions (>25), and dissemination of lesions suggest the patient may be immunocompromised. Impairment of cellular immunity may lead to widespread disease with marked systemic manifestations.

Differential Diagnosis

The differential diagnosis of "chest pain" is limited for patients presenting during the eruptive stage of herpes zoster, or for those presenting with a history of a typical zosteriform eruption. Few entities can be confused with a unilateral, dermatomal eruption that consists of blisters or erosions grouped on erythematous skin. Dermatomal herpes simplex, which may be painful and recurrent, can enter the differential. Early varicella may also appear dermatomal but is seldom painful. A very unusual occurrence is metastasis, particularly of carcinoma from the lung, to the chest wall in a dermatomal pattern. This may be painful but will not likely present confusion in the evaluation of "chest pain".

The differential diagnosis is more extensive when evidence of a unilateral, vesicular eruption is absent. Table 2–1 illustrates some of the differential diagnostic considerations.

Other Diagnostic Testing

Several laboratory procedures and research tools can be used to confirm the clinical diagnosis or assist in establishing the diagnosis in difficult cases of herpes zoster. The most common procedure used is the Tzanck

Table 2–1.		
Differential Diagnosis of "Chest Pain" in Herpes Zoster.		
Prodromal stage	*Eruptive stage*	*Post-herpetic neuralgia*
angina pectoris	varicella, early	Sensory involvement only
myocardial infarction	dermatomal herpes	myocardial infarction
pleurisy	simplex	pleurisy
gastroesophageal reflux	thermal or chemical burn	gastroesophageal reflux
duodenal ulcer	contact dermatitis	duodenal ulcer
cholecystitis	metastatic carcinoma	cholecystitis
bilary colic		bilary colic
renal colic		renal colic
appendicitis		appendicitis
musculoskeletal pain		musculoskeletal pain
intervertebral disk		intervertebral disk
disease		disease
dermatomal herpes		With motor involvement
simplex		cerebral vascular
		accident
		peripheral nerve
		damage

preparation, a cytologic examination of the blister contents for multinu-cleated giant cells. These cells are present in both herpes zoster and in her-pes simplex infections; thus, the test is most useful in differentiating her-pes zoster from nonviral entities. Alternatively, a direct fluorescent antibody test can be performed. It is rapid, reliable, and specific for herpes zoster, but more expensive and less available than the Tzanck preparation. A cutaneous biopsy can also be examined for multinucleated giant cells or viral antigens, but this is rarely needed. Finally, blister fluid or a biopsy specimen can be submitted for viral "culture" (cytopathic assay). These "cultures" are readily available to the clinician, but the results are often not available for more than a week.

Etiology and Basic Mechanisms Responsible for the "Pain"

The varicella-zoster virus is the etiologic agent for varicella (chicken pox) and herpes zoster (shingles). Although the pathogenesis of herpes zoster is not fully understood, the following model is currently accepted.[5] During the course of varicella, the virus is disseminated widely to the skin and mucous membranes. It gains access to the sensory nerve endings in the skin and mucous membranes and travels to the sensory ganglia where a la-tent infection is established. During this latent infection, the patient remains free of symptoms, usually for decades. The mechanisms involved in the re-activation of varicella-zoster virus are poorly understood but numerous as-sociations are recognized. Immunosuppression, particularly deficient cel-lular immunity, is associated with the occurrence of herpes zoster. Examples include infection with the human immunodeficiency virus, treat-ment with immunosuppressive agents, lymphoproliferative diseases, radi-ation exposure, and aging. Infections, local trauma, surgery, and emotional stress have also been associated with the onset of herpes zoster.

Regardless of the precipitating event, once reactivated, varicella-zoster virus multiplies in a sensory ganglion resulting in inflammation, neuronal necrosis, and neuralgia that is first experienced during the pro-dromal period. The virus travels distally to the skin where the infection produces inflammation and blisters in the skin served by the involved sen-sory nerves. The cutaneous inflammation activates sensory receptors in the skin and the patient may experience additional pain, burning, or itch-ing. Additionally, proximal spread of the virus may occur causing damage to neurons in the spinal cord resulting in the motor deficits occasionally as-sociated with herpes zoster. Damage to the spinal neurons, the ganglion and the peripheral nerves account for the pain, hyperesthesia and tender-ness of postherpetic neuralgia. This entire process is usually most intense in the dermatome served by a single sensory ganglion, but adjacent dermatomes may be involved to a lesser degree. The reasons for viral reactivation in a given ganglion and the immune mechanisms that confine the infection are not fully understood.

Treatment

Acute herpes zoster generally resolves spontaneously in approximately 3 weeks with or without treatment. Longer, more severe courses may be expected in immunosuppressed patients, and for this group of patients treatment may reduce the chance of dissemination. For immunocompetent patients the primary goals of therapy are to lessen the pain, limit the extent of the eruption and subsequent scarring, and reduce the risk of post herpetic neuralgia. Initial measures include rest, partial immobilization of the affected area, the application of cool compresses, and appropriate analgesia, which may range from acetominophen analgesics to narcotics. Oral corticosteroids, alone or in combination with systemic antiviral agents, can be useful in controlling inflammation and reducing the impact of the acute disease, but they have not been shown to significantly reduce the risk of developing post herpetic neuralgia.[6,7] The risks and benefits of using oral steroids must be assessed carefully in each patient. In addition to the nonspecific measures above, antiviral therapy is available but must be started during the first 3 to 4 days of active disease. Acyclovir, valacyclovir, and famciclovir are used orally in the treatment of immunocompetent patients. Valacyclovir must be used with caution in immunocompromised patients and dosing for all of these medications may need to be decreased in patients with renal disease. Immunosuppressed patients and those failing oral therapy may require intravenous acyclovir or vidarabine.[8] Current recommendations for the therapy of herpes zoster are detailed in *Fitzpatrick's Dermatology In General Medicine, Fifth Edition*.[2]

Postherpetic neuralgia is treated differently. The chronic pain of postherpetic neuralgia is not due to the persistence of virus; thus, antiviral agents have no affect on the course of the pain. Antidepressants, anticonvulsants, antiarrhythmics, oral and topical analgesics, physical modalities, nerve blocks, and destructive surgical procedures have all been used with variable success.[9]

References

1. Ragozzino MW, Melton III LJ, Kurland LT, et al. Population-based study of herpes zoster and its sequelae. *Medicine* 1982;61:310–316.
2. Straus SE, Oxman MN. Varicella and herpes zoster. In Freedberg IM, et al (ed):

Fitzpatrick's Dermatology In General Medicine, Fifth Edition. New York, NY, Mc-Graw-Hill, 1999, pp 2427–2450.

3. Brown GR. Herpes zoster: Correlation of age, sex, distribution, neuralgia, and associated disorders. *South Med J* 1976;69:576–578.
4. Gilden DH, Dueland AN, Devlin ME, et al. Varicella-zoster virus reactivation without rash. *J Infect Dis* 1992;166(Suppl 1):S30–34.
5. Meier JL, Straus SE. Comparative biology of latent varicella-zoster virus and herpes simplex virus infections. *J Infect Dis* 1992;166(Suppl 1):S13–23.
6. Whitley RJ, Weiss H, Gnann JW, et al. Acyclovir with and without prednisone for the treatment of herpes zoster. *Ann Intern Med* 1996;125:376–383.
7. Ernst ME, Santee JA, Klepser TB. Oral corticosteroids for pain associated with herpes zoster. *Ann Pharmacotherapy* 1998;32:1099–1103.
8. Whitley RJ, Soong S, Dolin R, et al. Early vidarabine therapy to control the complications of herpes zoster in immunosuppressed patients. *N Engl J Med* 1982;307:971–975.
9. Cluff RS, Rowbotham MC. Pain caused by herpes zoster infection. *Neurologic Clinics* 1998;16:813–832.

Part II

Musculoskeletal Diseases as a Cause for "Chest Pain"

Although the definition of "chest pain" → is discussed in Chapter 1, the definition is repeated here so that communication is clear.

The quotation marks around "chest" imply that different patients have different definitions of the word "chest." Here we use the word to indicate pain located above the waist. Then, too, *angina pectoris* is not always located in the pectoral region—it may be felt only in the jaw, neck, shoulder, elbow, or wrist. Therefore, the word "chest" implies that other parts of the upper body may also be involved with painful syndromes.

The quotation marks around "pain" imply that patients may assign other terms to their discomfort, such as indigestion, burning, ache, etc.

The arrow after "chest pain" implies that the physician initially may not know the cause of the symptom, so a differential diagnosis must be established that fits the available information.

3

"Chest Pain" in Patients with Costochondritis or Tietze's Syndrome

Byron R. Williams, MD

General Considerations

Costochondritis or Tietze's Syndrome is an inflammatory process involving the cartilage of the costochondral or costosternal joints that results in localized pain and tenderness. In contrast to myocardial infarction or aortic dissection, costochondritis is a benign condition causing chest discomfort.

Clinical Settings

Although it can occur at any age, costochondritis appears to be more common in young adults, usually before 40 years of age. There does not seem to be any sex preference for this condition. The true prevalence of the disease is not known, but in one study of patients referred for coronary angiography, 11% were diagnosed with costochondritis.[1] Another study in the emergency ward demonstrated that 30% of patients presenting with chest pain had costochondritis.[2] Costochondritis can be seen in the setting of trauma, infection, or a more generalized inflammatory disease, but most often there does not appear to be any specific etiology.

From: Hurst JW, Morris DC (eds): *"Chest Pain"* →. © Futura Publishing Co., Inc., Armonk, NY, 2001.

Characteristics of the "Pain"

Patient's characterization of the "chest pain"

The patient usually identifies a sharp pain that is knifelike in quality but aching, nagging, or a pressure sensation may also be described.

Common location of the "chest pain"

The pain is frequently well localized but can affect more than one joint space and may radiate extensively. The most common locations are the second through fifth costochondral junctions, and more than one junction is involved in 90% of cases (see Figures 3–1 and 3–2).

Uncommon location of the "chest pain"

When there is radiation of the pain, it is usually to the shoulder or arm on the involved side. These symptoms often make the patient think that they are having a heart attack (see Figures 3–3 and 3–4).

Size of the painful "area"

The more intense area of discomfort is located at the costochondral joints, but may be felt in the anterior portion of the chest and radiate to the shoulder and upper arm.

Duration of the "chest pain"

The duration of costochondritis can be quite variable. It most often is self-limiting and runs a benign course over several days or weeks. However, costochondritis has been reported to run the gamut from asymptomatic to chronic disabling pain.[3] Some patients are unaware of its presence until the chest is palpated during an examination, thus provoking the pain. Very few patients are disabled by costochondritis. In one study after 1 year follow-up, approximately one-half of the patients with costochondritis are completely free of pain. The remaining patients continue to have some pain but usually not severe or disabling. Interestingly, about one-third of these patients will continue to have tenderness to palpation on physical examination even though the majority of these patients lead a normal life without disability.[4]

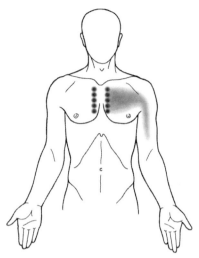

Figure 3–1. Location of the "chest pain" in patients with costochondritis. The second through fifth costochondrial joints are commonly involved. The pain may radiate to the left shoulder and arm.

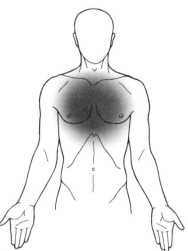

Figure 3–2. The pain of costochondritis may radiate widely over the precordium.

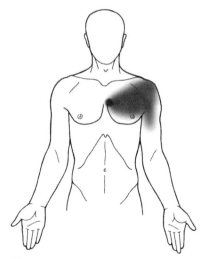

Figure 3–3. The pain may be localized to one costochondrial joint only (such as the third joint). The pain may radiate to the left shoulder and arm.

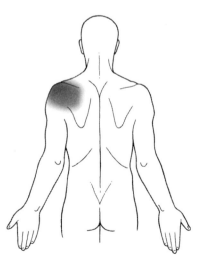

Figure 3–4. The pain of costochondritis may radiate to the shoulder.

Tenderness of the chest wall

The costochondral joints are usually tender; this is virtually diagnostic of the syndrome.

Precipitating causes of the "chest pain"

The pain of costochondritis may be precipitated most often by movement of the chest wall; thus turning the torso, lifting objects with the arms, or deep inspiration can be aggravating factors. The involved costochondral space is sensitive to touch and this property is very helpful in the diagnosis of costochondritis.

Relief of the "chest pain"

There are several solutions for pain relief from costschondritis. Local injection with lidocaine can result in prompt relief, which can be both therapeutic and diagnostic. Often the pain is self-limited and just the recognition that the condition causing the discomfort is benign is reassuring to the patient. This may be adequate in some cases for pain "relief." When reassurance alone is not adequate, costochondritis usually responds to anti-inflammatory therapy such as aspirin or nonsteroidal anti-inflammatory drugs, such as ibuprofen or indomethacin. Other local measures may also be beneficial to this condition. Application of heat, acupuncture, or local infiltration with corticosteroids may provide some measure of relief from pain. Biofeedback has been helpful in some patients not responding to simpler treatments.

Associated Symptoms

Often there are no other associated symptoms with costochondritis. Despite the fact that it is an inflammatory process, fever and chills are unusual. Clinical experience suggests that costochondritis occurs more frequently when patients have experienced upper respiratory infections. Thus, symptoms such as cough, sore throat, fever, etc. may be present either just before or during a bout of costochondritis. Furthermore, costochondritis can coexist with other disease processes. Wolf and co-workers reported that in over 300 patients referred for evaluation of precordial chest pain, the costosternal syndrome was present in approximately 10% and coexisted with definite coronary heart disease in 3% of these patients.[5] Another paper suggested that in patients diagnosed with normal coronary arteriograms, chest wall tenderness was present in over two-thirds of the patients, but only one-fourth of the patients with chest wall tenderness reported that it reproduced their pain.[6]

Associated Signs

Physical examination

Pain produced by palpation of the affected costochondral joints is a constant physical finding in patients with costochondritis. In fact, if there is absence of localized tenderness to examination of the chest wall, the diagnosis should be questioned and reconsidered. In the original description, Tietze's Syndrome was characterized by non-suppurative edema of the costosternal region, but most patients diagnosed with costochondritis in modern medicine lack localized chest wall edema.[7,8] In some of these patients there may be a generalized tenderness of the chest wall to palpation. Other than exhibiting anxiety about the cause of their pain and the aforementioned localized tenderness, patients should have a normal examination.

"Routine" laboratory tests

Routine laboratory tests are not usually required for this diagnosis. There are no specific studies that exist for costochondritis. The overall clinical setting coupled with the most likely differential diagnoses should guide requests for laboratory studies. Often laboratory tests are ordered on these patients and usually the complete blood count, biochemical profiles, cardiac enzymes, electrocardiogram, and chest x-ray film are all normal unless there is some coexistent disease process.

Exceptions to the Usual Manifestations

There are very few exceptions to the usual manifestations of costochondritis. Most often, no specific etiology is discovered for this condition. However, bacterial infections account for a small percentage of patients with costochondritis. Pyogenic infections are most frequently encountered following chest surgery or with intravenous drug abuse. Gram-negative bacilli are often the offending organism resulting in pyoarthritis in the setting of drug abuse.[9] These patients may appear toxic and have fever and leukocytosis.

Differential Diagnosis

All possible causes for chest pain should be considered when evaluating a patient who has costochondritis. Certainly, the diagnosis of myocardial infarction needs to be entertained, but often can be dismissed when the electrocardiogram is normal in a young patient and when the pain can be reproduced on physical examination by palpation of the affected area on the chest wall. Because of the positional and somewhat pleuritic nature of the pain, pericarditis, pneumonia, and pulmonary embolism are often considered. The differential diagnosis should also entertain other causes of neuromuscular chest pain including cervical spine disease, thoracic outlet syndrome, shingles (Herpes Zoster neuralgia), Mondor's syndrome (superficial thrombophlebitis of the chest wall), and various arthritides. Anxiety and hyperventilation may also mimic this condition or in fact coexist because of the patient's concern about a more serious illness such as acute myocardial infarction.

Other Diagnostic Testing

Once the diagnosis of costochondritis is considered and the physical findings are confirmatory, very little testing is usually necessary. Gallium scans may demonstrate uptake in the area of the affected costochondral joint, but are usually not needed and are not specific.

Occasionally, the physician may be concerned that another condition coexists with obvious costochondral tenderness or the patient cannot be certain that the pain elicited on palpation actually reproduces their presenting symptoms. In this scenario, additional laboratory testing may be needed and is guided by the differential that seems most likely. For example, if pneumonia or pericarditis are strong considerations, a complete blood count, chest x-ray film, electrocardiogram, and possibly an echocardiogram may be necessary to clarify the diagnosis. If myocardial infarction or myocardial ischemia are important to exclude, cardiac enzymes and perhaps stress nuclear imaging or even coronary arteriograms in selected cases may be necessary for the correct diagnosis.

Etiology and Basic Mechanisms Responsible for the Pain

The exact etiology of costochondritis is, for the most part, unknown. It appears to be an inflammatory process involving the costochondral or costosternal joints and is probably a non-specific response to previous repetitive minor trauma or unusual physical activity. It may also be an immune response to either viral or bacterial infections, often of the upper respiratory tract. Only in rare cases is it a true bacterial or fungal infection of the joint space, and this is primarily in the intravenous drug abuse setting. Costochondritis can be associated with other rheumatological conditions but most often is an isolated process.

Treatment

Since costochondritis is most often a benign and self-limiting process, treatment should be conservative. Avoidance of activities that may strain or cause trauma to the rib cage, along with other local measures such as application of heat, may be quite helpful. Adequate control of the pain is usually obtained by use of anti-inflammatory agents such as aspirin or nonsteriodal anti-inflammatory drugs. Mild analgesics may also be required in some instances. Often just reassuring the patient that the condition is not serious will provide a great deal of relief. In some more difficult cases, infiltration with local anesthetic or corticosteroids may provide excellent relief from the discomfort of costochondritis. Biofeedback and acupuncture have also been successfully used as treatment for this syndrome.[10,11]

References

1. Levine PR, Mascette AM. Musculoskeletal chest pain in patients with "angina": A prospective study. *South Med J* 1989;82(5):580–585,591.
2. Disla E, Rhim HR, Reddy A, et al. Costochondritis: A prospective analysis in an emergency department setting. *Arch Intern Med* 1994;154:2466–2469.
3. Ausubel H, Cohen BD, LaDue JS. Tietze's Disease of Eight Years Duration. *N Engl J Med* 1959;261:190.
4. Flowers LK, Wipperman BD, Chiang W, et al. Costochondritis. In *emedicine free online medical reference textbooks for doctors;* nttp.//www.emedicine.com/emerg/topic 116.ntm.
5. Wolf E, Stern S. Costosternal Syndrome: Its frequency and importance in differential diagnosis of coronary heart disease. *Arch Intern Med* 1976;136:189–191.
6. Wise CM, Semble EL, Dalton CB. Musculoskeletal chest wall syndrome in patients with non-cardiac chest pain: A study of 100 patients. *Arch Phys Med Rehab* 1992;73(2):147–149.
7. Kayser HL. Tietze's Syndrome. A Review of the Literature. *Am J Med* 1956;21:982.
8. Wadhwa SS, Phan T, Terei O. Anterior chest wall pain in postpartum costochondritis. *Clin Nucl Med* 1999;24(6):404–406.

9. Bayer AS, Chow AW, Louie JS. Sternoarticular Pyoarthrosis due to Gram-negative Bacilli. *Arch Intern Med* 1977;137:1036–1040.
10. van Peski-Oosteerbaan AS, Spinhoven P, van Rood Y. Cognitive-behavioral therapy for noncardiac chest pain—a randomized trial. *Am J Med* 1999;106(4): 424–429.
11. Baldry P. Cardiac and non-cardiac chest wall pain: Acupuncture in medicine. November 1997. Paper presented at the BMAS Spring Scientific Meeting in April 1997.

4

"Chest Pain" in Patients with Thoracic Outlet Syndromes

Vinod H. Thourani, MD and Joseph I. Miller, Jr., MD

General Considerations

Thoracic outlet syndrome is a condition that produces a constellation of neurovascular symptomology that is indicative of compression of nerves, arteries, or veins that traverse the thoracic outlet. This syndrome refers to compression of the subclavian vessels and brachial plexus at the superior aperture of the chest. Likewise, thoracic outlet syndrome can be subdivided into a neurogenic and/or vascular component (arterial or venous). Generally, the pain associated with thoracic outlet syndrome most commonly involves the neck, shoulder, arm, and hand. Patients who present with these symptoms are sometimes thought to have angina pectoris due to coronary artery disease.

Clinical Setting

Thoracic outlet syndrome is generally seen in young patients between the ages 25–40 years; rarely in the elderly or very young.[1-4] There is a female-to-male ratio of 4:1. It is also seen in muscular athletes, particularly weight lifters, swimmers, and baseball pitchers; and in patients who perform repetitive activity (e.g., assembly line workers, keyboardists, beauticians, typists, jack hammer operators). It is also seen in individuals who are constantly lifting objects above the level of the shoulder (e.g., painters and movers).

From: Hurst JW, Morris DC (eds): *"Chest Pain"* →. © Futura Publishing Co., Inc., Armonk, NY, 2001.

Characteristics of the "Pain"[5,6]

Patient's characterization of the "chest pain"

The characterization of pain in patients presenting with thoracic outlet syndrome depends on the etiology: neurogenic, arterial, or venous. Neurogenic manifestations of thoracic outlet syndrome are more frequent than vascular ones.

Neurologic complaints: Ninety-five percent of patients with neurogenic thoracic outlet syndrome complain of pain and paresthesias, while only 10% of the patients complain of motor weakness in the distal affected extremity. The pain and paresthesias are characteristically segmental in 75% of cases and 90% involve the ulnar nerve distribution. Correspondingly, 10% of the patients specifically complain of atrophy of hypothenar and interosseous muscles. Most commonly, patients report that paresthesias and numbness extend along the medial border of the forearm and hand. Sensory complaints vary in accordance with the differential compression of brachial plexus: involvement of the lower part of the brachial plexus leads to sensory complaints along the ulnar nerve distribution, while sensory complains in the thumb, index, and long finger are associated with involvement of the upper part of the brachial plexus or with associated carpal tunnel syndrome.

Complaints related to arterial obstruction: Patients presenting with thoracic outlet syndrome of arterial origin commonly note the affected extremity is cold, weak, easily fatigable, and that the pain is usually diffuse. Most patients with the arterial component of thoracic outlet syndrome seek treatment because they have noticed increasing difficulty in the functionality of their arm. They typically note that the arm is white and cold, and with sustained effort, it may begin to cramp and be painful (claudication). They often report that their affected extremity remains cold at night, even under covers. On attempts to use their affected arm, the patient notes that cramping occurs which progresses to pain severe enough to make all motion impossible, followed by the blanching of the digits. Cyanosis of the digits is followed by persistent rubor. Raynaud's phenomenon is noted in approximately 7.5% of patients with thoracic outlet syndrome. Unlike in patients with isolated Raynaud's, those with Raynaud's-thoracic outlet syndrome present with unilateral impairment which is more likely to be precipitated by hyperabduction of the involved arm, turning the head, or carrying heavy objects.

Complaints due to venous obstruction: Less frequently, the symptoms associated with thoracic outlet syndrome are those of venous obstruction or occlusion, commonly recognized as "effort thrombosis" or Paget-Schroetter syndrome. This results in symptoms of venous congestion, including edema, discoloration of the arm, distension of the superficial veins of the limb and shoulder, and aches and pains. For these patients, pain is not usually a major component of simple venous compression, but that the hand may become stiff and that the edema makes it hard to "work" the fingers and wrists.

Common location of the "chest pain"

While patients report that the pain associated with thoracic outlet syndrome may lead to discomfort radiating to the head and neck, the shoulder region (supra and subscapular), and/or the axilla, most note that the pain is directed along the somatic nerve distribution of the ulnar nerve (see Figures 4–1 and 4–2). The ulnar pain is secondary to pressure on the medial cord of the brachial plexus or the T1 root. Specifically, the symptoms occur most commonly along the medial aspects of the arm and hand, the fifth finger, and the lateral aspects of the fourth finger. The pain may also radiate to the posterior aspect of the upper arm and shoulder and occasionally seems to involve the entire arm.

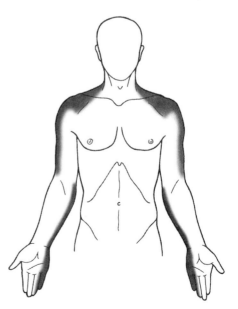

Figure 4–1. The common location of the "pain" caused by thoracic outlet syndrome (frontal view).

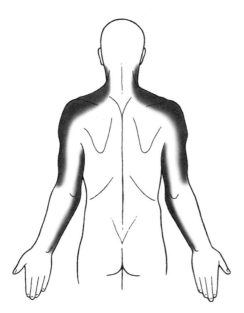

Figure 4–2. The common location of the "pain" due to thoracic outlet syndrome (viewed from the back).

Uncommon locations of the "chest pain"

A minority of the patients with thoracic outlet syndrome complain of pain involving the anterior chest wall (pectoral region), face, or parascapular area. Unlike angina pectoris, specific movements or positions elicit the "pain." Also, walking does not elicit the "pain" as it does with angina pectoris.

Physiologically, the compression of the superficial C8 to T1 cutaneous afferent (somatic) fibers by structural abnormalities in the thoracic outlet syndrome elicits transmission to the brain as pain or paresthesias in the ulnar nerve distribution. In contrast, compression of the predominantly deeper sensory (sympathetic) fibers elicits sensations that are regarded by the brain as deep pain originating from either the arm **or** chest wall; therefore, potentially simulating the "pain" of angina pectoris.

Size of the painful "area"

Most commonly, pain in patients associated with thoracic outlet syndrome extends from the cervical region to the medial aspects of the hand. Uncommonly, the pain may also be isolated to the axilla or pectoral regions (see Figures 4–1 and 4–2).

Duration of the "chest pain"

Most patients report that the pain associated with thoracic outlet has been increasing in severity over the last weeks to months and is beginning to interfere with their lifestyle. The duration of the pain most commonly endures the length of the offending motion, exercise, or repetitive motion.

Tenderness of the chest wall

Uncommonly, patients with thoracic outlet syndrome present with pain and paresthesias in the chest wall. On careful palpation of the axilla, some patients exhibit unusual sensitivity of the brachial plexus and/or of the pectoralis minor muscle, while others are tender along the scalene muscles or in the supraclavicular fossa.

Precipitating causes of the "chest pain"

The onset of pain for patients with thoracic outlet syndrome is usually insidious and commonly precipitated by strenuous exercises or sustained physical efforts. Initially, the symptoms for thoracic outlet syndrome may be appreciated by the patient after sleeping with the arms abducted and hands clasped behind the neck. Recent trauma to the shoulder or chest wall is characteristically a precipitating factor. Physical efforts that require overhead activity, heavy lifting, repetitive motions, or use of vibratory tools may also aggravate thoracic outlet syndrome. Downward pressure on the shoulder or abduction of the arm may potentially exacerbate the symptoms. Eventually, common activities such as menial housework, driving a car, lifting, or typing, may become so bothersome that the patient tries to avoid them.

In patients with venous thoracic outlet syndrome, the most pronounced upper extremity symptoms occur upon waking or following sustained efforts with the arm in abduction. Furthermore, rapid backward and downward movements of the shoulders, heavy lifting, or strenuous exercises involving the arm may constrict the vein and initiate vasospasm, potentially leading to venous thrombosis.

Relief of the "chest pain"

Alterations in physical efforts, exercises, or movements that precipitate the pain associated with thoracic outlet syndrome provide the best avenues for the amelioration of pain.

Associated Symptoms

Thoracic outlet syndrome can be characterized by two specific clinical symptomology patterns, or a combination of the two: the vascular or neurogenic components. Approximately 5% of patients with thoracic outlet syndrome will have vascular symptoms either as their presenting problem or along with the neuropathy. The vascular symptoms can be divided into the arterial or venous components. Symptoms most commonly characterized by the results of thrombosis or constriction of the subclavian artery include: loss of pulses, motor weakness, claudication, numbness of the extremity with repetitive motion or an elevation of the arm above the level of the shoulder, and upper extremity color, temperature, and trophic changes.

Symptoms characterized by venous changes are more frequently secondary to thrombosis or constriction of the subclavian vein: pain, cyanosis, collateralization of veins, upper extremity venous distension, edema, and Paget-Schroetter.

The majority of cases (~90%) of thoracic outlet syndrome involve the nerves exiting the thoracic outlet. Neurogenic symptoms of patients with thoracic outlet syndrome can be the result of peripheral or sympathetic nerve derangement. Associated symptoms of peripheral nerve abnormalities include: numbness, paresthesias, motor weakness, and pain patterns, particularly in the ulnar distribution. Those associated with sympathetic nerve abnormalities include: Raynaud's phenomena, pain, and upper extremity color, temperature, and trophic changes.

Associated Signs

Physical examination

The physician should examine the normal contour of arms, shoulder, forearms, and hands. Proximally, the brachial plexus may be tender on palpation at the supraclavicular or transaxillary anatomic areas. The tenderness is most likely secondary to the chronic stretching and irritation of the brachial plexus. The physician should to palpate for a cervical rib or bony abnormality at the base of the neck. The examiner should note any areas of hyperesthesia or anesthesia (particularly along the medial aspect of the forearm and hand) and any areas of muscular atrophy (usually in the hypothenar and interosseous muscles with clawing of the fourth and fifth fingers). The examiner should also note pallor of the hand or ischemic or gangrenous areas of the fingers, suggesting arterial insufficiency, or whether any venous engorgement is present to suggest compression of venous return. There are four classic maneuvers described for diagnosis of the thoracic outlet syndrome:

- Hyperabduction or Wright's test: When the arm is hyperabducted to 180°, the neurovascular bundle is pulled around the pectoralis minor tendon, the coracoid process, and the head of the humerus. If the radial pulse is decreased, thoracic outlet syndrome should be considered. It should be remembered that 15% of normal individuals will have a positive hyperabduction test.
- Costoclavicular or military position or Halsted's test: The shoulders are drawn downward and backward, which narrows the costoclavicular space by approximating the clavicle to the first rib, compressing the neurovascular bundle. Changes in the radial pulse and the appearance of symptoms indicate compression.
- Scalene or Adson's test: The patient is instructed to inspire and hold a deep breath, extend the neck fully, and turn the head toward the affected side (contralateral side for the reverse Adson's test); obliteration or diminution of the radial pulse suggests compression. This maneuver tightens the anterior and middle scalene muscles, decreasing the interscalene space and magnifying any pre-existing compression of the subclavian artery and brachial plexus.
- Elevated arm stress or Roos's test: The patient raises his or her arms over the head, with the shoulder abducted at 90° and maximally, rotated externally. The elbows should be flexed to 90° and the shoulders braced back with the hands intermittently clenching about once per second. If the patient's symptoms appear within 3 minutes, compression of the thoracic outlet syndrome should be considered.

"Routine" laboratory tests

The diagnosis of thoracic outlet syndrome depends upon the *history, physical and neurologic examination, and x-ray films of the chest and cervical spine.*

This approach commonly points the physician in the right direction, but other high-tech procedures are commonly needed to make the diagnosis and determine the exact cause of the problem.

There are no electrocardiographic changes due to the thoracic outlet syndrome. The electrocardiogram may be normal or abnormal depending on the patient's cardiac status.

Exceptions to the Usual Manifestations

There are few, if any, exceptions to manifestations discussed above.

Differential Diagnosis

The most common differential diagnosis for patients with thoracic outlet syndromes includes: cervical strain, herniated cervical intervertebral disk, brachial plexopathy secondary to trauma or inflammation, and video-terminal display syndrome. A more complete list of the differential diagnosis is listed in Table 4–1.

Other Diagnostic Testing

Magnetic resonance imaging of the cervical spine, doppler flow studies of the subclavian vessels, an electromyogram (EMG), and ulnar nerve conduction velocity (UNCV) studies are commonly needed (see Table 4–2). The studies listed in Table 4–2 constitute the standard work-up of thoracic outlet syndrome. Radiographs of the chest and the cervical ribs may indicate a superior sulcus tumor, osteophytic changes, cervical rib, elongated C7 transverse process, fractured callous of the clavicle or first rib, and intervertebal space narrowing. Loss of the normal lordotic cervical curve suggests cervical muscle spasm, which may be the underlying cause of the neurologic type of thoracic outlet syndrome. The most objective test is to measure the reduction of normal conduction velocities (85 m/sec) of the ulnar and median nerves across the thoracic outlet. In traumatic thoracic outlet syndrome, the ulnar nerve conduction studies may be normal. It is remarkable that the anatomic rearrangement by 1 to 3 mm may be enough to cause neurogenic compression.

Table 4–1.

Work-up for Patients with Thoracic Outlet Syndromes.

- Complete History and physical and neurologic examination
- Posterior-anterior and lateral chest x-ray film
- Cervical spine series
- Magnetic resonance imaging of the cervical spine (C4-T1)
- Doppler flow studies of the subclavian artery and vein
- Electromyogram
- Ulnar nerve conduction velocity studies

In atypical manifestations, other diagnostic procedures include:

- Cervical myelography
- Peripheral or coronary angiography
- Exercise stress testing
- Phlebography
- Somatosensory evoked potentials

Table 4–2.

Differential Diagnosis for Patients with Thoracic Outlet Syndromes.

Cervical spine:

- Cervical strain
- Herniated cervical intervertebral disk
- Cervical spondylosis
- Degenerative disease
- Osteoarthiritis
- Spinal cord tumors

Brachial plexopathy

- Superior pulmonary sulcus (Pancoast's) tumor
- Trauma/inflammation

Peripheral nerve abnormalities

- Entrapment neuropathy
- Neuritis
- Carpal tunnel syndrome-median nerve
- Ulnar nerve-elbow
- Radial nerve
- Suprascapular nerve
- Medical neuropathies
- Trauma
- Tumor

Arterial abnormalities

- Arteriosclerosis-aneurysm (occlusive)
- Thromboangiitis obliterans
- Embolism
- Functional (Raynaud's disease)
- Reflex (vasomotor dystrophy)
- Causalgia
- Vasculitis
- Collagen disease
- Panniculitis

Vascular abnormalities

- Thrombophlebitis
- Mediastinal venous obstruction/Paget-Schroetter syndrome (malignant or benign)

Inflammatory shoulder disorders

- Bursitis
- Fibrositis
- Pychoneurosis
- Myositis
- Tendinitis
- Video terminal display syndrome
- Angina pectoris
- Esophageal disorders
- Multiple sclerosis

In cases of atypical manifestations, other diagnostic procedures such as cervical myelography, arteriography, somatosensory evoked potential studies, or phlebography should be considered. Arteriograms and venograms are not indicated in the routine workup of patients with thoracic outlet syndrome and should be limited to those patients who have symptoms of arterial insufficiency or venous obstruction. Angiography is warranted in the presence of a paraclavicular pulsating mass, the absence of radial pulse, or the presence of supraclavicular or infraclavicular bruits. A phlebogram is often helpful in delineating the extent of the blockade and the status of the collateral venous circulation in circumstances where occlusion of the venous return is suspected.

Etiology and Basic Mechanisms Responsible for the "Pain"

The thoracic outlet is a triangular opening in which the superior boundary is the clavicle, the inferior boundary is represented by the first rib, and the posterior boundary by the medial scalene muscle. The anterior scalene muscle divides the thoracic outlet into the anterior space (containing the subclavian vein) and the posterior space (containing the subclavian artery and the brachial plexus). When the arm is abducted, the clavicle rotates backward towards the first rib and the insertion of the scalenus anticus muscle. Under normal conditions, the brachial plexus or subclavian artery or vein, which traverse the scalene triangle on the first rib, are not compressed. However, many factors may lead to compression at the thoracic outlet, leading to thoracic outlet syndrome. Although the true etiology of thoracic outlet syndrome has not been determined, factors which may potentially cause this abnormal anatomy include congenital abnormalities and traumatic conditions. Congenital bony abnormalities (present in approximately 30% of patients) include: a cervical rib, a bifid clavicle or first rib, exostosis of the clavicle or first rib, rudimentary first thoracic rib, fusion of the first and second rib into a bony abnormality, or enlarged transverse process of C7. Other congenital abnormalities include the appearance of a fibromuscular band usually starting at the neck of the first rib and compressing the T1 root of the brachial plexus or the subclavian artery. Traumatic injuries include the fracture of the clavicle or first rib, dislocation of head of the humerus, crushing injury to the upper thorax, sudden muscular shoulder girdle efforts, or cervical spondylosis.

Treatment

Conservative treatment should be the goal in all cases of thoracic outlet syndrome.[7] If possible, the offending exercise or activity should be stopped.

Multiple rest periods with the hands below the shoulder girdle should be practiced. Resting wrist splints at night to maintain the wrist in a neutral position and soft elbow pads to cushion the ulnar nerve and block elbow flexion are recommended. Obesity and large pendulous breasts will amplify thoracic outlet syndrome and weight loss plans or bilateral mammoplasty may be considered. Physiotherapy (heat massages, active neck exercises, stretching of the scalenus muscles, strengthening of the upper trapezuis muscle, and posture instruction) aimed at strengthening the shoulder girdle and other neck muscles is suggested. Furthermore, patients should begin muscle-strengthening and postural exercises designed to elevate the shoulders and slightly abduct them. These exercises may help relax the compressive force on the neurovascular bundle. Conservative modalities including, physiotherapy, anti-inflammatory drugs, exercises, and correct posture should be implemented for at least 3 months. The majority of cases due to neurogenic compression will respond, while the majority of vascular cases do not.

Although 80% to 85% of all patients improve with conservative treatment modalities, some patients with thoracic outlet syndrome ultimately require surgical intervention. Most patients with thoracic outlet syndrome who have ulnar nerve conduction velocities of more than 60 m/s improve with conservative management. If the conduction velocity is below that level, most patients, despite physiotherapy, will remain symptomatic, and surgical resection of the first rib and correction of other bony abnormalities may be needed. If an arteriogram demonstrates intrinsic arterial injury (e.g., post-stenotic dilatation, distal embolization, or intimal ulceration), surgery is indicated without a trial of conservative treatment. For patients with Paget-Schroetter syndrome (effort thrombosis of the axillary vein), definitive early surgical intervention following thrombolysis of clot is warranted.

Since the first rib forms the rigid base of the thoracic outlet, surgical treatment involves resection of the first rib and cervical rib (when present). The fibrous bands that are attached to the first rib and impinge on the brachial plexus are resected as well. Surgical approach for patients with thoracic outlet syndrome can be performed through several approaches: transaxillary (preferred route), supraclavicular and infraclavicular, transthoracic, or high posterior paravertebral. Dorsal sympathectomy is helpful for patients with sympathetic maintained pain syndrome associated with thoracic outlet syndrome. Surgical risks are minimal in the hands of well-trained surgeons. Symptomatic recurrence occurs in approximately 25% of patients within 3 to 5 years.

References

1. Atasoy E. Thoracic outlet compression syndrome. *Orthopedic Clin North Am* 1996;27(2):265–303.

2. Mackinnon S, Patterson GA, Urschel HC Jr. Thoracic outlet syndromes. In Pearson FG, Deslauriers J, Ginsberg RJ, et al. (eds). *Thoracic Surgery*. New York, NY, Churchill Livingstone, 1995, pp 1211–1235.
3. Urshcel HC Jr. Thoracic outlet syndromes. In Baue AE, Geha AS, Hammond GL, et al. (eds). *Glenn's Thoracic and Cardiovascular Surgery*. Stamford, CT, Appleton and Lange, 1996, pp 567–580.
4. Urschel HC Jr. Thoracic outlet syndrome. In Shields TW (ed). *General Thoracic Surgery*. Malvern, PA, Williams & Wilkins, 1994, pp 564–571.
5. Mackinnon SE and Novak CB. Evaluation of the patient with thoracic outlet syndrome. *Seminars Thorac Cardiovasc Surg* 1996;8(2):190–200.
6. Roos DB. Diagnosis of thoracic outlet syndrome. In Ernst CB, Stanley JC (eds). *Current Therapy in Vascular Surgery*. Philadelphia, PA, B.C. Decker, Inc, 1991, pp 217–223.
7. Urschel HC Jr, Razzuk MA. Neurovascular compression in the thoracic outlet: Changing management over 50 years. *Ann Surg* 1998;228(4):609–617.

$$\boxed{5}$$

"Chest Pain" in Patients with Chest Wall Syndromes

J. Willis Hurst, MD

General Considerations

There are several causes of chest wall pain. "Chest pain" due to herpes zoster is discussed in Chapter 2. "Chest pain" in patients with costochondritis is discussed in Chapter 3. The thoracic outlet syndrome is discussed in Chapter 4. "Chest pain" in patients with osteoarthritis of the cervical spine is discussed in Chapter 9. "Chest pain" due to Mondor syndrome is discussed in Chapter 10. "Chest pain" due to herniation of a cervical disc is discussed in Chapter 11. There are, however, several causes of "chest pain" due to chest wall syndrome in addition to those mentioned above. *Polymyocytis rheumatica* may produce pain in the shoulder and upper arm (as well as elsewhere) and *fibromyalgia* may cause pain at multiple sites including the neck, shoulder, and the parasternal areas.[1,2] Finally, Epstein, et al. identified a group of patients with chest wall pain that simulated the pain of myocardial ischemia that fell outside of the list of conditions mentioned above.[3]

Clinical Setting

Polymyositis occurs more often in women who are more than 50 to 60 years of age. The mean age of onset is about 70 years.[1] *Fibromyalgia* occurs at any age in both sexes, but is more common in women between the ages 20 and 50 years.[2] Epstein's patients were from 20 to 66 years of age.[3]

From: Hurst JW, Morris DC (eds): *"Chest Pain"* →. © Futura Publishing Co., Inc., Armonk, NY, 2001.

Characteristics of the "Pain"

Patient's characterization of the "chest pain"

The patient may describe mild to severe pain or ache that may occur abruptly or gradually. Many of the patients are concerned about the pain and some of them believe they are having a "heart attack."[3]

Common location of the "chest pain"

The pain of *polymyalgia rheumatica* is usually located in the upper arm as well as the pelvic girdle and knees. The pain of *fibromyalgia* may be located in the neck, shoulders, upper back, upper portion of the anterior chest, hip area and knees. The "chest pain" in Epstein's patients was located in the areas shown in Figure 5–1.

Uncommon locations of the "chest pain"

The "pain" due to *polymyalgia rheumatica* and *fibromyalgia* occurs in multiple locations in the body.[1,2] It is actually uncommon to be located solely in the arms, shoulders, or anterior chest area (see Figure 5–2). The

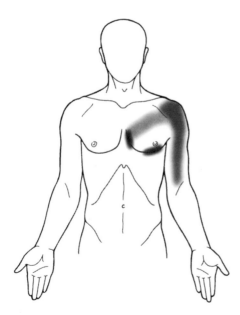

Figure 5–1. Most patients with chest wall "pain" as described by Epstein, et al. have pain in the precordial area. The pain may also be located in the left third and fourth intercostal spaces near the sternum and radiate toward the left shoulder and left arm. These areas are also tender when firm pressure is applied.

This diagram was created using the information described by the authors in the text of reference 3.

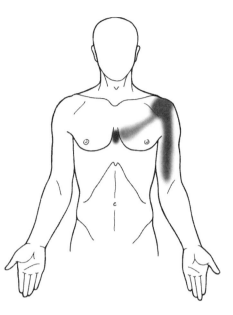

Figure 5–2. Uncommonly, the chest wall pain as described by Epstein is located only in the retrosternal area and radiates to the left shoulder and arm.[3] The area of retrosternal pain is also tender when firm pressure is applied.

This diagram was created using the information described by the authors in the text of reference 3.

location of the pain in Epstein's patients was limited to the anterior chest wall and left arm, as described above.[3]

Size of the painful "area"

The size of the painful area varies from patient to patient and ranges from a few centimeters to the size of the hand (see Figure 5–1 which shows the size of the painful area in Epstein's patients.)[3]

Duration of the "chest pain"

The pain of *polymyalgia rheumatica* and *fibromyalgia* may last days or weeks. Epstein reported that the "pain" of some of his patients lasted no longer than 3 to 5 minutes, while some of the patients had pain for 15 to 20 minutes and two had "pain" for an hour.[3] Therefore, in some patients the pain can be confused with angina pectoris and in others it can be confused with infarction.

Tenderness of the chest wall

Chest wall tenderness in the area of the "pain" is almost always present in each of the three conditions described here. In fact, exquisite tenderness of the chest wall is almost diagnostic for one cause of chest wall "pain."

Precipitating causes of the "chest pain"

The pain of *polymyositis rheumatica* may come on abruptly without apparent cause or it may develop gradually. There are no obvious precipitating causes.[1] It is not directly related to effort.

The pain of *fibromyalgia* usually occurs without apparent cause. It may occur after a stressful event, like an automobile accident without body injury. The patient may have other conditions, such as depression, migraine headache, or pain in the mandibulo-temporal joint.[2]

A few of *Epstein's patients* described "pain" associated with effort. Epstein's group believed that in such patients that the change in posture played a role in producing the "pain."[3]

Relief of the "chest pain"

The pain of *polymyalgia rheumatica* is usually relieved with low-dose prednisone. Nonsteroidal anti-inflammatory drugs, including aspirin, may be helpful. The pain is not relieved with nitroglycerin.

Fibromyalgia is difficult to relieve with prednisone or nonsteroidal anti-inflammatory drugs. Therefore, many "treatments" are tried including acupuncture, physical therapy, and the treatment of co-morbid illnesses such as depression. Nitroglycerin is not helpful.

The pain in eight of twelve of *Epstein's patients* was relieved by nitroglycerin. It was not tried in two patients and offered no relief in two patients. One would suspect, because the pain lasted only 2 to 5 minutes in some of the patients, that it was difficult to determine if the nitroglycerin caused the relief or if the pain self-limited.

Associated Symptoms

Patients with *polymyalgia rheumatica* have multiple complaints related to the musculoskeletal system, including the complaint of stiffness and aching in the shoulders, upper extremities, and pelvic girdle, especially when they get up in the morning. They may have difficulty raising their arms above their head. In addition, they do not feel well generally, sleep poorly, lose weight, and complain of fatigue and of depression.[1]

Patients with *fibromyalgia* have pain in many musculoskeletal areas of the body including the neck, shoulders, hip areas, and knees. The patient may have complaints suggesting anxiety or depression.[2]

Epstein's patients were referred to his team at the *National Heart, Lung and Blood Institute* because of "chest pain." The authors did not mention if their patients had multiple musculoskeletal sites of pain. If they did not, this virtually excludes the likelihood that their patients had *polymyalgia rheumatica* or *fibromyalgia*.[3]

Associated Signs

Physical examination

The patients with *polymyalgia* and *fibromyalgia* complain of tenderness of the multiple painful areas.[1,2] The patients reported by Epstein have tender areas of the chest wall only.[3] The tenderness is evoked when the physician applies firm, steady pressure to the third and fourth intercostal spaces or the precordium. The pain may radiate to the left arm and shoulder. Rarely, Epstein reports, the patient may have retrosternal pain and tenderness with radiation to the left arm and shoulder.[3]

Epstein and his coworkers used four maneuvers to precipitate the chest wall pain in their patients. They suggest: palpation of the chest wall, horizontal flexion of the arm with the head rotated toward the opposite shoulder, having the patient extend his or her neck toward the ceiling while pulling the upper arms backwards and superiorly, and pressure exerted on top of the head.[3]

"Routine" laboratory tests

The Westergren sedimentation rate is almost always elevated in patients with polymyalgia rheumatica. The routine laboratory tests are normal in patients with fibromyalgia.

Epstein made no mention of the routine laboratory tests in his patients. The patients were referred to his team because of chest pain and the studies that were performed were used to assess the status of the coronary arteries.

Exceptions to the Usual Manifestations

There are no known exceptions to the manifestations mentioned above.

Differential Diagnosis

The diagnosis of chest wall pain due to musculoskeletal disorder requires the consideration and exclusion of: herpes zoster (see Chapter 2), costochondritis (see Chapter 3), the thoracic outlet syndrome (see Chapter

4), osteoarthritis of the cervical spine (see Chapter 9), Mondor's syndrome (see Chapter 10), and herniation of a cervical disc (see Chapter 11).

Patients with *polymyalgia rheumatica* and *fibromyalgia* are easily excluded, because multiple areas of the body are almost always affected with these conditions. In addition, the sedimentation rate is almost always elevated in patients with polymyalgia rheumatica.

Patients with chest wall pain similar to that described by Epstein are more commonly thought to have coronary atherosclerotic heart disease. Accordingly, it will be necessary to have coronary arteriograms or nuclear studies in some patients.

Some patients have pain due to coronary atherosclerotic heart disease and chest wall pain. Accordingly, the diagnosis of chest wall pain must be made by positive finding rather than assuming that the presence of coronary disease always implies that the chest pain is solely due to myocardial ischemia.

Other Diagnostic Testing

No additional testing is needed to diagnose polymyalgia or fibromyalgia.

It is impossible to always exclude coronary atherosclerotic heart disease as a cause of "chest pain" in all patients with what is later believed to be musculoskeletal pain. Accordingly, studies to identify the presence of obstructive coronary disease or myocardial ischemia may be needed in some patients. But, as emphasized earlier, the presence of chest wall pain as described by Epstein must be diagnosed by positive finding, such as chest wall tenderness, because the coexistence of angina and chest wall pain is common.

Etiology and Basic Mechanisms Responsible for the "Pain"

The etiology of polymyalgia rheumatica, fibromyalgia, and the chest pain of the patients described by Epstein is unknown.[1–3]

Treatment

The treatment of the pain due to thoracic outlet syndrome, osteoarthritis of the cervical spine, herniated cervical disc, costochondritis, and Mondor's syndrome is discussed in the chapters devoted to them.

Corticosteroids, such as prednisone, or nonsteroidal anti-inflammatory drugs are usually of considerable benefit to patients with polymyalgia rheumatica. Some patients, however, are resistant to such drugs and continue to be plagued with symptoms of the condition.[1]

The treatment of fibromyalgia is not satisfactory; the painful areas are not usually relieved by prednisone or nonsteroidal anti-inflammatory agents. Many approaches to treatment have been used, but none are totally satisfactory.[2]

Physical therapy was useful in some of the patients reported by Epstein, but the relief was often temporary.[3] He concludes that the physician's greatest contribution to the patient is the reassurance that the pain is not due to serious coronary atherosclerotic heart disease, and when the patient also has coronary atherosclerotic heart disease, to help the patient distinguish between the "pain" of the two conditions.[3]

References

1. Gonzalez EB. Polymyalgia rheumatica. In Hurst JW (ed): *Medicine for the Practicing Physician*, 4*th* ed. Stamford, Connecticut, Appleton & Lange, 1996, pp. 240–244.
2. Moldofsky H. Fibromyalgia. In Hurst JW (ed): *Medicine for the Practicing Physician*, 4*th* ed. Stamford, Connecticut, Appleton & Lange, 1996, pp. 242–245.
3. Epstein SE, Gerber LH, Borer JS. Chest wall syndrome. *JAMA* 1979;241(26): 2793–2797.

6

"Chest Pain" in Patients with The Shoulder-Hand Syndrome

Mark E. Silverman, MD

General Considerations

Reports of a painful, stiff shoulder in association with acute myocardial infarction date back to the 1930's.[1] Shoulder involvement combined with swelling and trophic changes of the hand was first noted in 1940.[2] At one time, this syndrome was well known and said to occur in 10% to 20% of patients postinfarction;[1] however, it has virtually disappeared in the setting of coronary disease, and most cardiologists have never seen an example.

Clinical Setting

Originally called the "shoulder-hand syndrome" and "reflex sympathetic dystrophy," it is now classified under "Complex Regional Pain Syndrome, type I."[3-6] The 1997 International Association for the Study of Pain established the following diagnostic criteria:[3]

- The presence of an initiating noxious event or a cause of immobilization
- Continuing pain, allodynia, or hyperalgesia in which the pain is disproportionate to the exciting event
- Evidence at some time of edema, changes in skin blood flow, or abnormal sudomotor activity in the painful region

The diagnosis is excluded by the existence of conditions that would otherwise account for the degree of pain and dysfunction. The age and sex distribution mirrors the coronary population.[1]

From: Hurst JW, Morris DC (eds): *"Chest Pain"* →. © Futura Publishing Co., Inc., Armonk, NY, 2001.

Characteristics of the "Pain"

Three stages have been described, though the course may vary considerably.[7]

Patient's characterization of the "chest pain"

The first stage usually begins with bitter complaints of tenderness in the shoulder, described by the patient as burning, aching, or agonizing, particularly with abduction. The severity can vary from mild to severe, and may closely simulate the pain of myocardial infarction. Bursitis or arthritis is often initially considered. The hand signs may develop before the shoulder problem, or not at all.[2,8] Typically, several months after the onset of the shoulder pain, a second stage of unilateral or bilateral hand involvement begins with painful swelling of the hand and fingers.

Common location of the "chest pain"

Either or both shoulders or hands can be affected; however the pain may be hard to localize[7] (see Figures 6–1, 6–2, and 6–3). The symptoms and findings on examination do not follow a dermatome or arterial distribution, but rather involve the entire anatomic region.

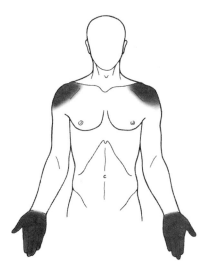 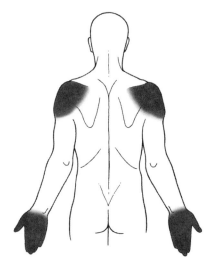

Figure 6–1. Diagram (frontal view) showing possible locations of the pain and physical findings of patients with shoulder-hand syndrome.

Figure 6–2. Diagram (dorsal view) showing possible locations of the pain and physical findings of patients with shoulder-hand syndrome.

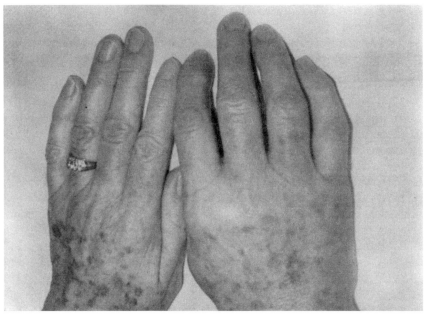

Figure 6–3. Shoulder-hand syndrome. Painful, swollen right hand compared with left hand.

Uncommon locations of the "chest pain"

There are no uncommon locations—the incidence of right, left, and bilateral involvement is fairly equal in several series.[1,7]

Size of the painful "area"

The area of involvement encompasses either or both shoulders and the hands below the wrist.

Duration of the "chest pain"

The shoulder and hand symptoms may persist from weeks to months, to several years. The hand changes may become irreversible.

Tenderness of chest wall

The chest wall is not involved.

Precipitating causes of the "chest pain"

The onset of symptoms in the shoulder-hand syndrome begins from shortly after to as late as 7 months post-myocardial infarction. The site or radiation of the chest pain and the severity of the myocardial infarction bear no relationship to the development of the syndrome. Although myocardial infarction has been by far the most common inciting cardiac etiology, prolonged or repetitive attacks of angina pectoris, atrial fibrillation, and aortic stenosis have also been implicated.[1]

Relief of the "chest pain"

Analgesics are usually tried, but are minimally helpful. Physiotherapy, including heat, may afford partial relief. Cortisone is sometimes effective.

Associated Symptoms

A psychologic disturbance, including depression, anxiety, withdrawal, and suicidal ideation, has been described in patients with this syndrome.[3] It is unclear whether this is a result of the chronic pain that these patients often endure.

Associated Signs

Physical examination

The shoulder is tender to the touch, and trigger spots may be found.[1] The area may be hypersensitive (allodynia) to air and clothing. Movement of the shoulder girdle, especially abduction and external rotation, is painful, and the patient keeps the affected limb immobile or splinted. The affected hand and fingers become diffusely swollen, painful, and stiff (see Figure 6–2). The hand and fingers may be cold to the touch, though the arterial circulation seems normal by palpation of the radial or brachial arteries. The swollen fingers may become glossy with loss of normal skin creases. Discoloration of the palm or dorsum of the hand, varying from erythema to a purplish or cyanotic hue, may be noticeable and can change from moment to moment.[2] Gangrene and ulcerations of the skin are not present. The hand signs may resolve or progress to a third stage, with the development of interosseous atrophy, thickening of the palmar tissue, and flexion deformities of the fingers, similar to Dupuytren's contractures. The hand findings may suggest the diagnosis of sclerodactyly.[8] Ridging and thickening of the nails can develop.

"Routine" laboratory tests

Routine laboratory tests have not been specific or helpful. The electrocardiogram, of course, shows evidence for a myocardial infarction. The erythrocyte sedimentation rate may or may not be elevated. X-ray films of the affected region may show patchy demineralization or, eventually, marked osteoporosis.

Exceptions to the Usual Manifestations

The shoulder and/or hand involvement may be right-sided, left-sided, or bilateral. The hand pain may precede the shoulder pain by several months.[2] Rarely, the shoulder pain occurs before the myocardial infarction.[1]

Differential Diagnosis

The differential diagnosis of the shoulder or hand pain includes myocardial infarction, cardiac causalgia (which may be a variant of this disorder),[9] bursitis, tendonitis or rotator cuff tear of the shoulder, a scalenus anticus syndrome, atypical rheumatoid arthritis, or gout. There are many causes of the complex regional pain syndrome.[2,5,7] These include traumatic injury (which does not have to be severe), vascular disease (thrombophlebitis, vasculitis, Raynaud's disease), neurologic disorders (post stroke, peripheral neuropathy, postherpetic neuralgia, multiple sclerosis, radiculopathy), infections (cellulitis, infectious arthritis), rheumatic disease (rheumatoid arthritis, systemic lupus erythematosus), and psychiatric disorders (factitious disorder, hysterical conversion reaction).

Other Diagnostic Testing

Roentgenograms or a computed tomography (CT) scan of the shoulder might be indicated to evaluate for local pathology. Thermography has been used to document a temperature difference, usually hypothermia, between the painful area and the opposite side.[4]

Etiology and Basic Mechanisms Responsible for the "Pain"

The etiology is unknown. The theory that the sympathetic nervous system is abnormally activated remains controversial, despite intensive investigation. An increased sensitivity of peripheral pain receptors to circulating catecholamines or sensitization of central pain neurons to pain perception has been postulated.[4–6]

Treatment

Since the shoulder-hand syndrome related to coronary atherosclerotic heart disease no longer seems to occur, it is difficult to state how it should be treated currently. Therapy in the past, including peripheral nerve block and sympathectomy, was never satisfactory; the pain often recurred even when relief was initially obtained.[1] Early physiotherapy has always been advised. Treatment regimens for current causes of complex regional pain syndrome include: regional sympathetic blockade with lidocaine and guanethidine; oral drugs (including alpha blocking, beta blocking, and calcium channel blocking agents, muscle relaxants, narcotics and other analgesics, antidepressants, corticosteroids, gabapentin, and placebos); and topical anesthetic agents.[3–5,10] These approaches have generally been of limited or transient effectiveness. A transcutaneous electrical nerve stimulating unit may be tried. Psychotherapy for the individual or family, biofeedback, and relaxation therapy may be indicated in selected patients. Patients with this frustrating disorder can be referred to the Reflex Sympathetic Dystrophy Syndrome Association of America, P.O. Box 821, Haddonfield, NJ 08033, telephone 1-609-795-8845. A web site is also available (www.cyboard.com/rsds/)

Classic Description

"We wish to describe a syndrome of painful disability of both the shoulder and hand which persists for several months to one or two years after coronary occlusion. The syndrome of combined shoulder and hand disability has not been described, although we feel that it is not a rare sequel of coronary occlusion. We do not refer to the left arm and hand pain after a paroxysm of angina pectoris, when the extremity is held immobile for fear of exciting more pain, but to a persistent, painful disability which is associated with restriction of shoulder movement and swelling of the fingers."[2]

References

1. Russek HI. Shoulder-hand syndrome following myocardial infarction. *Med Clin North Am* 1958;42:1555–1566.
2. Askey JM. The syndrome of painful disability of the shoulder and hand complicating coronary occlusion. *Am Heart J* 1941;22:1–12.

3. Pittman DM, Belgrade MJ. Complex regional pain syndrome. *Am Fam Phys* 1997;56:2265–2270.
4. Raj PP. Complex regional pain syndromes—reflex sympathetic dystrophy and causalgia. *Current Review of Pain* 1998;2:242–253.
5. Mandel S, Rothrock RW. Sympathetic dystrophies: Recognizing and managing a puzzling group of syndromes. *Postgrad Med* 1990;87:213–218.
6. Hooshmand H. *Chronic Pain: Reflex Sympathetic Dystrophy: Prevention and Management.* Boca Raton, Fl, CRC Press, Inc, 1993, pp 3–65.
7. Rosen PS, Graham W. The shoulder-hand syndrome: Historical review with observations on seventy-three patients. *Canad M A J* 1957;77:86–91.
8. Johnson AC. Disabling changes in the hands resembling sclerodactylia following myocardial infarction. *Ann Int Med* 1943;19:433–455.
9. Burch GE, Phillips JH, DePasquale NP. Cardiac causalgia. *Am Heart J* 1968; 76:725–727.
10. Schwartzman RJ. New treatment for reflex sympathetic dystrophy. *N Engl J Med* 2000;343:654–656.

<table>
<tr><td>7</td></tr>
</table>

"Chest Pain" in Patients with Bursitis of the Shoulder

Stephen B. Miller, MD

General Considerations

There are many causes of shoulder pain and, because angina pectoris and myocardial infarction are among them, the other causes, including bursitis deserves emphasis.[1]

Clinical Setting

Bursitis of the shoulder occurs commonly in people over 30 years of age, reportedly with a greater incidence for females. Younger and middle-aged patients are much more likely to experience acute bursitis than older patients with chronic rotator cuff syndrome (see Chapter 8). Occupational risks are greater among those with chronic overhead use of the arms such as painters, wallpaper hangers, etc.

Characteristics of the "Pain"

Patient's characterization of the "chest pain"

The typical episode of acute bursitis of the shoulder is abrupt in onset and often excruciating. It is described variably as severe burning, "like a knife" or a "hot poker."

From: Hurst JW, Morris DC (eds): *"Chest Pain"* →. © Futura Publishing Co., Inc., Armonk, NY, 2001.

Common location of the "chest pain"

Most patients cannot localize the pain more specifically than in the "whole shoulder" (see Figure 7–1).

Uncommon locations of the "chest pain"

Pain is sometimes felt in the upper arm, but radiation beyond the elbow into the forearm or fingers is rare. Likewise, radiation in the anterior chest or upper back is rare.

Size of the painful "area"

The area of pain is usually about the size of a clinched fist.

Duration of the "chest pain"

The pain does not usually subside spontaneously. With appropriate treatment, resolution of the acute pain may be anticipated in 1 to 2 days, with complete relief expected in most cases in a week.

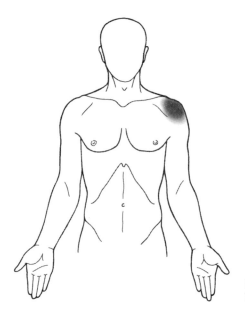

Figure 7–1. Location of pain due to bursitis.

Tenderness of the chest wall

There is no tenderness of the chest wall, but the afflicted shoulder is exquisitely tender.

Precipitating causes of the "chest pain"

Most often there is no obvious event or change in routine that triggered the episode. However, it sometimes begins during or soon after intensive overhead work, such as painting, wallpapering, or scrubbing walls. Recreational activities, particularly swimming and weightlifting, can sometimes be incriminated.

It is particularly important to determine if the shoulder pain is precipitated by walking or stressful emotional events because; should this be the case, one would have to consider that the pain could possibly be due to myocardial ischemia. However, in patients with bursitis, shoulder movement in any direction causes pain particularly abduction and elevation. In severe cases patients cannot sleep or dress without help.

Relief of the "chest pain"

Self-administered trials of locally applied heat, cold, non-narcotic analgesics, over-the-counter non-steroidal anti-inflammatory drugs, and rest are helpful. However, the majority of patients still seek medical care for persistent and disabling pain.

Associated Symptoms

There may be no additional symptoms.

Associated Signs

Physical examination

The patient is in considerable pain, holding the involved arm rigidly at the side and as motionless as possible. Although all shoulder movements are uncomfortable, the pain is most intense on active abduction, particularly approaching the horizontal plane and above. Increased pain elicited by the examiner on resisting abduction is the primary confirmatory test for bursitis. Additional diagnostic accuracy is obtained by a positive impingement test, in which the subacromial bursa and rotator cuff are forced against the undersurface of the overhanging acromion. Sometimes tendeness is localized primarily to the tip of the shoulder, but most often it is diffuse. Swelling, increased temperature, or systemic signs of inflammation are absent.

"Routine" laboratory tests

Routine laboratory testing, as well as any other specific lab tests, are normal and therefore not required. Similarly, x-rays of the shoulders are usually normal, but may be helpful in a minority of patients when the diagnosis is unclear. The finding of calcification in the rotator cuff tendons, and less often the subacromial bursa, strongly supports the diagnosis.

Exceptions to the Usual Manifestations

The pain may radiate down into the upper arm where the deltoid muscle inserts. This suggests the cervical spine as the source of radicular pain. However, the physical examination will clearly differentiate the shoulder as the primary source.

Differential Diagnosis

- Acute Synovitis (eg., rheumatoid arthritis). These conditions produce diffuse tenderness without localization, often with swelling due to an effusion. Multiple joint involvement and other stigmata of rheumatoid arthritis present.
- Acute Rotator Cuff Tear. This condition is more common in the younger end of the age group, i.e., under 40. It is often preceded by an injury (falling on outstretched arm or hyperabduction). The severity of pain, loss of active range of motion, and weakness are quite variable depending on a partial or complete tear (see Chapter 8).

Other Diagnostic Testing

Specialized diagnostic procedures are usually unnecessary. If the response to the appropriate treatment is poor, an arthrogram is the imaging study of choice to diagnose a rotator cuff tear, and in the overall assessment of underlying shoulder pathology.

Etiology and Basic Mechanisms Responsible for the "Pain"

Bursitis of the shoulder is actually a secondary event due to inflammation arising in the rotator cuff. This inflammation arises in the supraspinatus tendon, which forms the floor of the subacromial bursa. This rotator cuff tendonitis is a result of impingement of the rotator cuff and subacromial bursa between the humeral head and overlying coracoacromial arch. It is this close anatomical relationship between the subacromial bursa and the supraspinatus tendon that is the basis for the pathology.

There are two layers of muscles about the shoulder, superficial and deep. The deep group comprises the rotator cuff muscles (supraspinatus, subscapularis, infraspinatus, and teres minor).

The deltoid is the major muscle in the superficial group. It is larger and more powerful than the rotator cuff. During shoulder abduction and elevation, the deltoid pulls the humeral head superiorly towards the overhanging acromion. The main function of the cuff muscles is to stabilize the humeral head in its socket (glenoid), thereby counterbalancing the deltoids' actions. Therefore, dysfunction of the rotator cuff muscles due to tears or weakness can lead to impingement and reactive tendonitis and bursitis. The bursitis can be acute or chronic, and sometimes associated with calcium deposits in the rotator cuff tendons, i.e., calcific tendonitis. In summary, the complex shoulder anatomy and its extensive mobility contribute to the spectrum of acute or chronic tendonitis and bursitis secondary to impingement.

Treatment

In most acute cases, rest with the arm in a sling, analgesics, and physical modalities such as hot packs or cold applications are very beneficial. Often though, injection of the subacromial bursa with a corticosteroid will produce rapid pain relief. Once past the acute stage, specific range of motion exercises should be begun to avoid a potential for developing a frozen shoulder. Nonsteroidal drugs (NSAIDS) may be useful adjunctive medications.

Reference

1. Steinfeld R, Valente R, Stuart MJ. A commonsense approach to shoulder problems. *Mayo Clinic Proc* 1999;74:785–794.

8

"Chest Pain" in Patients with Rotator Cuff Tendonitis or Arthritis of the Shoulder

Andrew P. Gutow, MD

General Considerations

Pain of the shoulder area due to musculoskeletal causes is a common disorder in the same patient population frequently affected by angina pectoris. The two major causes of musculoskeletal-induced pain in the shoulder are *tendonitis* (most commonly *rotator cuff* or *bicipetal*) and *arthritis* (of the *glenohumeral joint* or the *acromioclavicular joint*). These disorders can occur either immediately after an acute trauma, in a delayed manner (a few hours to a day after strenuous activity), or insidiously. Although the pain can be confusing to the patient as it may be diffuse, nonfocal and referred, its musculoskeletal origins can always be proven on physical examination, where palpation or provocative maneuvers can reproduce or increase the pain.[1-6]

Clinical Setting

Musculoskeletal-caused pain of the shoulder area can occur in patients of any age or sex. The incidence of *rotator cuff tendonitis* increases with age, and is more common among those in the fifth and sixth decades of life than in younger individuals. In the younger patient population tendonitis occurs more frequently in individuals who engage in overhead sports such as tennis, or physically vigorous occupations such as painters, automobile mechanics, or janitors. Arthritis of *the acromioclavicular joint* is more common in individuals with a history of shoulder injury, contact

From: Hurst JW, Morris DC (eds): *"Chest Pain"* →. © Futura Publishing Co., Inc., Armonk, NY, 2001.

sports or weightlifting. *Glenohumeral arthritis* is mainly a disorder of individuals in the fifth decade and beyond, but may occur in younger individuals with history of trauma or dislocation.

Rotator Cuff Tendonitis

Characteristics of the "Pain"

Patient's characterization of the "chest pain"

Patients with tendonitis of the rotator cuff or proximal biceps tendon report a deep pain in the shoulder area. The pain may change from dull to sharp with certain motions of the shoulder. The pain may awaken the patient from a sound sleep, especially after rolling onto the shoulder.

Common location of the "chest pain"

The pain most commonly is described as directly in the shoulder area under the lateral acromion (see Figure 8–1). Patients may not specifically describe "shoulder" pain, but instead may describe deep "arm" pain which may be similar to the referred pain of angina pectoris.

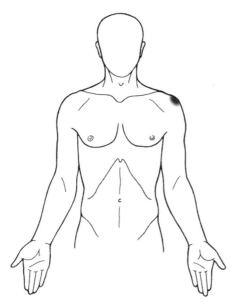

Figure 8–1. Common location of the "pain" due to rotator cuff tendonitis.

Uncommon location of the "chest pain"

Less frequently it may be referred more distally to the middle arm near the deltoid insertion laterally (see Figure 8–2). Rarely the pain may be referred down to the middle third of the arm without pain in the shoulder. In patients with this pattern of radiation, the patient is frequently dubious that shoulder tendonitis is the cause of the pain. Some patients have pain going up towards the neck over the belly of the supraspinatus muscle more proximally.

Size of the painful "area"

The area of pain is usually between the size of a golf ball and a tennis ball. In severe situations the patient will describe it as enveloping the whole shoulder area.

Duration of the "chest pain"

The sharp pain which comes with activity may last from seconds to minutes. The deep burning or aching pain may last constantly for hours or days, and intermittently for months to years.

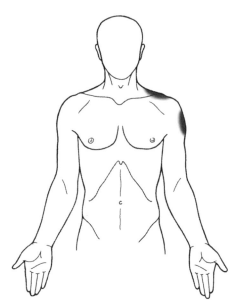

Figure 8–2. Uncommon location of the "pain" due to rotator cuff tendonitis. The "pain" may be located in either of the areas shown in the diagram.

Tenderness of the area

There may be pain to direct palpation over the inflamed rotator cuff tendons on the anterior lateral shoulder, just inferior to the acromion. Pain may also be found over the proximal biceps tendon on the anterior inferior aspect of the shoulder in the bicipetal groove between the greater and lesser tuberosities of the shoulder. In some cases it is not possible to induce pain with direct palpation, but pain can be induced with a provocative maneuver.

Precipitating causes of the "chest pain"

The pain may be activity-related, directly following or a few hours after overhead activity or strenuous use, such as raking the lawn. A traumatic event, such as a catching oneself with the arm while falling, may be another cause of the pain. The pain may also come on insidiously, without a discrete precipitating cause.

Sharp pain is usually related to some specific activity such as reaching overhead, or reaching behind one's back to remove a wallet, tuck in a shirt, or fasten a brassiere strap.

Patients often describe pain with attempting to sleep on the shoulder, or after rolling onto the shoulder while sleeping.

Relief of "chest pain"

Patients find most relief resting the arm motionless at their side.

Acromioclavicular Joint Arthritis

Characteristics of the "Pain"

Patient's characterization of the "chest pain"

Patients with arthritis of the acromioclavicular joint have deep aching pain in the area of the joint on the anterior-superior aspect of the shoulder area. The pain may change from dull to sharp with certain motions of the shoulder, such as reaching across the front of the body to touch the other shoulder or reach the opposite axilla.

Common location of the "chest pain"

The pain most commonly is described as directly on the anterior-superior aspect of the shoulder around the acromioclavicular joint (see

Figure 8–3). Less frequently, it may be referred more deeply into the shoulder inferior to the acromioclavicular joint.

Uncommon location of the "chest pain"

The pain may be referred down to the middle third of the arm, or radiate up towards the neck (see Figure 8–4).

Size of the "painful" area

The area of pain is usually the size of a golf ball. In severe situations the patient will describe it as enveloping the whole shoulder area.

Duration of the "chest pain"

The sharp pain which comes with activity may last for seconds to minutes. The deep aching pain may be permanently present.

Tenderness of the area

The pain is elicited with direct palpation over the acromioclavicular joint on the superior-anterior aspect of the shoulder. The joint can be located

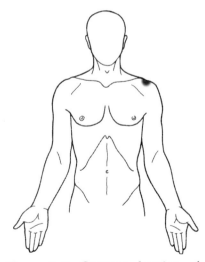

Figure 8–3. Common location of the "pain" due to acromioclavicular arthritis.

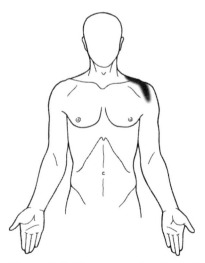

Figure 8–4. Uncommon location of the "pain" due to acromioclavicular arthritis.

by palpating from medial to lateral along the anterior-superior border of the clavicle until the slight bulge of the joint is palpated at the junction of the clavicle and the acromion.

Precipitating causes of the "chest pain"

The pain of acromioclavicular arthritis may be brought out by activity, following directly or a few hours after use. A traumatic event such as a direct blow to the shoulder (a low grade acromioclavicular or shoulder separation) may also precipitate the pain. The pain may also come on insidiously without a discrete cause.

Sharp pain is usually related to some specific activity, such as reaching out to pick up a heavy item, or reaching across ones chest as a patient may do to apply antiperspirant to the opposite axilla.

Relief of the "chest pain"

Patients find most relief resting the arm motionless at their side.

Glenohumeral ("Shoulder") Arthritis

Characteristics of the "Pain"

Patient's characterization of the "chest pain"

Patients with arthritis of the glenohumeral joint (true shoulder joint arthritis) have deep aching pain in the shoulder area. The pain may change from dull to sharp with almost any motions of the shoulder.

Common location of the "chest pain"

The pain most commonly is described as directly in the shoulder area inferior to the acromioclavicular joint (see Figure 8–5).

Uncommon location of the "chest pain"

Less frequently it may be referred more distally to the middle arm near the deltoid insertion laterally. The pain may even be referred down to the middle third of the arm (see Figure 8–6).

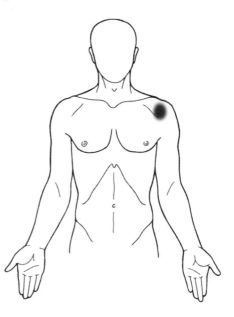

Figure 8–5. Common location of the "pain" due to glenohumeral arthritis.

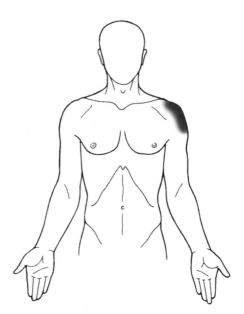

Figure 8–6. Uncommon location of the "pain" due to glenohumeral arthritis.

Size of the "painful" area

The area of pain is usually the size of a tennis ball. In severe situations the patient will describe it as enveloping the whole shoulder area.

Duration of the "chest pain"

The sharp pain which comes with activity may last for seconds to minutes. The deep aching pain may be constantly and permanently present.

Tenderness of the area

It is usually not possible to elicit pain with palpation, but pain can be induced with a provocative maneuver. In some cases of arthritis co-occurring rotator cuff tendonitis or tears may be present, and pain can be elicited from palpation of the rotator cuff.

Precipitating causes of the "chest pain"

The deep aching pain of shoulder arthritis may be brought out by low grade trauma or activity. It may occur directly following the insult or a few hours later. The pain may also come on insidiously without a discrete cause. The acute sharp pain is usually related to some specific activity, such as reaching overhead or out to the side.

Relief of the "chest pain"

Patients find most relief resting the arm motionless at their side.

Associated Symptoms

Most of the symptoms have been listed under the description of pain that characterizes each of the three conditions.

Associated Signs

Physical examination

The most important physical finding in the diagnosis of musculoskeletal-caused shoulder pain is reproduction or enhancement of the patient's pain with active or passive motion of the shoulder. In longstanding rotator cuff tendonitis or glenohumeral arthritis, the patient's shoulder may have limitations of overhead elevation, internal rotation (reaching behind the back), and external rotation.

In *rotator cuff tendonitis* the patient may describe pain in the "arc of impingement" as the arm is raised to near 90° of abduction. Pain may be induced by the "impingement maneuver" described by Charles Neer, where the physician applies passive forward flexion of the arm.[2] As the arm reaches 90° to 100° of forward flexion, the patient may experience pain. In this maneuver the supraspinatus tendon is being rubbed against the undersurface of the medial acromion.[6] Pain may be induced by the "impingement maneuver" described by Richard Hawkins, where the physician apples passive forward flexion of the arm with 90° internal rotation of the shoulder (the forearm held parallel to the floor.[1] In this maneuver the supraspinatus tendon is being rubbed against the undersurface of the coracoacromial ligament.[6]

In patients with *acromioclavicular arthritis,* the cross body adduction test reproduces the patient's pain and is diagnostic for acromioclavicular arthritis.[5] The physician grasps the patient's elbow, bends the elbow to 90° of flexion, elevates the patient's arm to 90° of forward flexion, and then adducts the arm across the patient's chest. Having the patient resist this motion with abduction augments this test. Pain with direct palpation of the joint is sensitive for acromioclavicular arthritis but not specific, as this palpation may also cause pain in patient with rotator cuff disease.[5] Most patients with acromioclavicular arthritis do not have limitations of shoulder motion.

Patients with arthritic shoulders often have limitation of motion compared to the opposite side. Loss of overhead elevation and of external rotation are frequently present. In severe cases pain can be induced with passive internal and external rotation of the arm with the elbow at the side. In less severe cases pain occurs with abduction and extremes of rotation.[3]

"Routine" laboratory tests

Diagnosis of these conditions is mainly based on history and physical examination.[1,2] Plain x-rays may show changes of a beaked or curved acromion in cases of rotator cuff tendonitis, or even a high-riding humeral head in cases of a complete rotator cuff tear. In many cases of rotator cuff tendonitis the x-rays are normal , although in some chronic cases of tendonitis there may be cystic changes present at the insertion of the supraspinatus tendon into the greater tuberosity.[2,4] Plain x-rays can show arthritic changes in the glenohumeral joint as well as in the acromioclavicular joint.[3,5] The true anterior posterior view of the shoulder joint (as opposed to an anterior posterior view of the lateral aspect of the thorax) should be taken with beam angled 40° across the chest so as to be parallel to the glenohumeral joint is most helpful in visualizing joint space narrowing and changes of arthritis. The axillary lateral view is also helpful for diagnosing glenohumeral arthritis. For diagnosis of acromioclavicular arthritis the joint can be best visualized with a Zanca view of the shoulder shot with the beam aimed 15° superior and at 50% of normal kilovoltage.[5]

Exceptions to the Usual Manifestations

None.

Differential Diagnosis

Other, rarer musculoskeletal causes of pain of the shoulder girdle include infection (septic arthritis), gout, inflammatory arthritis, chronic instability (subluxation) of the shoulder, tear of the glenoid labrum ("SLAP" lesion), adhesive capsulitis ("frozen shoulder"), primary tumor of the bone or soft tissue, metastatic tumor, and traumatic or pathologic fracture of the shoulder girdle.[1]

Other Diagnostic Testing

Magnetic Resonance Imaging (MRI) can confirm rotator cuff tendonitis or rotator cuff tear and help to plan for surgical treatment, but is not needed to make the diagnosis. With improved MRI resolution, arthrograms of the shoulder should be reserved for the assessment of recurrent rotator cuff tears and suspected labral lesions. CT scans can be used to define the arthritic changes of the glenohumeral joint, but are not indicated as a screening study.

Etiology and Basic Mechanisms Responsible for the "Pain"

The pain of *rotator cuff tendonitis* comes from inflammation or tearing of the distal aspect of the supraspinatus tendon and from secondary inflammation of the overlying subacromial bursa. This occurs with age and repetitive overhead use. As the arm is brought up into abduction and forward flexion, the distal aspect of the supraspinatus tendon rubs against ("impinges") the overlying coracoacromial arch, which consists of the coroid acromial ligament and the anterior inferior aspect of the acromion. This distal aspect of the supraspinatus tendon is poorly vascularized and is therefore prone to attritional tearing. As the process advances, the rotator cuff muscles are used less due to pain and therefore weaken. This weakness increases the symptoms as the overlying deltoid pulls the humeral head and attached tendon up against the acromion as the rotator cuff can no longer adequately depress the humeral head.

The pain from arthritis of the *acromioclavicular* or *glenohumeral joint* comes from loading of an arthritic joint, with the exposed bone bearing a load which should be borne by cartilage. Usually the acromioclavicular joint has only 5° to 8° of motion as the shoulder runs through a range of motion. In low grade acromioclavicular separations, the joint surface is injured, and the capsule is damaged enough to allow increased motion, but the articular surfaces remain in contact causing cartilage degradation.[5]

In primary glenohumeral arthritis the articular cartilage is first lost in the area of the humeral head which contacts the glenoid at 60° to 100° of abduction. This is the area of greatest contact pressure between the humeral head and the glenoid.[3] In patients with arthritis secondary to dislocations, the initial cartilage injury occurs from the shearing which occurs with the dislocations or subluxations.

Treatment

For both arthritis and tendonitis treatment consists initially of rest, activity alteration, anti-inflammatory medication, physical therapy and sometimes cortisone injection. For those patients who fail to find relief with these treatments, surgical intervention may be necessary.

For relief of acute symptoms patients should avoid use of the arm, and may use a sling for several days. Sling immobilization should not be used for more than 1 to 2 weeks due to the risk of iatrogenically creating a stiff shoulder. Oral non-steroidal anti-inflammatories provide some relief, but may take days to months to work.

The pain of rotator cuff tendonitis can be aided and often cured by a directed program of physical therapy to strengthen the rotator cuff muscles and correct the dynamic imbalance of the shoulder muscles which led to the impingement.[1] Therapy is less effective in treating acromioclavicular arthritis, and may have moderate benefit in patients with glenoid humeral arthritis.

Temporary complete relief and a confirmation of diagnosis can be provided by injection of a local anesthetic (e.g. xylocaine) into the affected area. The addition of a corticosteroid (e.g. betamethasone acetate) to the injection can provide longer lasting relief. In cases of rotator cuff tendonitis without a rotator cuff tear, subacromial steroid injection can sometimes provide permanent relief.[7] For arthritis of the acromioclavicular joint and the glenohumeral joint, steroid injection can provide long lasting, but rarely permanent, relief of the arthritis pain.[8]

For diagnosis and treatment of rotator cuff tendonitis, the subacromial space can be approached from a anterior, lateral or posterior direction with the placement of a 25-gauge, 1.5-inch needle just inferior to the edge of the acromion. The acromioclavicular joint[5] is approached from above. For glenohumeral arthritis, the injection of local steroid is into the shoulder joint itself (not into the subacromial bursa) from a posterior approach, and requires a long needle (e.g. 22-gauge, 2.5-inch spinal needle).

Chronic rotator cuff tendonitis may be treated with either open or arthroscopic subacromial decompression with removal of the coracoacromial ligament, the subacromial bursa and the anterio-inferior undersurface of the acromion.[1,2] Arthritis of the acromioclavicular may be treated surgically by the excision of the distal 1.5 cm of the clavicle either in an open manner or arthroscopically.[5] The pain of glenohumeral arthritis can be effectively relieved by shoulder replacement.[3]

References

1. Hawkins RJ, Kennedy JC. Impingement syndrome in athletes. *Am J Sports Med* 1980;8(3):151–158.
2. Neer CS II. Anterior acromioplasty for the chronic impingement syndrome in the shoulder. A preliminary report. *J Bone Joint Surg* 1972;54-A(1):41–50.
3. Neer CS II. Replacement arthroplasty for glenohumeral osteoarthritis. *J Bone Joint Surg* 1974;56-A(1):1–13.
4. Rockwood CA, Lyons FR. Diagnosis, Radiographic evaluation, and treatment with a modified Neer Acromioplasty. *J Bone Joint Surg* 1993;75-A(3):409–424.
5. Shaffer BS. Painful conditions of the acromioclavicular joint. *J Am Acad Orthop Surg* 1999;7(3)176–188.
6. Valadie AL, Jobe CM, Pink MM, et al. Anatomy of provocative tests for impingement syndrome of the shoulder. *J Shoulder Elbow Surgery* 2000;9(1):36–46.
7. Blair B, Rokito AS, Cuomo F, et al. Efficacy of injections of corticosteroids for subacromial impingement syndrome. *J Bone Joint Surg* 1996;78-A(11):1685–1689.
8. Jacob AK, Sallay PI. Therapeutic efficacy of corticosteroid injections in the acromioclavicular joint. *Biomed Sci Instrum* 1997;34:380–385.

9

"Chest Pain" in Patients with Joint Disease of the Cervical or Thoracic Spine

Stephen B. Miller, MD

General Considerations

There are multiple causes of joint disease of the cervical and thoracic spine.[1]

Clinical Setting

Patients with pain of the cervical and/or thoracic spine are generally in an older age group. The conditions occur equally in males and females, and are unrelated to a specific occupation.

Characteristics of the "Pain"

Patient's characterization of the "chest pain"

The pain of cervical (neck) arthritis is chronic, with exacerbations and periods of improvement. Patient descriptions are highly variable. Patients feel "uncomfortable" and have twinges of pain, particularly with rapid head movements. Sometimes the patient will describe a "cracking or crunching" sound on neck movement.

From: Hurst JW, Morris DC (eds): *"Chest Pain"* →. © Futura Publishing Co., Inc., Armonk, NY, 2001.

Common location of the "chest pain"

Pain is usually felt posteriorly overlying the vertebrae from the base of the skull, inferiorly to the lower cervical region, and lower when the diseases involve the thoracic spine (see Figure 9–1).

Uncommon locations of the "chest pain"

Radiation of pain to the shoulder and/or down the arm (radicular pain) is infrequent, unless the predominant clinical problem is degenerative intervertebral disc disease.

Size of the painful "area"

The size of the painful area is usually confined to the midline overlying the involved joints (see Figure 9–1).

Duration of the "chest pain"

The pain is usually present at a low intensity throughout the day but often worsens at night. Shorter, but more intense, painful episodes punctuate the chronic background discomfort.

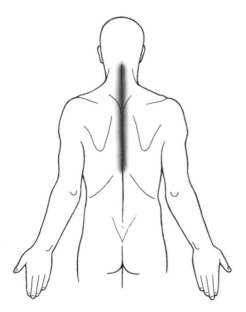

Figure 9–1. Location of the "pain" caused by joint disease of the cervical or thoracic spine.

Tenderness of the chest wall

There is no chest wall tenderness.

Precipitating causes of the "chest pain"

A precipitating cause of an increase in pain is not usually obvious. Sometimes, however, a cause seems definable, such as after driving a long distance or working long hours in tight quarters. The pain is not directly related to walking up an incline or precipitated by emotional disturbances such as anger.

Relief of the "chest pain"

The chronic pain can be relieved with non-steroidal anti-inflammatory medications (NSAIDs), hot packs and rest periods as needed. A soft cervical collar may be helpful particularly during exacerbations. Pain in the thoracic spine due to osteoarthritis is much less frequent than cervical pain, and other etiologies should be more intensively pursued (see below, "Differential Diagnosis").

Associated Symptoms

None, other than the symptoms related to the intensity of the pain.

Associated Signs

Physical examination

Examination of the cervical spine (neck) may show great variability depending on the degree of arthritic involvement. Flexion and extension, left and right rotation, and left and right lateral flexion is tested. With mild disease the range of motion may be full and painless. More severe arthritis will reflect itself most prominently with an asymmetric decrease in lateral flexion. Flexion/extension and rotation become limited as the arthritis progresses in severity. Muscle weakness and localized adenopathy are absent.

Examination of the thoracic spine may show an obvious kyphosis or scoliosis. Rotation with the trunk fixed from the waist down may be accompanied by pain. Otherwise there are no other significant abnormalities.

"Routine" laboratory tests

Routine laboratory tests are not helpful. Standard antero-posterior and lateral radiographs of the cervical or thoracic spine are indicated.

Exceptions to the Usual Manifestations

None.

Differential Diagnosis

Diseases of the Cervical Spine

Degenerative disc disease without radiculopathy must be excluded (see Chapter 11). Although arthritis (usually osteoarthritis) of the true spinal joints, namely the apophyseal or facet joints, is a different process than disc degeneration, they are very closely linked and usually accompany each other. X-ray films of the cervical and upper thoracic spine will establish the presence of either or both conditions.

Spondyloarthropathies must be excluded. Ankylosing spondylitis and its variants commonly involve the neck. Severe restriction in range of motion out of proportion to pain is characteristic. X-ray films of the cervical and upper thoracic spine confirm the diagnosis.

Rheumatoid arthritis produces severe pain often with radicular symptoms. An x-ray film of the thoracic spine will usually confirm the diagnosis.

Diseases of the Thoracic Spine

Osteoporotic compression fractures can be confirmed by an x-ray film made of the cervical and thoracic spine.

Metastatic cancer to the spine can be confirmed by an x-ray film made of the cervical and thoracic spine.

Other Diagnostic Testing

Computed tomography and magnetic resonance imaging are valuable radiographic procedures and are particularly useful in diagnosing spinal stenosis.

Etiology and Basic Mechanisms Responsible for the "Pain"

Vertebral articulation is accomplished by the only true synovial joints of the spine, namely, the apophyseal joints. Osteoarthritis affects these joints in a similar manner as peripheral joints producing identical pathologic changes. The actual cause of osteoarthritis remains unknown. Many local factors contribute to the pain. These include an elevated intraosseous pressure in subchondral bone, periosteal elevation, stretching on the joint capsule, and a secondary mild synovitis. In advanced cases, destructive changes of the cartilage cause instability and incongruity with "bone on bone" contact.

Treatment

Treatment is symptomatic, and directed primarily at chronic pain. Acetaminophen, salicylates, and other NSAIDs are used empirically. The goal is to gain maximum effectiveness with the least toxicity, which usually manifests as gastric intolerance. Application of local heat, creams, and ointments, and intermittent use of a soft cervical collar, are all helpful.

References

1. Borenstein DG, Wiesel SW, Boden SD. *Neck Pain in Medical Diagnosis and Comprehensive Management.* Philadelphia, WB Saunders, 1996, pp 161–437.

Part III

Thrombophlebitis as a Cause for "Chest Pain"

Although the definition of "chest pain"→ is discussed in Chapter 1, the definition is repeated here so that communication is clear.

The quotation marks around "chest" imply that different patients have different definitions of the word "chest." Here we use the word to indicate pain located above the waist. Then, too, *angina pectoris* is not always located in the pectoral region—it may be felt only in the jaw, neck, shoulder, elbow, or wrist. Therefore, the word "chest" implies that other parts of the upper body may also be involved with painful syndromes.

The quotation marks around "pain" imply that patients may assign other terms to their discomfort, such as indigestion, burning, ache, etc.

The arrow after "chest pain" implies that the physician initially may not know the cause of the symptom, so a differential diagnosis must be established that fits the available information.

10

"Chest Pain" in Patients with Mondor's Syndrome

Stephen D. Clements, Jr., MD

General Considerations

Superficial thrombophlebitis of the breast and anterior chest wall is known as Mondor's syndrome. Henri Mondor, a French surgeon, described this entity in 1939, referring to the clinical finding of "string phlebitis of the chest wall."[1]

Flagge had also described the entity with particular attention to the groove-like retracted area on the lateral aspect of the breast.[2] Since these original descriptions were published, many cases have been reported.[3,4] The syndrome is of interest to clinicians since it can cause left precordial pain and cause concern about myocardial ischemia or cancer of the breast.

Clinical Setting

Although Mondor's disease occurs most frequently in women, it has been reported in men. The age of those affected ranges from 25 to 55 years[2] and patients from all walks of life are affected.

Characteristics of the "Pain"

Patient's characterization of the "chest pain"

Those affected may describe the pain as a soreness, tightness, tautness, or bruise-like discomfort that may have a gradual or sudden onset. Occasionally, the problem is not painful.

From: Hurst JW, Morris DC (eds): *"Chest Pain"* →. © Futura Publishing Co., Inc., Armonk, NY, 2001.

Common location of the "chest pain"

The most common location of the pain is in the anterolateral area of the left breast extending vertically toward the axilla (see Figure 10–1).

Uncommon location of the "chest pain"

Uncommon locations of the chest discomfort are: the right breast extending toward the axilla, the upper abdomen on either side and rarely, the upper arms. All of these areas follow the distribution of a superficial vein.

Size of the pain "area"

The painful area consists of a firm, tender subcutaneous chord-like area measuring 3 to 5 mm in diameter and extending up to 30 cm in length. From the painful, tender stage, a more chronic retracted area develops in a band-like fashion, contracting and causing a furrowed area in the skin or a deep puckered groove. The veins commonly involved are the lateral thoracic vein, the thoracoepigastric vein, and the superior epigastric vein. Rarely, even the veins of the upper arm and shoulder are involved.[2]

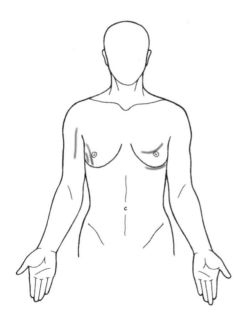

Figure 10–1. Mondor's syndrome results in painful lines across the anterolateral aspect of the breast extending superiorly toward the axilla, or laterally to the epigastrium, or more rarely on the anterior aspect of the arms. This is more likely to be the distribution of pain in females.

Duration of the "chest pain"

The pain usually lasts from a few days to (rarely) a few months.

Tenderness of the chest wall

Tenderness in the affected area is usually present initially, and less so as the area becomes more retracted or fibrous.

Precipitating causes of the "chest pain"

The precipitating causes of the chest discomfort and disease process are often obscure or idiopathic; however, trauma, surgery (such as breast biopsy or resection) and even infection in a breast can precede Mondor's disease. Rarely, breast cancer can precede this abnormality.

Elevation of the arm, such as when writing on a blackboard, deep breathing, or abdominal wall stretching, will aggravate the discomfort.

Relief of the "chest pain"

Relief is usually spontaneous, requiring no specific treatment. Warm compresses may help. Anticoagulants, steroids and antibiotics have not proven of any value. Rarely, with biopsy, through severing or excising the fibrous cord and thereby relieving tension on the breast, relief is obtained. At the time of interruption of the cord, an audible snap, like a cut bow string, has been recorded.

Associated Symptoms

There are no associated symptoms, unless the condition follows trauma or surgery.

Associated Signs

Physical examination

There are no associated signs unless the condition is caused by trauma, cancer of the breast, or biopsy of the breast.

"Routine" laboratory tests

Routine laboratory examination is not revealing. The chest x-ray film is normal unless the condition is caused by trauma or cancer that could, under severe circumstances, reveal the cause of the syndrome.

Exceptions to the Usual Manifestations

There are no exceptions to the clinical findings described above.

Differential Diagnosis

Knowing that such a condition exists will allow one to make the diagnosis. Herpes zoster (prevesicular phase) and costochondritis should be considered.

Other Diagnostic Testing

The clinical findings are sufficient. No other tests are needed.

Etiology and Basic Mechanisms Responsible for the "Pain"

The exact etiology of the phlebitis and periphlebitis is uncertain. Thrombus and endophlebitis are present, in addition to a periphlebitic reaction that encircles the vessel in a cuff-like manner. Histocytes and epithelioid-type cells are present, with the healing process leading to obliterative endophlebitis and a fibrous band. The etiology of this vascular reaction is not clear, but trauma often is associated. The inflammatory reaction results in initial symptoms; later the fibrous band, furrowed skin, and retracted subcutaneous tissue produce the pulling and tight, taut-like sensation.

Treatment

No specific treatment has been shown to alter the disease significantly. Anti-inflammatory agents and steroids may decrease the pain, but do not alter the basic natural history. Biopsy and cutting of the "bow string" may relieve the pulling sensation. Warm compresses may ease the early symptoms of pain and signs of tenderness.

References

1. Mondor H. Tronculite sous-cutanée subaiguë de la paroi thoracique antéro-latérale. *Med Acad Chir (Paris)* 1939;65:1271–1278.
2. Hogan G. Mondor's disease. *Arch Int Med* 1964;113:881–885.
3. Honig C, Rado R. Mondor's disease-superficial phlebitis of the chest wall. *Ann Surg* 1961;153:589–591.
4. Winslow SB. Superficial phlebitis of the breast and chest wall: Mondor's disease. *J Mich Med Soc* 1961;60:1523–1524.

Part IV

Neurologic Disease as a Cause for "Chest Pain"

Although the definition of "chest pain"→ is discussed in Chapter 1, the definition is repeated here so that communication is clear.

The quotation marks around "chest" imply that different patients have different definitions of the word "chest." Here we use the word to indicate pain located above the waist. Then, too, *angina pectoris* is not always located in the pectoral region—it may be felt only in the jaw, neck, shoulder, elbow, or wrist. Therefore, the word "chest" implies that other parts of the upper body may also be involved with painful syndromes.

The quotation marks around "pain" imply that patients may assign other terms to their discomfort, such as indigestion, burning, ache, etc.

The arrow after "chest pain" implies that the physician initially may not know the cause of the symptom, so a differential diagnosis must be established that fits the available information.

11

"Chest Pain" in Patients with Cervical Disc Syndromes

David J. Hewitt, MD

General Considerations

Cervical disc herniation leads to pain down an arm in a recognizable distribution with associated sensory, motor, and reflex changes and can occur spontaneously or as a result of trauma. Acute onset of neck pain and radicular symptoms can be a neurologic emergency if associated with corticospinal tract involvement.

Clinical Setting

The cervical disc syndrome occurs in male and female adults who are middle-aged and older.

Characteristics of the "Pain"

Cervical disc syndromes occur more frequently as people age. Degenerative changes involve bony and ligamentous structures of the spine as well as the disc. Gender is not a predisposing factor, but women are more susceptible to osteoporosis. Jobs that require physical labor with repetitive stresses increase the risk for the development of disc herniations.

Patient's characterization of the "chest pain"

Patients describe the pain as a shooting or lancinating pain that starts in the neck and runs down the arm. Areas of pain in the arm can be de-

From: Hurst JW, Morris DC (eds): *"Chest Pain"* →. © Futura Publishing Co., Inc., Armonk, NY, 2001.

scribed as shooting, lancinating, electrical, a burning or tingling, and as an aching pain similar to a toothache.

Common location of the "chest pain"

Radicular pain follows along a dermatomal distribution (see Figures 11–1 and 11–2).

Uncommon locations of the "chest pain"

Scalp pain and headache can occur, as the C2 dermatome supplies the posterior scalp. Also, since the nucleus and spinal tract of the trigeminal nerve descend to the third or fourth cervical spinal cord level, lesions affecting the upper cervical cord can result in ipsilateral facial analgesia, hypesthesia, and thermoanesthesia involving the peripheral (lateral) forehead, cheek, and jaw.

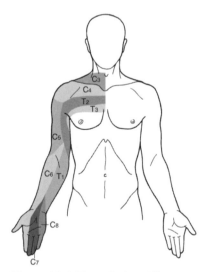

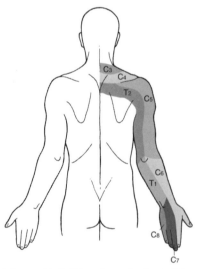

Figure 11–1. Frontal view. The common location of the radicular pain due to cervical disc syndromes follows along a dermatomal distribution. The cervical nerve roots are labeled with a C and the number of the root. The thoracic nerve roots are labeled with a T and the number of the root.

Figure 11–2. View from the back. The common location of the radicular pain due to cervical disc syndromes follows along a dermatomal distribution. The cervical nerve roots are labeled with a C and the number of the root. The thoracic nerve roots are labeled with a T and the number of the root.

The size of the painful "area"

The size of the painful area can be limited to the distribution of the dermatome involved, but tender points and muscle spasms can occur outside the area of the nerve distribution.

Duration of the "chest pain"

The pain can last as long as the disc protrusion is present and pressing against a nerve root. Frequently, the disc herniation and pain resolve within weeks. Pain can occur as a continuous baseline pain, but may also involve times of breakthrough pain with significant worsening of pain intensity. Moving the limb or neck produces a type of "breakthrough" pain.

Tenderness of the chest wall

Muscles can become tender due to changes in body mechanics that occur in an effort to relieve pain in the arm. Muscle spasms and muscle tenderness frequently occurs.

Precipitating causes of the "chest pain"

Maneuvers that decrease the diameter of the spinal foramen or stretch the roots can precipitate pain. Flexion, extension, or rotation of the head can increase pain. Valsalva's maneuver can increase intraspinal pressure and also increase pain.

Relief of the "chest pain"

Pain commonly occurs upon changing the position of the arm and neck. Accordingly, the patient usually finds a position of the arm and neck that relieves their pain to some degree. Medications can also be helpful in relieving pain and associated symptoms.

Associated Symptoms

Compression of spinal roots result in motor weakness, sensory segmental deficits, and a decrease or absence of stretch reflexes. Weakness and atrophy in a myotomal distribution are the results of injury to the ventral root. Patients themselves may be aware of the muscle fasciculations in their weak muscles.

Symptoms that may result from central disc herniation include weakness in the arms or legs, changes in coordination gait or balance, and changes in bowel, bladder or sexual function.

Associated Signs

Physical examination

Sensory changes commonly occur in a dermatomal distribution. Motor changes involve myotomes that refer to the anterior root involved. Reflexes can be decreased or absent in the setting of compression of the dorsal or ventral root interrupting either the afferent or efferent arc of a muscle stretch reflex.

Compression of C1: Compression of C1 produces purely motor symptoms because there is no dorsal root from C1. Involvement of C1 results in minor motor difficulties. Motor weakness occurs in muscles that support the head and fix the neck, assist in neck flexion and extension, and control tilt of the head to one side (longus capitis, rectus capitis, obliquus capitis, longissimus capitis, and cervicis, multifidi, intertransversarii, rotatores, semispinalis, and infrahyoid muscles).

Compression of C2: Compression of C2 produces sensory symptoms and signs posterior to the interauaral line on the scalp (C2 dermatome). Muscles supplied by this root are the same as those innervated by C1, as well as the sternocleidomastoid muscle (head rotation and flexion), a muscle that is predominantly innervated by the spinal accessory nerve (cranial nerve XI).

Compression of C3: Compression of C3 results in sensory changes over the lower occiput, the angle of the jaw, and the upper neck. Weakness involving the scalene and levator scapulae muscles of the neck (infrahyoids, semispinalis capitis and cervicis, longissimus capitis and cervicis, intertransversarii, rotatores, multifidi) and the trapezius (shoulder elevation) may occur. The trapezius is predominantly innervated by the spinal accessory nerve. Since the phrenic nerve receives some of its fibers from the C3 segment, diaphragmatic weakness may occur.

Compression of C4: Compression of C4 produces sensory changes in the lower neck and weakness in the scalene (lateral neck flexion) and levator scapulae muscles (scapular rotation), rhomboid muscles (scapular elevation and adduction), trapezius muscle (shoulder elevation), and some muscles of the neck. As with C3, diaphragmatic weakness may occur since C3 supplies some fibers of the phrenic nerve.

Compression of C5: Compression of C5 nerve root results in pain in the neck, shoulder, and upper anterior arm; sensory changes involve the lateral arm. Weakness occurs predominantly and to varying degrees in the levator scapulae, rhomboids, serratis anterior, supraspinatus, infraspinatus, deltoid, biceps, and brachioradialis. Rarely, diaphragmatic weakness can occur due to C5 supply of the phrenic nerve. The biceps reflex and the brachioradialis reflexes may be depressed since it is supplied by segments C5-C6.

Compression of C6: Compression of C6 nerve root occurs as a result of disc herniation at the C5-C6 vertebral level. The monoradiculopathy affecting the C6 nerve root is the second most common level of cervical radiculopathy. Pain occurs in the lateral arm and dorsal forearm, with sensory changes occurring in the lateral forearm, lateral hand, and the first and second digits. Weakness predominantly involves the serratus anterior, biceps, pronator teres, flexor carpi radialis, brachioradialis, extensor carpi radialis longus, supinator, and extensor carpi radialis brevis. Decreased reflexes occur in the biceps and brachioradialis (C5-C6). An important sign to look for is the "inverted radial reflex" which results when the lesion compresses the spinal cord at the C5-C6 level. This finding is often the result of a central disc prolapse or a horizontal bar due to degenerative disc disease. Also, involvement of the corticospinal tract at the C5-C6 level results in hyper-reflexia in the lower levels. While the brachioradialis reflex might be absent percussion to elicit this reflex may produce a brisk contraction of the finger flexors which are innervated by a lower segment, C7-C8.

Compression of C7: Compression of C7 nerve root by disc herniation at the C6-C7 vertebral level is the most common level of disc herniation.[1,2] Pain occurs in the dorsal forearm and sensory changes involve the third and fourth digits. Weakness may be variable, occurring in the serratus anterior, pectoralis major, latissimus dorsi, pronator teres, flexor carpi radialis, triceps, extensor carpi radialis longus, extensor carpi radialis brevis, and extensor digitorum. The triceps reflex may be depressed.

Compression of the C8: Compression of C8 nerve root is the result of disc herniation at the C7-T1 vertebral level. Pain occurs in the medial arm and forearm. Sensory changes occur on the medial forearm and hand and on the fifth digit. Weakness involves flexor digitorum superficialis, flexor pollicis longus, flexor digitorum profundus I to IV, pronator quadratus, abductor pollicis brevis, opponens pollicis, flexor pollicis brevis, all lumbricals, flexor carpi ulnaris, abductor digitiminimi, opponens digiti minimi, flexor digiti minimi, all interossei, adductor pollicis, extensor digiti minimi, extensor carpi ulnaris, abductor pollicis longus, extensor pollicis longus and brevis and extensor indicis. The finger flexor deep tendon reflex (C8-T1) may be depressed. Sympathetic fibers ascending to the superior cervical ganglia are interrupted, producing a Horners syndrome.

Compression of the T1: Compression of the T1 nerve root produces sensory changes in the medial forearm and weakness in the abductor pollicis brevis, opponens pollicis, flexor pollicis brevis, all lumbricals and interossei, abductor digiti minimi, opponens digiti minimi, flexor digiti minimi and adductor pollicis. Depressed finger flexor reflexes may occur (C8-T1) and sympathetic fibers may get interrupted resulting in an ipsilateral Horner syndrome.

Long tract signs should be evaluated if the history obtained is suggestive of a process affecting the cord. Increased reflexes in the lower extremities, and increase in motor tone, increase in deep tendon reflexes, and the presence of a sensory level at the cervical levels are concerning and worthy of further evaluation.

"Routine laboratory tests"

The x-ray films of the chest and neck are very good at assessing bony structures and abnormalities including degenerative disease, congenital abnormalities, primary and metastatic tumors, metabolic bone disease, vertebral body fractures, and osteophytes. Structural and functional integrity can be assessed using flexion and extension films of the cervical spine. Due to the overlap of bony structures, certain areas cannot be evaluated well; these include C2, C7, and T1.

Exceptions to the Usual Manifestations

It is not uncommon for patients to have involvement of more than one nerve root and a more complicated set of signs and symptoms. Also, a patient's complaints may be due to nerve entrapments (e.g., carpal tunnel syndrome) or two areas of nerve involvement (double crush injury).

Differential Diagnosis

Foraminal stenosis, degenerative disease, facet arthrosis, spondylosis, a hypertrophied ligamentum flavum, primary tumors involving nerves, panus formation, mononeuritis from diabetes mellitus, and compression or infiltration of nerve by tumor should be considered on the differential diagnosis. Trauma to the spinal roots may result from missile or penetrating wounds. Compression neuropathies should also be considered. Involvement of C6 and C7 produces sensory symptoms in the thumb, index, and middle fingers, mimicking symptoms of carpal tunnel syndrome. Unlike carpal tunnel syndrome, pain frequently involves the neck and can be made worse with neck movement. The sensory changes and pain can radiate down the along the lateral forearm and occasionally the radial portion of the dorsum of the hand. Worsening of the pain can occur at nighttime, but this is more common with carpal tunnel syndrome. Weakness involves C6,7 innervated muscles, and not median innervated C8 muscles. Patients with radiculopathy keep their arm and neck still, which contrasts with patients with carpal tunnel syndrome who will often shake their arms and rub their hands to relieve the pain.

Other Diagnostic Testing

Magnetic resonance imaging

Magnetic resonance imaging (MRI) provides resolution of the spinal cord, subarachnoid space, discs, and the vertebral anatomy. Gadolinium is needed to distinguish recurrent disc from post-operative scar. Sagittal combined with axial images provides an excellent assessment for disc herniation. The water content in the nucleus pulposus and the inner annular fibers produce high signal intensity on T-2 weighted images. MRI can detect small radial tears, and is also better at differentiating sequestered disc fragment from other degenerative changes.[3,4]

Computed tomography

Computed tomography (CT) can assess bone and soft tissues contiguous with neural structures. CT through evaluation of bone windows can detect bone changes before plain radiography and bone scan. CT can evaluate both vertebral bodies and disc disease. Contrast is added to distinguish scarring from past surgeries from recurrent disc herniations of intervertebral discs. Axial images are helpful in assessing disc protrusion and the impingement of other elements on the disc.

CT-myelography

CT-myelography can detect subtle nerve root displacement secondary to posterior lateral herniations of intervertebral discs and osteophytes.

Myelography

Myelography can be used to assess the patency of the cerebral spinal fluid space after spinal stabilization.

CT and CT-myelography

Computed tomography and CT-myelography are used when MRI cannot be performed due to the presence of a magnetically active substance from trauma or surgery or after pacemaker placement.

Electromyography and nerve conduction are usually performed. Muscles may have spontaneous activity, particularly fibrillation potentials, positive sharp waves, and complex repetitive discharges. Cervical radiculopathy is characterized by involvement of paraspinal muscles, as well as limb muscles. The H reflex and F waves can be used to evaluate the proximal segment of nerves.

Nerve blocks can be diagnostic as well as therapeutic. When pain relief occurs following a block, it is suggestive of a diagnosis. Multiple blocks can be used to break the cycle of pain. CT-guided facet blocks can also be effective to determine if the symptoms are arising from the facet joint.

Etiology and Basic Mechanisms Responsible for the "Pain"

Pain is usually the direct result of compression of neural structures. Pain can also arise from somatic tissues that are innervated by nerves and are involved in a degenerative process.

Treatment

When weakness is present, surgical referral is warranted. If significant neurologic compromise is not present, then a conservative approach is recommended. In a prospective evaluation of cervical disc herniation with radicular type symptoms and objective neurologic findings, 12 of 13 patients demonstrated regression of the cervical disc herniation and improved symptoms.[5]

Treatment of pain may include multiple nerve blocks, physical therapy, cervical traction, and rest. Use of analgesic medications include nonsteroidal anti-inflammatory drugs, muscle relaxants, adjuvant analgesic medications such as anticonvulsants (e.g. gabapentin, phenytoin, carbamazepine) or tricyclic antidepressants (e.g. amitriptyline, nortriptyline, desipramine).

References

1. Marinacci, AA. A correlation between operative findings in cervical herniated disc with the electromyograms and opaque myelograms. *Electromyography* 1966;6:5.
2. Radhakrishnan K, et al. Epidemiology of cervical radiculopathy, a population-based study from Rochester, Minnesota, 1976 through 1990. *Brain* 1994;117:325.
3. Masaryk TJ, Ross JS, Modic MT, et al. High resolution MR imaging of the sequestered lumbar intervertebral disks. *Am J Roentgenol* 1998;150:1155–1162.
4. Greiner N, Kressel HY, Schiebler ML, et al. Normal and degenerative posterior spinal structures: MR imaging. *Radiology* 1989;170:489–493.
5. Bush K, Chaudhuri R, Hiller S. The pathomorphologic changes that accompany the resolution of cervical radiculopathy: A prospective study with repeat magnetic resonance imaging. *Spine* 1997;22:183–186.

12

"Chest Pain" in Patients with Brachial Plexus Neuropathy

David J. Hewitt, MD

General Considerations

Brachial plexus neuropathy may produce severe pain in the shoulders or arms which, at the beginning, may lead the physician to consider the diagnoses of myocardial infarction or dissection of the aorta.

Clinical Setting

Brachial plexus lesions can occur at any age from birth onward, and the patient's sex is not a risk factor. Most of the plexus injuries in North America are caused by motor vehicle accidents involving motorcycles. Birth injury to the plexus[1] may be the result of pressure in breech deliveries; traction associated with shoulder dystocia in cephalic deliveries,[2] or associated clavicular fractures or shoulder dislocation.[3] Later in life, brachial plexopathy can be the result of trauma, cancer, radiation therapy, and in the case of idiopathic plexitis ("neuralgic amyotrophy" or Parsonage-Turner syndrome) from no antecedent cause, or it can be related to sera or vaccines.[4] Traction injury to the plexus results from improper positioning during anesthesia, excessive sternal retraction during intracardiac operations, prolonged compression during narcotic-induced coma, excessive supraclavicular pressure from the weight of heavy knapsacks (e.g., knapsack paralysis), firearm recoil,[5] axillary catheterization causing hematoma, and using a crutch to ambulate. A familial brachial neuritis can occur with recurrent attacks.[6]

From: Hurst JW, Morris DC (eds): *"Chest Pain"* →. © Futura Publishing Co., Inc., Armonk, NY, 2001.

Characteristics of the "Pain"

Patient's characterization of the "chest pain"

Pain associated with brachial plexopathy is described as burning, tingling, sharp, shooting, well localized, electrical, freezing, and lancinating. The pain may be severe. Unusual sensory disturbances called dysesthesias can be felt by the patient. The patient may complain that non-noxious stimuli produce painful sensations (allodynia) over the affected area. Patients also complain that noxious stimuli produce an unusually painful response (hyperalgesia). Areas with decreased sensation can be very sensitive to stimuli (hyperpathia). Pain can occur as a constant underlying, or "baseline," pain. Breakthrough pain occurs superimposed upon the constant pain. It can occur either spontaneously, or as the result of action that increases stress on the limb (incident pain). Pain can start gradually, or occur with an acute onset.

During contact sports, a sudden forceful depression of the shoulder can produce a transient episode of abrupt, intense burning dysesthesia and anesthesia encompassing the entire upper extremity and accompanied by generalized limb weakness ("burners" or "stingers"). Within minutes, the symptoms resolve without any residual weakness. While the entire arm is involved, findings most prominently involve the upper plexus.

Parsonage-Turner syndrome,[7] also known as neuralgic amyotrophy, occurs with acute, severe pain in the shoulder radiating into the arm neck, and back. The arm is held in a position of flexion at the elbow and adduction at the shoulder, in an effort to avoid movement that causes pain. Within several hours to days the pain is followed by paresis of the shoulder and proximal arm musculature. The most commonly affected muscles are those innervated by the axillary, suprascapular, and long thoracic nerves. The condition is usually unilateral, bilateral involvement can occur. The cause is thought to be brachial plexitis or multiple mononeuritis and can follow viral illness or immunizations.

Common location of the "chest pain"

The pain of brachial plexus lesions can involve the entire limb or parts of the limb. Involvement of the upper plexus produces pain in the thumb and medial aspect of the arm; involvement of the lower plexus can produce pain in the lateral aspect of the arm (see Figures 12–1 and 12–2). Tumor infiltration produces severe pain in the shoulder, upper arm, and elbow radiating into the fourth and fifth fingers.

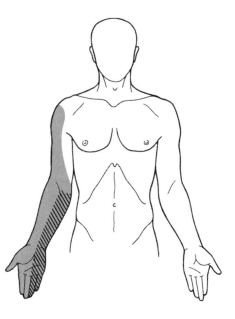

Figure 12–1. Frontal view. The location of the sensory changes produced by lesions of the brachial plexus (C5, C6, C7, C8, T1) are shown in the solid gray color. The location of the sensory changes produced by lesions of the lower roots of the brachial plexus (C8, T1) are illustrated by the diagonal lines.

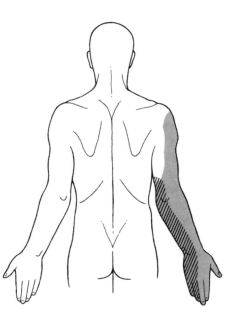

Figure 12–2. View from the back illustrating the location of the sensory changes associated with lesions of the nerve roots described above.

Uncommon locations of the "chest pain"

The pain associated with the Parsonage-Turner syndrome may be felt in the posterior portion of the upper part of the chest before it is felt in one of the arms.

Size of the painful "area"

The size of the painful area depends upon which nerves are involved and the stage of the disease. Initially, the pain may be the size of the hand, while later the pain may involve the entire arm.

Duration of the "chest pain"

The duration depends upon the cause and the availability of treatment and the use of ongoing analgesic medication. The pain may last a few minutes when due to depression of the shoulder during a contact sport or for a week or two as occurs with the Parsonage-Turner syndrome.

Tenderness of the chest wall

Distal paresthesias produced by supraclavicular percussion indicates that the nerve roots have retained continuity with the spinal cord. Axonal regeneration can be assessed by checking Tinel's sign, moving distally.

Precipitating causes of the "chest pain"

Pain increases with movement of the arm, but can occur spontaneously as the nerves die or grow back. The pain is not produced by walking.

Relief of the "chest pain"

Relief can be hard to obtain. The pain may be so intense and persistent that it prevents sleep. The patient will frequently place the arm in a position that is most comfortable, but movement can make the pain worse. Splints can be used to relieve pain and increase function. Analgesia is often needed.

Associated Symptoms

Weakness, alterations in sensation, and other symptoms correspond to the part of the plexus that is involved. Weakness of the periscapular and proximal arm muscles is the most common presentation of brachial plexus dysfunction, since the upper plexus is commonly involved in most traumatic and inflammatory lesions. While the hand can function normally, the proximal muscles of the arm cannot position it for effective use. Middle plexus paralysis involves the radial nerve producing weakness in the extensors of the forearm, hand, and fingers. Lower plexus paralysis is the result of injury to C8 and T1 roots or the lower trunk of the plexus and results in a decrease in distal arm function.

Edema may result from loss of sympathetic tone after root avulsion, pooling of venous blood (resulting from loss of the pumping action supplied by the paralyzed muscles), from the pull of gravity on the dependent arm, or when lymphatics are blocked by tumor. Disuse produces severe limitations in shoulder and elbow joint mobility that can interfere with functional recovery.

Associated Signs

Physical examination

Abnormalities in motor function include decreased strength, decreased tone, and muscle atrophy. Sensation is decreased to primary modalities. Deep tendon reflexes can be decreased. Examination requires assessing whether the distribution of the muscular weakness is consistent with an innervation pattern of a trunk, cord, or individual peripheral nerve.

Total plexus paralysis results in a paralyzed arm that hangs limp at the patient's side. All the muscles in the arm may undergo rapid atrophy. Complete anesthesia occurs distal to a line extending obliquely from the tip of the shoulder to the medial arm half way to the elbow. The entire limb is areflexic.

When the upper plexus is involved, paralysis or paresis occurs in muscles supplied by C5-C6 roots. The limb assumes a characteristic position often referred to as the so-called policeman's tip or porter's tip position: the limb is internally rotated and adducted and the forearm extended and pronated, with the palm facing out and backward. There is impaired shoulder abduction (deltoid and supraspinatus), elbow flexion (biceps, brachioradialis, brachialis), external rotation of the arm (infraspinatus), and forearm supination (biceps). Weakness in the rhomboids, levator scapulae, serratus anterior, and scalene muscles occur with more proximal lesions. Sensation is typically intact, with possible sensory loss over the outer surface of the upper arm, especially over the deltoid muscle. Biceps and brachioradialis reflexes are decreased or absent.

Middle plexus weakness involves the triceps, anconeus, extensor carpi radialis and ulnaris, extensor digitorum, extensor digiti minimi, extensor pollicis longus and brevis, abductor pollicis longus, and extensor indicis. Flexion of the forearm is spared, since the brachioradialis and brachialis are innervated predominantly by C5 and C6 segments. Decreased sensation is inconsistent and patchy and may occur over the extensor surface of the forearm and the radial aspect of the dorsum of the hand. The triceps reflex may be depressed or absent.

Lower plexus injury leads to paralysis and atrophy of muscles supplied by the C8 and T1 roots. Weakness involves wrist and finger flexion and the intrinsic muscles of the hand producing a claw-hand deformity. Sensation can be lost on the medial arm, medial forearm, and ulnar aspect of the hand, but can be intact. The finger flexor reflex (C8-T1) is either depressed or down. Autonomic signs occur because of involvement of sympathetic fibers ascending to the superior cervical ganglion and ultimately the eye, upper lid, and face producing an ipsilateral Horner syndrome (ptosis, miosis, and anhidrosis).

Lateral cord, medial cord, and posterior cord lesions produce distinctive patterns of weakness and sensory changes that help in localizing the part of the brachial plexus involved.[8]

"Routine" laboratory tests

The use of the ordinary chest x-ray film can be helpful as an initial screen when a Pancoast tumor is suspected. No other routine laboratory tests are helpful in making the diagnosis.

Exceptions to the Usual Manifestations

Brachial plexopathy can be quite variable depending on the cause of the brachial plexopathy and the part of the brachial plexus that is involved.

Accordingly, in the beginning, it is not uncommon for the physician to be confused. But as the course of the condition unfolds, the diagnosis is usually made.

Differential Diagnosis

Nerve root avulsions, multiple disc herniations, degenerative disease of the spine, peripheral neuropathy, complex regional pain syndromes, and injuries that effect a combination of the radial, ulnar, or median nerves should be considered as alternative diagnoses.

Other Diagnostic Testing

X-ray film of the cervical spine

Such x-ray films are usually ordered, but even if the films reveal cervical disc protrusion, it is the physical examination that is all important in diagnosing brachial plexus neuropathy.

Magnetic resonance imaging

Magnetic resonance (MR) imaging provides sagittal, coronal, and oblique views, and is very helpful in establishing the diagnosis. Nerves can be distinguished from other soft tissues and followed from the spinal cord through the plexus and to peripheral nerves.[9,10] Magnetic resonance imaging can also distinguish radiation fibrosis from recurrent tumor.

Three dimensional MR myelography

This procedure can show the majority of traumatic lesions that involve the proximal portion of the brachial plexus and has 89% sensitivity, 95% specificity, and 92% diagnostic accuracy in the evaluation of nerve root integrity.[11]

Computed tomography

This procedure can help distinguish a tumor from radiation fibrosis.

CT-myelography

This technique can distinguish nerve root avulsions from injury to the brachial plexus.

Electrodiagnostic study

This procedure can confirm the diagnosis of brachial plexopathy. Paraspinal muscles are spared when the lesion involves the plexus, but are affected when the root or a preganglionic lesion is involved.[12] Conduction studies on distal segments of the nerves may reveal a low or absent motor or sensory response. Slowing may be detected using the F response or H reflex. Tumor infiltration produces segmental slowing. Myokymia is suggestive of radiation fibrosis.

Etiology and Basic Mechanisms Responsible for the "Pain"

Pain is often the result of direct compression to the nerve. When the nerve is severed, a deafferentation-type pain syndrome can occur. The superficial location of the brachial plexus and the close relationship to bony structures and the mobility of the shoulder girdle and neck make it vulnerable to injury. Traction injuries occur when the head, neck, shoulder, and arm are forced in opposite directions, as commonly occurs in motorcycle accidents.

The types of trauma that commonly cause brachial plexus neuropathy are listed in the introduction to this chapter. A glaring exception to traumatic causes is the Parsonage-Turner syndrome, which can develop spontaneously or occur after receiving a vaccine or having a viral infection. This syndrome, more than the other causes, is the one that may simulate dissection of the aorta or myocardial infarction.

Treatment

Due to the long distance that nerves must traverse before reinnervating the distal arm and hand muscles, infraclavicular injuries have poor spontaneous recovery.[13] Chemotherapy or radiation can treat plexopathy due to tumor and resolve the pain. In the setting of trauma, surgical techniques can sometimes be used including nerve grafts, but commonly the injury is too extensive and surgery is not an option. When myelin sheaths are maintained, nerves can grow back and function can be obtained. Range of motion exercises should be performed to prevent the development of contractures. Recovery is more likely to reach a satisfactory level with infraclavicular plexus lesions from fractures and dislocations around the shoulder. Onset of recovery ranges from 3 to 9 months with intrinsic muscles of the hand recovering last. With supraclavicular lesions, if the distance from the site of injury to proximal muscles is not too great, improvement can occur. Peripheral nerve surgeons may explore traumatic brachial plexus injuries after 3 to 6 months of observation. Since adequate recovery of hand muscles is rare after severe lower plexus lesions, reinnervation of the proximal arm and shoulder muscles utilizing neuroma resection, end-to-end anastomosis if possible, and nerve grafts can be performed if needed. Splints can be used to protect the arm and encourage function.

Adjuvant analgesics such as antidepressants and anticonvulsants can be effective for the management of neuropathic pain associated with brachial plexopathy. Common anticonvulsants used are gabapentin, phenytoin, and carbamazepine. The tricyclic antidepressants imipramine, amitriptyline, nortriptyline and desipramine can also be effective. Corticosteroids, baclofen, and mexilitine can sometime be useful. The Parsonage-Turner syndrome is commonly relieved by the use of corticosteroids. The severe pain associated with plexopathy may necessitate the use of opioid analgesia. Experience from the treatment of cancer pain supports the use of opioid analgesia for the treatment of brachial plexopathy pain. Transcutaneous nerve stimulation can be effective in treating the pain associated with brachial plexopathy. Dorsal root-entry zone lesions can provide relief in some patients.

References

1. Eng GD, Koch B, Smokvina MD. Brachial plexus palsy in neonates and children. *Arch Phys Med Rehabil* 1978;59:458.
2. Rubin A. Birth injuries: Incidence, mechanisms, and end results. *Obstet Gynecol* 1964;23:218.
3. Eng GD. Brachial plexus palsy in newborn infants. *Pediatrics* 1971;48:18.
4. Liveson JA. *Peripheral Neurology: Case Studies in Electrodiagnosis.* Philadelphia, PA, F.A. Davis Company, 1979, pp. 36–43.
5. Wanamaberg WM. Firearm recoil palsey: *Arch Neurol* 1974;31:208.
6. Wiederholdt WC. Hereditary brachial neuropathy: Report of two families. *Arch Neurol* 1974;30:252.
7. England JD, Sumner AJ. Neurologic amyotrophy: An increasingly diverse entity. *Muscle Nerve* 1987;10:60.
8. Brazis PW, Masdeu JC, Biller J. *Localization in Clinical Neurology, 3rd ed.,* Boston, MA, Little, Brown, and Co. Inc., 1985, pp 54–62.
9. Rapaport S, Blair DN, McCarthy SM, et al. Brachial plexus: Correlation of MR imaging with CT and pathologic findings. *Radiology* 1988;167:161–165.
10. Fishman EK, Campbell JN, Kuhlman JE, et al. Multiplanar CT evaluation of brachial plexopathy in breast cancer. *J Comput Assist Tomogr* 1991;15:790–795.
11. Gasparotti R, Ferraresi S, Ginelli L. Three-dimensional MR myelography of traumatic injuries of the brachial plexus. *Am J Neuroradiol* 1997;18:1733–1742.
12. Bufanlini C, Pescatori G. Posterior cervical electromyography in the diagnosis and prognosis of brachial plexus injuries. *J Bone Joint Surg (Br)* 1969;51B:627.
13. Schaumburg HH, Berger AR, Thomas PK. *Diagnosis of Peripheral Nerves, 2nd ed.,* Philadelphia, PA, F.A. Davis Company, 1992, pp 216–221.

Part V

Mediastinal Disease as a Cause for "Chest Pain"

Although the definition of "chest pain" → is discussed in Chapter 1, the definition is repeated here so that communication is clear.

The quotation marks around "chest" imply that different patients have different definitions of the word "chest." Here we use the word to indicate pain located above the waist. Then, too, *angina pectoris* is not always located in the pectoral region—it may be felt only in the jaw, neck, shoulder, elbow, or wrist. Therefore, the word "chest" implies that other parts of the upper body may also be involved with painful syndromes.

The quotation marks around "pain" imply that patients may assign other terms to their discomfort, such as indigestion, burning, ache, etc.

The arrow after "chest pain" implies that the physician initially may not know the cause of the symptom, so a differential diagnosis must be established that fits the available information.

13

"Chest Pain" in Patients with Mediastinal Emphysema

Michelle M. Freemer, MD and Talmadge E. King, Jr., MD

General Considerations

The mediastinum consists of those structures and organs separating the two lungs, between the sternum in front and the vertebral column behind, and from the thoracic inlet above to the diaphragm below. Pneumomediastinum is defined as aberrant air or gas in the mediastinum. Mediastinitis is defined as infection or inflammation in the mediastinum. Although both pneumomediastinum and mediastinitis can occur together (for example, in esophageal rupture) they often present separately and have different patterns of illness. This chapter will focus on pneumomediastinum, also known as mediastinal emphysema.[1] Pneumothorax, an important life-threatening form of extra-alveolar air, will be discussed in Chapter 15.

Clinical Setting

Pneumomediastinum may occur in patients of any age, from the newborn to the elderly. Although mediastinal emphysema has historically been described in primipara women,[2] there is male predominance in most patient series.[3–6] The incidence of spontaneous pneumomediastinum varies widely in the literature from 2.5 in 100,000 to 13.7 in 100,000 hospital admissions.[3–5]

Mediastinal air may result from a variety of causes that may be either intrathoracic or extrathoracic. Many procedures can cause pneumomediastinum, including dental procedures, intubation with positive pressure

From: Hurst JW, Morris DC (eds): *"Chest Pain"* →. © Futura Publishing Co., Inc., Armonk, NY, 2001.

ventilation, tracheotomy, esophageal dilation, performance of the Heimlich maneuver or cardiopulmonary resuscitation, bronchoscopy, and esophagosopy. *Spontaneous pneumomediastinum* (also referred to as medical pneumomediastinum) has been used to designate patients with pneumomediastinum arising outside the setting of trauma, surgery, or other procedures (such as positive pressure ventilation). Medical pneumomediastinum may be precipitated by airway obstruction such as in asthma,[7] bronchitis/bronchiolitis, foreign body inhalation, or inhalation of meconium in neonates. Any maneuver increasing intra-alveolar pressure may also precede pneumomediastinum, including coughing, straining (e.g., in vomiting or labor),[2,8] valsalva (e.g., inhalational drug use,[5,6,9] athletic competition,[10] and Kussmaul's breathing in diabetic ketoacidosis.)[11,12] Rapid ascent or descent causing changes in pressure can also preciptate pneumomediastinum.[7] Infections, such as influenza, military tuberculosis, or retropharyngeal soft tissue infections have also been reported to cause pneumomediastinum.[3,13] Importantly, pneumomediastinum may truly be spontaneous, arising in an otherwise healthy individual at rest. Any cause of retroperitoneal air may also produce pneumomediastinum, with air dissecting cephalad (for example, gastric or intestinal perforation, diverticulitis, pneumatosis cystoides intestinalis).

Characteristics of the "Pain"

Patient's characterization of the "chest pain"

The patient usually states that the onset of the "pain" is sudden. The pain is described as stabbing or sharp in quality.

Common location of the "chest pain"

The pain is frequently localized to the retrosternal area or precordial region (see Figure 13–1). The "pain" may radiate to the back, neck, and left arm or shoulder (see Figure 13–2).

Uncommon locations of the "pain"

The pain may be felt only in the neck.[6]

Size of the pain "area"

The "painful" area is usually larger than the hand.

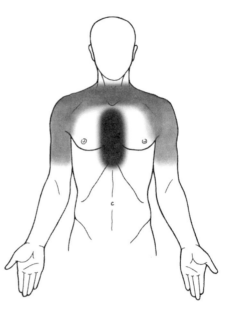

Figure 13–1. Frontal view. Common location of the "pain" due to mediastinal emphysema. The pain is usually located in the retrosternal area (black area) but may be located in the precordial area. The pain may radiate to the back, neck, shoulder, and arm (gray area). Subcutaneous emphysema (crepitance) may be found in the neck, face, and/or arms, or in the retrosternal area.

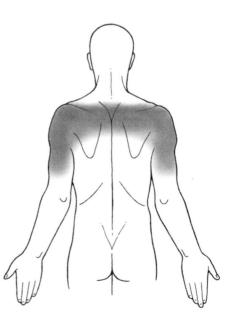

Figure 13–2. View from the back. The "pain" and crepitation may be located in the area shown in gray.

Duration of the "chest pain"

The pain generally lasts a few hours, but may return with changes of position (for example, when reclining).[12] A few days of intermittent symptoms is the usual course, with one recent series describing a mean duration of symptoms to be 48 hours.[3] Earlier studies, such as the case reported by Bodey,[3] provides details of symptoms as lasting over a period of weeks to months with intermittent worsening.

Tenderness of the chest wall

The chest wall is not tender, but crepitation of the chest, face and arms may be present.

Precipitating causes of the "chest pain"

Inspiration, coughing, swallowing and reclining may cause worsening of the pain.

Relief of the "chest pain"

Typically, assuming the upright position and leaning forward provides some relief of the discomfort.

Associated Symptoms

In addition to the chest pain which is the most frequent symptom of pneumomediastinum, patients may also experience dyspnea in about 50 percent of patients,[4,6] cough, neck, back or shoulder pain,[5] abdominal pain,[7] dysphagia,[5] odynophagia,[13] changes in voice quality,[13,14] as well as anxiety and "psychiatric symptoms."[4,7]

Associated Signs

Physical examination

The classic sign of pneumomediastinum is Hamman's crunch: a crackling sound auscultated over the precordium, synchronous with systole.[12] The sound can be accentuated when auscultation is carried out in the left lateral decubitus position or upon expiration. Upright posture and inspiration will diminish the "crunch" to the point that it may be inaudible in these positions. This finding, once considered pathognomonic of mediastinal emphysema, is neither sensitive nor specific (noting that the same finding may also be heard in pneumothorax or pneumopericardium, for example).[15]

In addition, subcutaneous emphysema (crepitance) is also frequently found in the neck, chest, face, and/or arms. Signs of pneumothorax may also be present, as pneumothoraces may be a concomitant finding. Finally, loss of cardiac dullness or hyperresonance over the precordium may also be present on examination. Importantly, not all patients with pneumomediastinum have an abnormal physical examination.[6] Fever has been variably reported.[2,3,7]

"Routine" laboratory tests

Chest radiographs are the diagnostic test of choice. Most importantly, a lateral projection is necessary or pneumomediastinum may be undetected. The radiographic signs of pneumomediastinum depend on the depiction of normal anatomic structures that are outlined by the air as they leave the mediastinum. Findings on radiograph include pneumopericardium with the border of the heart outlined on the anterior-posterior projection and air present between the heart and sternum on the lateral projection. Air may also be seen in the pulmonary interstitium as well as extrapleurally (between the parietal pleura and the diaphragm). Pneumomediastinum may be difficult to differentiate from medial pneumothorax and pneumopericardium. Decubitus projections may be useful to distinguish air within the pericardium (which will move with alterations in position) from air within the mediastinum (which will remain unaltered with change in position).

Exceptions to the Usual Manifestations

As previously noted, neck pain and even airway obstruction[16,17] may be the predominant manifestation of pneumomediastinum. This diagnosis should always be a consideration in young, healthy patients presenting with sudden onset of chest pain.

Differential Diagnosis

Given the primary symptom of chest pain, which may resemble angina, myocardial infarction would be in the differential diagnosis of mediastinal emphysema. Similarly, cardiac inflammation including pericarditis or myocarditis would also be considered. The pleuritic component of the pain in pneumomediastinum may be reminiscent of pulmonary embolism, pneumonia, or pneumothorax (noting that these diagnoses are not mutually exclusive). Based on the retrosternal location of the pain, esophageal dysfunction (spasm, esophagitis, and tear) may present in a manner similar to pneumomediastinum. Pathology of other mediastinal structures, including aortic dissection, may also present with similar pain to that of pneumomediastinum. The potential for chest wall involvement may suggest musculoskeletal pain or inflammation. Inflammation of the mediastinum from infection should also be considered.

Other Diagnostic Testing

Additional routine tests, such as arterial blood gas evaluation and electrocardiogram, are nondiagnostic. Arterial blood gas tests usually reveal no abnormality. Electrocardiographic changes (e.g., diffusely low voltage, nonspecific axis shifts, ST-T wave changes, and ST segment elevation in the lateral precordial leads) may be found in some cases in the absence of other cardiac abnormalities.[1] Leukocytosis may also be present, though likely as a result of underlying illness.[2,3,7]

Computed tomographic (CT) digital radiography and conventional CT can also be helpful in establishing or confirming the diagnosis.[18]

Etiology and Basic Mechanisms Responsible for the "Pain"

Macklin[19] described the importance of intra-alveolar pressure gradients causing rupture of marginal alveoli into underlying perivascular sheaths following animal experimentation. Additional animal studies by Caldwell[20] emphasized the importance of increased intrapulmonary pressure leading to perivascular interstitial emphysema. Recent clinical observations in a patient with pneumomediatsinum receiving partial liquid ventilation provided evidence that the air dissects not only along perivascular, but also peribronchial connective tissue planes.[21] After marginal alveolar rupture, air dissects following a pressure gradient (maintained by subsequent respiration) from the alveoli to the mediastinum.[19] Pain presumably results from stimulation of the mediastinal viscera and dissection of air along connective tissue planes.

Treatment

Treatment of spontaneous pneumomediastinum is conservative, with observation alone a reasonable approach. The use of high concentration of oxygen to promote air reabsorption is not of benefit if the point of rupture is significant or remains patent.[22,23] Serious sequelae may result from *"malignant"* pneumomediastinum, including: 1) vascular collapse due to compression of vessels (pulmonary and cardiac) by air within the mediastinum, 2) respiratory failure from pressure imposed on the airway by extrapulmonary air, or 3) pneumothorax (including tension pneumothorax) if mediastinal pressure rises without exit through connective tissue of adjacent structures. Such circumstances would necessitate surgical intervention to allow escape of the air within the mediastinum.[14,24] It remains controversial whether all patients with pneumomediastinum merit hospitalization (the level of care can also be subject to debate, e.g., the need for intensive care monitoring and frequency of follow up radiographs). Another area of controversy relates to the need for additional diagnostic work-up in order to exclude the need for emergent intervention. Specifically, in a patient presenting without apparent cause for pneumomediastinum, the question of the need to further image in order to exclude disruption of the aerodigestive tract arises. Some studies have demonstrated that, in spontaneous pneumomediastinum occurring in a patient without clinical information suggestive of a lesion of the alimentary or respiratory tract, additional imaging is of low yield. CT scanning of the chest or abdomen may be the best next step if concern exists regarding the etiology.

Classic Description

"On the morning of February 8, while shaving he was suddenly seized with intense pain under the sternum radiating to the left shoulder. The pain lasted about half an hour then gradually passed . . . On the morning of February 11, the patient reported to Dr. Moore that during the evening before, when lying on the left side, he heard a curious loud bubbling, crackling sound synchronous with the heart beat. His wife, sitting on the bed beside him, had heard the sound very plainly . . . I put my stethoscope over the apex of the heart and with each impulse there occurred the most extraordinary crunching, bubbling sound. It is difficult to describe. Crunching is the best adjective I can think of though it is far from apt. . . It certainly conveyed the impression of air being churned or squeezed about in the tissues. When the patient turned on his back the sound at once disappeared."[12]

References

1. Park DR, Pierson DJ. Pneumomediastinum and mediastinitis. In: Murray JF, Nadel JA, Mason RJ, et al., (eds). *Textbook of Respiratory Medicine, 3rd ed.* Philadelphia: W.B. Saunders, 2000, pp. 2095–2121.

2. Gordon CA. Respiratory emphysema in labor: With two new cases and a review of 130 cases in the literature. *Am J Obstet Gynec* 1917;14:633–646.
3. Bodey GP. Medical mediastinal emphysema. *Ann Intern Med* 1961;54:46–56.
4. Yellin A, Gapany-Gapanavivius M, Lieberman Y. Spontaneous pneumomediastinum: Is it a rare cause of chest pain? *Thorax* 1983;38:383–385.
5. Abolnik I, Lossos IS, Breuer R. Spontaneous pneumomediastinum. A report of 25 cases [see comments]. *Chest* 1991;100:93–95.
6. Panacek EA, Singer AJ, Sherman BW, et al. Spontaneous pneumomediastinum: Clinical and natural history. *Ann Emerg Med* 1992;21:1222–1227.
7. Munsell WP. Pneumomediastinum: A report of 28 cases and review of the literature. *JAMA* 1967;202:129–133.
8. Millard CE. Pneumomediastinum. *Dis Chest* 1969;56:297–300.
9. Riccio JC, Abbott J. A simple sore throat? Retropharyngeal emphysema secondary to free-basing cocaine. *J Emerg Med* 1990;8:709–712.
10. Morgan EJ, Henderson DA. Pneumomediastinum as a complication of athletic competition. *Thorax* 1981;36:155–156.
11. Caramori ML, Gross JL, Friedman R, et al. Pneumomediastinum and subcutaneous emphysema in diabetic ketoacidosis [letter]. *Diabetes Care* 1995;18:1311–1312.
12. Hamman L. Spontaneous mediastinal emphysema. *Bull Johns Hopkins Hosp* 1939;64:1–21.
13. Holmes KD, McGuirt WF. Spontaneous pneumomediastinum: Evaluation and treatment [see comments]. *J Family Practice* 1990;31:422–429.
14. Kirchner JA. Cervical mediastinal emphysema. *Arch Otolaryngology* 1980;106:368–375.
15. Baumann MH, Sahn SA. Hamman's sign revisited. Pneumothorax or pneumomediastinum? *Chest* 1992;102:1281–1282.
16. Caraballo V, Barish RA, Floccare DJ. Pneumomediastinum presenting as acute airway obstruction. *J Emerg Med* 1996;14:159–163.
17. Rose WD, Veach JS, Tehranzdeh J. Spontaneous pneumomediastinum as a cause of neck pain, dysphagia, and chest pain. *Arch Intern Med* 1984;144:392–393.
18. Zylak CM, Standen JR, Barnes GR, et al. Pneumomediastinum revisited. *Radiographics* 2000;20:1043–1057.
19. Macklin CC. Transport of air along sheaths of pulmonic blood vessels from alveoli to mediastinum: Clinical implications. *Arch Int Med* 1939;64:913–926.
20. Caldwell EJ, Powell RD, Jr., Mullooly JP. Interstitial emphysema: A study of physiologic factors involved in experimental induction of the lesion. *Am Rev Resp Dis* 1970;102:516–525.
21. Jamadar DA, Kazerooni EA, Hirschl RB. Pneumomediastinum: Elucidation of the anatomic pathway by liquid ventilation. *J Comp Ass Tom* 1996;20:309–311.
22. Fine J, Frehling S, Starr A. Experimental observations on the effect of 95 per cent oxygen on the absorption of air from the body tissues. *J Thoracic Surg* 1935;4:635–642.
23. Fine J, Hermanson L, Frehling S. Further clinical experiences with ninety-five per cent oxygen for the absorption of air from body tissues. *Ann Surg* 1938;107:1–13.
24. Gray JM, Hanson GC. Mediastinal emphysema: Aetiology, diagnosis, and treatment. *Thorax* 1966;21:325–332.

Part VI

Pulmonary Causes of Chest Pain

Although the definition of "chest pain"→ is discussed in Chapter 1, the definition is repeated here so that communication is clear.

The quotation marks around "chest" imply that different patients have different definitions of the word "chest." Here we use the word to indicate pain located above the waist. Then, too, *angina pectoris* is not always located in the pectoral region—it may be felt only in the jaw, neck, shoulder, elbow, or wrist. Therefore, the word "chest" implies that other parts of the upper body may also be involved with painful syndromes.

The quotation marks around "pain" imply that patients may assign other terms to their discomfort, such as indigestion, burning, ache, etc.

The arrow after "chest pain" implies that the physician initially may not know the cause of the symptom, so a differential diagnosis must be established that fits the available information.

14

"Chest Pain" in Patients with Pleuritis

Michelle M. Freemer, MD and Talmadge E. King, Jr., MD

General Considerations

The pleura is a thin, smooth semitransparent membrane that covers the surface of the lung (visceral pleura) and lines the inside of the chest wall, diaphragm, and mediastinum (parietal pleura). Normally, these two surfaces are in close contact but are separated by a small amount of fluid (5 to 10 mL) that lubricates them, making it possible for the lung to expand and glide over the chest wall with the least amount of friction. Pleuritis or pleurisy is an inflammation of the pleura. Fluid may accumulate in the pleural space (pleural effusion) or it may remain dry (e.g., "dry pleurisy"). The process may be self-limited, or the fibrinous exudate that develops on the pleural surface may organize into fibrous tissue, resulting in pleural adhesions. The term "pleurisy" is often used to describe a self-limited viral or idiopathic illness characterized by pleuritic pain without pleural effusion.

Clinical Setting

Pleuritis may occur in patients of any age and sex. Inflammation of the pleural surface occurs in a variety of clinical situations (see Table 14–1). Most often pleuritis results from an underlying parenchymal lung process (e.g., pneumonia, infarction, or tuberculosis). Infectious agents or other irritating substance may directly enter the pleural space (e.g., with esophageal rupture, pancreatitis or other cause of intra-abdominal inflammation). In patients with infection, the onset of pleuritis may be acute or chronic. Tuberculosis is the classic example of an infection inciting pleurisy as it produces

From: Hurst JW, Morris DC (eds): *"Chest Pain"* →. © Futura Publishing Co., Inc., Armonk, NY, 2001.

Table 14–1.

Causes of Pleural Inflammation

Infection

Parapneumonic/empyema
  Bacterial
  Atypical pneumonia
  Mycobacterium
  Fungal
  Viral
Abdominal

Immune mediated

Systemic lupus erythematosus
Rheumatoid arthritis
Sjogren's syndrome
Sarcoidosis
Wegener's granulomatosis
Post-cardiac injury

Drug mediated (see table 14–2)

Malignancy

Primary (mesothelioma) or metastatic
Radiation

Anatomic aberrations (lymphatics)

Chylothorax
Yellow Nail Syndrome

Vascular

Pulmonary embolism/infarction

Miscellaneous

Pancreatitis
Esophageal rupture
Uremia
Asbestos exposure

erythematous inflammation of the parietal pleura with multiple nodules.[1] In tuberculosis, the pleurisy often precedes the development of an effusion (and diagnosis).[1] In young patients (less than 40 years old) presenting with pleurisy, the most common etiologies are idiopathic (presumably "viral" infection, in 53% of the cases), infectious pneumonitis (18%) and pulmonary embolism (21%).[2] Immunologic causes of pleurisy are also common. Pleural involvement in the connective tissue diseases may occur in previously diagnosed patients, or may be a presenting manifestation and does not correlate with other signs of systemic disease activity.[3] In systemic lupus erythematosis (SLE) pleural involvement, pleural effusion, or pleuritic chest pain occurs in up to 70% during the clinical course. Pleural involvement occurs in about 5% of patients with rheumatoid arthritis (RA); 20% of patients give a history of pleuritic chest pain. Pleural thickening is found at postmortem examination in 38%–70% of patients with RA.[3] In the post-cardiac injury syndrome, the pleurisy usually begins approximately 3 weeks following cardiac injury.[4] Such pain may be recurrent over the course of several months.[5] While carcinomas may involve the pleura extensively, chest pain is experienced in a minority of patients.[6,7] Drug-induced pleural disease is relatively uncommon compared to drug-induced parenchymal lung disease (see Table 14–2).[8] Many drugs have been associated with the development of pleuritis (especially chemotherapeutic agents or drugs associated with a lupus-like syndrome).[8] Radiation therapy can produce pleurisy (with and without associated effusions), usually occurring within 6 months of therapy.[9] Pleuritis associated with pulmonary embolism is discussed elsewhere in this monograph. Other events or illnesses that may precipitate pleurisy include asbestos related pleural disease, uremia, Yellow Nail Syndrome, and lymphangiomyomatosis.[9]

Characteristics of the "Pain"

Patient's characteristics of the "chest pain"

The "pain" may be described as vague discomfort or intense sharp, burning or stabbing. "Pleuritic pain" has become accepted as a descriptive term as this pain is universally recognized to be a sharp, localized pain intensified by inspiration.

Common location of the "chest pain"

The location of the pain is variable, but is typically localized to the site of pleuritis, usually the lateral chest wall. The "pain" may be referred to the back, or neck (see Figures 14–1 and 14–2).

Uncommon locations of the "chest pain"

There are no uncommon locations of the pain.

Size of the painful "area"

The size of the painful area is about the size of the hand.

Table 14–2.

Drugs Associated with Pleural Disease[8]

Cardiovascular agents

Amiodarone
Minoxidil
Practolol

Sclerotherapy agents

Absolute alcohol
Sodium morrhuate

Ergoline drugs

Methysergide
Bromocriptine

Pleural fluid eosinophia

Dantrolene
Nitrofurantoin
Valproic acid
Propylthiouracil
Isotretinoin

Chemotherapeutic Agents

Bleomycin
Cyclophosphamide
Methotrexate
Mitomycin
Procarbazine

Other agents

Acyclovir
Clozapine
D-Penicillamine
Granulocyte colony stimulating factor
Itraconazole
L-Tryptophan
Simvastin

Drug-induced lupus-like pleuritis

Procainamide
Hydralazine
Isoniazid
Chlopromazine
Mesalamine
Quinidine

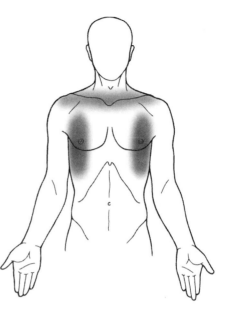

Figure 14–1. Frontal view. "Chest pain" in patients with pleuritis. The dark shaded areas indicate the common sites of "pain." The light shaded areas indicate the areas where the pain radiates.

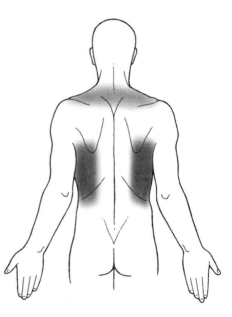

Figure 14–2. View from the back. "Chest pain" in patients with pleuritis. The dark shaded areas indicate the common sites of "pain." The light shaded areas indicate the areas where the pain radiates.

Duration of the "chest pain"

The severe pain usually subsides in few hours, although it may recur. Conversely, the dull discomfort of chronic pleurisy may persist for months.

Tenderness of the chest wall

The affected area may be tender.

Precipitating causes of the "chest pain"

Characteristically, the "pain" varies with the respiratory cycle. In fact, it is the intensification of the "chest pain" with inspiration that is the hallmark of pleuritic "pain." The "pain" may be exacerbated by coughing, yawning, laughing, or other movements of the chest wall.

Relief of the "chest pain"

Pleuritic "chest pain" may be relieved by maintaining shallow (often grunting) respirations and limited chest wall motion. Some patients find that the pain eases with lying on the affected side.

Associated Symptoms

Given the variety of inciting factors for pleurisy, the associated symptoms may also be quite variable. In general, however, other markers of inflammation are present such as fever, myalgias, or arthralgias. Dyspnea and cough may also be present. Diseases and other manifestations of serositis may be evident in the connective tissue. In a patient with a large pleural effusion dyspnea, or vague chest discomfort are more common symptoms than typical "pleuritic" chest pain.

Associated Signs

Physical examination

Based on the degree of inflammation, varying signs may be present. Observation may reveal rapid shallow breathing with decreased diaphragmatic excursion, because deep breathing induces pain. A pleural friction rub (squeaky rubbing sound) may be auscultated, particularly in late inspiration—this may be confused with localized pulmonary crackles. Usually the rub has two components, an inspiratory and an expiratory phase. A pleuropericardial rub may be heard if the pleuritis is adjacent to the heart. Occasionally, the affected area is tender to palpation or a coarse vibration may be felt on the chest wall. In the cases of pleural effusion, the characteristic findings of dullness on percussion with diminution of tactile fremitus and vesicular breath sounds may be present. Egophony and bronchial sounds may be appreciated at the top of an effusion.

"Routine" laboratory tests

Radiographic evaluation includes chest radiographs in the upright and decubitus positions. The main importance of chest radiographs is to reveal the presence of parenchymal lung inflammation or pleural effusion. The earliest detection of pleural fluid may be in the posterior costophrenic sulcus on the lateral view.[10]

Exceptions to the Usual Manifestations

There are few, if any, exceptions to the manifestations described above.

Differential Diagnosis

The differential diagnosis of pleurisy involves distinction of the various precipitating causes noted above. In addition, the chest pain must be distinguished from other processes such as pneumothorax, pneumomediastinum, chest wall inflammation (myositis, neuritis, rib pathology, pleurodynia), and pericardial inflammation. Epidemic pleurodynia (Bornholm disease, the devil's grip) is severe pain in the side generally associated with the coxsackie B viral infection.[11] It occurs at any age but is seen most commonly in children and young adults, usually as part of an epidemic. Pleurodynia is a disease of skeletal muscle. The pain is usually accompanied by sudden onset of fever, with sharp, severe pleuritic paroxysmal pain over the lower ribs and sternum. The pain may radiate to the shoulders, neck, and back. Abdominal muscular pain and spasm can be present in about 50% of cases.

With regards to distinguishing between the many potential etiologies of pleural inflammation, in addition to the clinical presentation (e.g., signs of infection, connective tissue disease, or an intra-abdominal process), thoracentesis is mandatory for the diagnosis of pleural effusions as three conditions are associated with need for emergency treatment: pulmonary embolism, hemothorax, and empyema. If the fluid is a transudate, no further invasive studies are usually necessary.

Other Diagnostic Testing

In addition to radiographs and pleural fluid analysis, other tests may be indicated depending on the clinical situation. Serologic evaluation in connective tissue diseases, imaging to exclude an intra-abdominal process or pulmonary embolus, cultures/serologies for infectious diseases, and biopsies to evaluate for malignancies may all provide useful information. Pleural biopsy/thorascopy may also be indicated in situations in which preliminary evaluation (as described above) does not yield a diagnosis. Following pleural biopsy or thorascopy less than 10% of the cases remain unexplained. Careful follow-up of these patients is required because a diagnosis will become apparent in one-third of the patients: malignancy (72% of cases) and collagen vascular disease (17%).[11]

Etiology and Basic Mechanisms Responsible for the "Pain"

Pleuritic pain arises from inflammation involving the parietal pleura (as the visceral pleura lacks innervation) and is localized directly over the affected area. If the central diaphragmatic surface is affected, the pain may be referred to the shoulder or neck via the phrenic nerve. Irritation of the posterior and peripheral portions of the diaphragmatic pleura (supplied by the lower six intercostal nerves) will result in pain referred to the epigastric region of the lower chest wall and may simulate intra-abdominal disease.

The specific pathogenesis of the inflammatory response varies with the inciting process. The inflammation may arise in the pleura itself, as in the case of infections of the pleura (e.g., tuberculosis). Alternatively, it may be immunologically mediated, as is possibly true in fungal lung infections with associated pleural thickening[12] or as is presumed in post-myocardial-infarction syndrome.[5] Increased capillary permeability is the major cause of pleural involvement in the connective tissue disorders.[3] However, an immune mechanism is important in many connective tissue disorders (especially RA, SLE, Churg-Strauss syndrome, and possibly Sjogren syndrome).[3] Circulating immune complexes have been shown in the blood and pleural fluid of these patients. These immune complexes can localize either to the subpleural or pleural capillaries, and can activate the complement system leading to endothelial injury and the accumulation of protein-rich fluid in the lung interstitium or pleural space.[3] The mechanisms underlying chemically-induced pneumonitis remain unexplained, although hypersensitivity is a possible explanation.[13] Radiation therapy can cause pleural effusions by three mechanisms: radiation pleuritis, systemic venous hypertension, or lymphatic obstruction from mediastinal fibrosis.[9]

Treatment

The primary treatment for pleurisy is to treat the underlying disease process (for example, antibiotics for infection). Anti-inflammatory agents for pain relief may be of benefit while awaiting resolution of the primary disease process. Indomethacin has been shown to be efficacious in treating the pleurisy associated with infectious, embolic, and traumatically induced disease.[14] Steroids can produce dramatic improvement in patients with post-myocardial-infarction syndrome[4,5] although they are of no proven benefit in tuberculous disease.[15] Codeine or other narcotics may be required but should be avoided because suppression of the cough reflex and hypoventilation may increase the risk of pneumonia. In patients with severe pain intradermal lidocaine around the site of pain may provide dramatic pain relief. Rarely, intercostal nerve blocks may be placed with local anesthesia.

Classic Description

"Pleurisy is inflammation of the pleura. It derives its name from the stitch in the side which is generally its most characteristic symptom. . . . By the term pleurisy, however, we now almost universally mean inflammation of the pleura alone. . . . It is, nevertheless, true, that, in many instances, pleurisy and peripneumony exist together. . . . Pleurisy is either chronic or acute.

Inflammation of the pleura is always accompanied by an extravasation on its internal surface, and which may be considered as the species of suppuration proper to serous membranes. This extravasation appears to commence with the inflammation itself. It consists of two very different matters. The one, of a firmer, semi-concrete consistence, is usually termed *false membrane*, or coaguable lymph; the other, very thin and watery, is called *serosity* or *sero-purulent effusion*. Both of these exhibit great variation in character."[16]

References

1. Sibley JC. A study of 200 cases of tuberculous pleurisy with effusion. *Am Rev Tuberc* 1950;62:314–323.
2. Branch WT, McNeil BJ. Analysis of the differential diagnosis and assessment of pleuritic chest pain in young adults. *Am J Med* 1983;75:671–679.

3. Joseph J, Sahn SA. Connective tissue diseases and the pleura. *Chest* 1993;104 (1):262–270.
4. Stelzner TJ, King TE, Antony VB, et al. The pleuropulmonary manifestations of the postcardiac injury syndrome. *Chest* 1983;84:383–387.
5. Dressler W. The post-myocardial-infarction syndrome. *Arch Int Med* 1959;103: 28–42.
6. Chernow B, Sahn SA. Carcinomatous involvement of the pleura: An analysis of 96 patients. *Am J Med* 1977;63(5):695–702.
7. Weick JK, Kiely JM, Harrison EG, Jr., et al. Pleural effusion in lymphoma. *Cancer* 1973;31(4):848–853.
8. Morelock SY, Sahn SA. Drugs and the pleura. *Chest* 1999;116(1):212–221.
9. Sahn SA. State of the art. The pleura. *Am Rev Respir Dis* 1988;138(1):184–234.
10. Rudikoff JC. Early detection of pleural fluid. *Chest* 1980;77(1):109–111.
11. Oxman MN. Enteroviruses. In: Goldman L, Bennett JC (eds): *Cecil Textbook of Medicine, 21st ed.* Philadelphia, W.B. Saunders, 2000, pp. 1829–1830.
12. Hillerdal G. Pulmonary aspergillus infection invading the pleura. *Thorax* 1981;36(10):745–751.
13. Urban C, Nirenberg A, Caparros B, et al. Chemical pleuritis as the cause of acute chest pain following high-dose methotrexate treatment. *Cancer* 1983;51 (1):34–37.
14. Sacks PV, Kanarek D. Treatment of acute pleuritic pain. Comparison between indomethacin and a placebo. *Am Rev Respir Dis* 1973;108(3):666–669.
15. Wyser C, Walzl G, Smedema JP, et al. Corticosteroids in the treatment of tuberculous pleurisy. A double-blind, placebo-controlled, randomized study [see comments]. *Chest* 1996;110(2):333–338.
16. Laennec RTH. *A Treatise on the Disease of the Chest.* New York, Hafner Publishing Co, 1962, pp. 145–147.

15

"Chest Pain" in Patients with a Pneumothorax

Michelle M. Freemer, MD and Talmadge E. King, Jr., MD

General Considerations

Pneumothorax is defined as air in the pleural space—between the visceral and parietal pleurae. Spontaneous pneumothorax may be primary (i.e., occurring in patients without pre-existing lung disease or when there is no apparent provoking factor) or secondary (i.e., those with known lung disease). Iatrogenic pneumothorax can result from diagnostic interventions, e.g., transthoracic-needle aspiration, placement of a catheter in the subclavian vein, thoracentesis, and pleural biopsy or barotrauma. Traumatic pneumothorax is the result of penetrating or blunt trauma to the chest, with air entering the pleural space directly through the chest wall; visceral pleural penetration; or alveolar rupture due to sudden compression of the chest.[1]

Clinical Setting

Primary and secondary pneumothoraces occur more frequently in men. In one series of patients (Olmstead County, Minnesota cases between 1950–1974), the male:female was 6:1 for primary pneumothorax compared to 3:1 for secondary pneumothorax.[2] Overall, the incidence of spontaneous pneumothorax was 7.9/100,000 person-years. A more recent review in England (1991–1995) described incidences of 16.8/100,000 for outpatients and 11.1/100,000 for emergency admissions.[3] Some series have described a bimodal distribution, between 20–24 years and 80–84 years for men with the early peak in women ages 30–34. Pneumothoraces are very rare in children.

From: Hurst JW, Morris DC (eds): *"Chest Pain"* →. © Futura Publishing Co., Inc., Armonk, NY, 2001.

Cigarette smoking dramatically increases the risk of spontaneous pneumothorax—by a factor of 22 times for men and 8 times for women.[4] The risk is dose related. However, during a 10-year period, the rate of pneumothoraces among all smokers followed at the Mayo Clinic for COPD was only 0.003%.[5] Young, otherwise healthy patients tend to have primary pneumothoraces thought to be due to subpleural apical bleb or congenital abnormality of the pleura.[6–8] Older patients are more likely to have secondary pneumothoraces associated with emphysema or lung fibrosis.[9–12] Body habitus, specifically that of thin, tall males, is thought to be the prototypic patient with pneumothoraces. However, a series of Japanese patients demonstrated the association with low body weight/obesity indices and lung height, rather than body height.[13] Activity level at the onset of symptoms has also been evaluated. Specifically, Bense and coworkers demonstrated that pneumothoraces did not occur in the setting of heavy physical exercise, but, in fact, 61% of patients had the onset of symptoms between 5 AM and 8 AM with inactivity or low activity.[14] In addition, bronchial anomalies, found on bronchoscopy, increase the risk of spontaneous pneumothorax by greater than 200-fold.[15] Conditions which predispose to patients to developing secondary pneumothoraces are shown in Table 15–1.[1,11,12,16]

Characteristics of the "Pain"

Patient's characterization of the "chest pain"

Patients generally experience a sudden onset of pain. In fact, patients are often able to document the onset of pain with reasonable accuracy. The pain may be pleuritic. The patient may describe it as "cutting."

The symptoms are more severe in patients with secondary pneumothorax when compared to patients with spontaneous pneumothorax.

Common location of the "chest pain"

The "chest pain" usually lateralizes to the side of the pneumothorax (See Figure 15–1). It is rare for spontaneous pneumothorax to be bilateral (about 5% of cases).[2]

Uncommon locations of the "chest pain"

The pain is almost always as described above.

Table 15–1.

Causes of Secondary Spontaneous Pneumothorax[1,12,16]

Airway disease

Emphysema
Cystic fibrosis
Status asthmaticus

Infectious lung disease

Acquired immunodeficiency syndrome (AIDS) (usually have history of *Pneumo-cystis carinii* infection, prophylactic inhaled pentamidine, or have a recurrence of their P. carinii infection, often difficult to treat)
Pneumocystis carinii pneumonia
Tuberculosis
Necrotizing pneumonias (caused by anaerobic, gram-negative bacteria or staphylococcus)

Interstitial lung disease

Sarcoidosis
Idiopathic pulmonary fibrosis
Pulmonary histiocytosis X (Langerhans'-cell granulomatosis)
Lymphangioleimyomatosis
Tuberous sclerosis

Connective-tissue disease

Rheumatoid arthritis (causes pyopneumothorax)
Ankylosing spondylitis
Polymyositis and dermatomyositis
Scleroderma
Marfan's syndrome
Ehlers-Danlos syndrome

Cancer

Sarcoma
Primary and metastatic cancer
Nonpulmonary (e.g., lymphoma, Hodgkin's disease)

Miscellaneous

Infarction
Pneumonitis (chemical, radiation)
Toxic drug effect (e.g., oxygen, pentamidine)
Drug abuse (e.g., cocaine, marijuana)
Pneumoperitoneum (via diaphragm defects)
Esophageal rupture

Thoracic endometriosis (related to menses; causes catamenial pneumothorax)

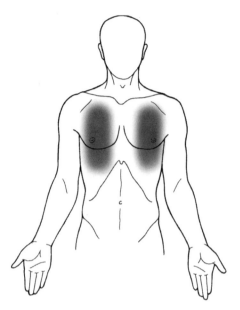

Figure 15–1. Frontal view. The "chest pain" of pneumothorax is usually located in the lateral portion of the chest.

Size of the painful "area"

The painful area is about the size of a hand.

Duration of the "chest pain"

The "pain" usually lasts less than 24 hours (usually 1–2 hours).

Tenderness of the chest wall

The chest wall is not tender.

Precipitating causes of the "chest pain"

When pleuritic pain is present, it typically increases with respiration.

Relief of the "chest pain"

The primary symptom, "chest pain," is usually relieved partially with splinting of the chest.

Associated Symptoms

Shortness of breath was present in 21%–64% of military recruits at the time of presentation.[17,18] Less common symptoms include cough[18,19] and generalized malaise.[18] Of note, however, patients may also be completely asymptomatic (6% of patients in one series from the military).[18]

Associated Signs

Physical examination

Inspection may reveal decreased chest wall movement on the side of the pneumothorax. Tachypnea and tachycardia are common. Auscultation may demonstrate diminished or absent breath sounds and hyperresonance on percussion.[19] Subcutaneous emphysema may be present. Uncommonly, cyanosis, hypotension, or shock may occur. Tracheal shift away from the side of the pneumothorax occurs in the setting of tension pneumothorax. Tension pneumothorax is present when the intrapleural pressure exceeds the atmospheric pressure throughout expiration, and often during inspiration as well. This is a medical emergency seen most often in patients receiving mechanical ventilation and is characterized by sudden deterioration in their cardiopulmonary status.

"Routine" laboratory tests

Chest radiograph is usually sufficient to make the diagnosis. The characteristic frontal upright radiograph demonstrates a visible visceral pleural line outlining the edge of the lung and its interface with air in the pleural space. Apical pneumothoraces may be seen with full expiratory films; lateral decubitus films may also aid in demonstrating a pneumothorax. However, in patients with underlying bullous disease the distinction between bullae and pneumothoraces may be a difficult one.[20] Computed tomography scan of the chest is the most sensitive diagnostic tool.[12]

Exceptions to the
Usual Manifestations

Despite the usually abrupt onset of severe symptoms, about 30% of patients may be asymptomatic or have minor, nonspecific complaints with the pneumothorax being incidentally found on examination/radiographic evaluation.[12] In addition, given that symptoms are not always severe, some patients may present with symptoms of several days duration.[18] Unilateral pulmonary edema (re-expansion pulmonary edema) may occur following rapid expansion of a lung that has been collapsed for several days.[18]

Differential Diagnosis

Other considerations in the differential diagnosis of patients with pneumothorax would include pulmonary embolism and/or infarction, pericarditis, tracheal/esophageal perforation, pleural effusion, and pneumonia. While the former three conditions generally are of sudden onset, similar to the presentation of pneumothoraces, the latter two are generally more subtle in onset. Pulmonary embolism can produce symptoms and signs similar to those of pneumothorax, although the lung examination in patients with pulmonary embolism does not usually reveal asymmetry of breath sounds or hyperresonance. Likewise, pericarditis may produce sudden pleuritic pain, yet the pain is not usually unilateral in location. Esophageal or trachea disruption may, in fact, be associated with a pneumothorax (or pneumomediastinum), and can cause similar symptoms though the pain may be localized to the upper chest/neck with a central distribution. Pleural effusions, though usually not sudden in onset, may produce unilateral pleuritic pain. Following a gradual onset, however, the pain associated with a pleural effusion typically persists beyond the duration expected (less than 24 hours, usually 1–2 hours) in a pneumothorax. Similarly, pneumonia may produce unilateral pleuritic chest pain, although it is usually slow to evolve and resolve. Large cysts or emphysematous bulla, skin folds, the inner border of the scapula, chest bandages, and a large diaphragmatic hernia with herniated air-filled viscus may simulate a pneumothorax on chest x-ray.[12]

Other Diagnostic Testing

Ancillary tests are not often indicated. Arterial blood gases may reveal hypoxemia with an abnormally increased alveolar-arterial gradient and no change in $PaCO_2$.[21,22] Patients with more severe cardiopulmonary disease are more likely to develop secondary spontaneous pneumothorax. Therefore, arterial blood gases are frequently abnormal in these patients. For example, among patients in the Veterans Administration cooperative study the arterial PO_2 was below 55 mmHg in 17% and below 45 mmHg in 4%. The arterial PCO_2 exceeded 50 mmHg in 16% and exceeded 60 mmHg in 4%. In the Veterans Administration cooperative study, 30% (51 of 171 patients) had an FEV1 of less than 1.0 L and 33% had an FEV1/FVC less than 40%.[23]

Etiology and Basic Mechanisms Responsible for the "Pain"

The chest pain associated with a pneumothorax is of undetermined etiology. The lung parenchyma, visceral pleura, and inner surface of the parietal pleura are insensitive. The sensory supply of the outer parietal surface is from the brachial plexus (C5-T1) in the apical region and the intercostal nerves (T2–8) for all other levels of the lung. While a pneumothorax indicates a rupture of the insensitive visceral pleura, it is presumed that bleeding causes irritation of the parietal pleura.[24] Such tears in the pleura are from ruptured subpleural blebs in most patients, with blebs being visible in 66%–90% patients when taken to surgery[12,18] even if not visible radiographically.

Treatment

The goals of therapy in any pneumothorax are to remove air from the pleural space to restore normal lung function as quickly as possible and to prevent recurrence and mortality. Options for therapy depend on the clinical situation and are beyond the scope of this discussion.[1,25,26] Important considerations include the stability of the patient, the size of the pneumothorax, the presence (and persistence of) an air leak, number of prior pneumothoraces, and the predicted risk of recurrence (and patient's reserve to tolerate such a recurrence). Death from spontaneous pneumothorax is rare and usually due to tension pneumothorax. The most conservative approach would be observation alone. This would be appropriate for a small pneumothorax (less than 20%), in a stable patient. With observation alone, air absorption occurs at a rate of 1.25% of the volume of the hemithorax per day.[27] Additional intervention is recommended for patients with pneumothoraces of greater than 20% (given the prolonged time for resolution) despite successful management of stable patients with larger pneumothoraces.[27]

The next potential intervention is supplemental oxygen therapy that accelerates the rate of pleural air absorption by at least four times.[25,27,28] Additional therapeutic options include: simple aspiration of air (thoracentesis with a small needle, about 16 gauge); tube drainage with a tube placed in the pleural space; pleurodesis (tube thoracostomy with the instillation of sclerosant, for example either talc in a slurry or a tetracycline derivative such as doxycycline or minocycline); thorascopy (with/without pleurodesis); and parietal pleurectomy. Importantly, intrapleural injection of talc has resulted in the acute respiratory distress syndrome in some patients treated for malignant pleural effusion.[29] The presence of a bronchopleural fistula (persistent air leak) necessitates surgical management. There is insufficient evidence on the effects of surgical pleurodesis compared to chemical pleurodesis.[26]

In a series of 120 patients with primary pneumothorax, the rate of recurrence was approximately 50%.[6] Of the patients with a second spontaneous pneumothorax, the rate of recurrence was approximately 60%. In those with a third pneumothorax, the recurrence rate was approximately 80%. In terms of the reduction of recurrence, the Veterans Administration Cooperative study demonstrated that pleurodesis with tetracycline (parenteral tetracycline is no longer available) reduced the rate of recurrence from 41% to 25%.[23] Additional studies have also demonstrated a reduction in recurrence with more invasive interventions.[9,18] Most recurrences occur within the first 6 months of the initial pneumothorax.[23]

References

1. Sahn SA, Heffner JE. Spontaneous pneumothorax. *N Engl J Med* 2000;342 868–874.
2. Melton LJ, Hepper NG, Offord KP. Incidence of spontaneous pneumothorax in Olmsted County, Minnesota: 1950 to 1974. *Am Rev Respir Dis* 1979;120:1379–1382.
3. Gupta D, Hansell A, Nichols T, et al. Epidemiology of pneumothorax in England. *Thorax* 2000;55:666–671.
4. Bense L, Eklund G, Wiman LG. Smoking and the increased risk of contracting spontaneous pneumothorax. *Chest* 1987;92:1009–1012.
5. Dines DE, Clagett OT, Payne WS. Spontaneous pneumothorax in emphysema. *Mayo Clinic Proceedings* 1970;45:481–487.
6. Gobbel WG, Rhea WG, Jr., Nelson IA, et al. Spontaneous pneumothorax. *J Thorac Cardiovasc Surg* 1963:331–345.
7. Lesur O, Delorme N, Fromaget JM, et al. Computed tomography in the etiologic assessment of idiopathic spontaneous pneumothorax. *Chest* 1990;98:341–347.
8. Bense L, Lewander R, Eklund G, et al. Nonsmoking, non-alpha 1-antitrypsin deficiency-induced emphysema in nonsmokers with healed spontaneous pneumothorax, identified by computed tomography of the lungs [see comments]. *Chest* 1993;103:433–438.
9. O'Rourke JP, Yee ES. Civilian spontaneous pneumothorax. Treatment options and long-term results [see comments]. *Chest* 1989;96:1302–1306.
10. Watt AG. Spontaneous pneumothorax. A review of 210 consecutive admissions to Royal Perth Hospital. *Med J Australia* 1978;1:186–188.
11. Wait MA, Estrera A. Changing clinical spectrum of spontaneous pneumothorax. *Am J Surg* 1992;164:528–531.
12. Weissberg D, Refaely Y. Pneumothorax. *Chest* 2000;117:1279–1285.
13. Kawakami Y, Irie T, Kamishima K. Stature, lung height, and spontaneous pneumothorax. *Respiration* 1982;43:35–40.
14. Bense L, Wiman LG, Hedenstierna G. Onset of symptoms in spontaneous pneumothorax: Correlations to physical activity. *Eur J Respir Dis* 1987;71:181–186.

15. Bense L, Eklund G, Wiman LG. Bilateral bronchial anomaly. A pathogenetic factor in spontaneous pneumothorax. *Am Rev Respir Dis* 1992;146:513–516.

16. McEwen J. Pleural disease. In: Rosen P (ed): *Emergency Medicine: Concepts and Clinical Practice, 4th ed.* St. Louis, Mosby-Year Book Inc., 1998, pp. 1511–1528.

17. Vail MW, Always AE, England NJ. Spontaneous pneumothorax. *Dis Chest* 1960;38:512–515.

18. Seremetis MG. The management of spontaneous pneumothorax. *Chest* 1970;57: 65–68.

19. Lippert HL, Lund O, Blegvad S, et al. Independent risk factors for cumulative recurrence rate after first spontaneous pneumothorax. *Eur Respir J* 1991;4: 324–331.

20. Waitches GM, Stern EJ, Dubinsky TJ. Usefulness of the double-wall sign in detecting pneumothorax in patients with giant bullous emphysema. *Am J Roent* 2000;174:1765–1768.

21. Norris RM, Jones JG, Bishop JM. Respiratory gas exchange in patients with spontaneous pneumothorax. *Thorax* 1968;23:427–433.

22. Moran JF, Jones RH, Wolfe WG. Regional pulmonary function during experimental unilateral pneumothorax in the awake state. *J Thorac Cardiovasc Surg* 1977;74:396–402.

23. Light RW, O'Hara VS, Moritz TE, et al. Intrapleural tetracycline for the prevention of recurrent spontaneous pneumothorax. Results of a Department of Veterans Affairs cooperative study. *JAMA* 1990;264:2224–2230.

24. Levene DL. Chest pain arising from intrathoracic structures. In: Levene DL, (ed): *Chest Pain: An Integrated Diagnostic Approach.* Philadelphia, Lea & Febiger, 1977, pp.83–84.

25. Light RW. Management of spontaneous pneumothorax. *Am Rev Respir Dis* 1993;148:245–248.

26. Cunnington J. Spontaneous pneumothorax. In: Godlee F (ed). *Clinical Evidence, 3rd ed.* London: BMJ Publishing Group, 2000, pp. 731–736.

27. Northfield TC. Oxygen therapy for spontaneous pneumothorax. *Brit Med J* 1971;4:86–88.

28. Hill RC, DeCarlo DP, Jr., Hill JF, et al. Resolution of experimental pneumothorax in rabbits by oxygen therapy. *Ann Thorac Surg* 1995;59:825–828.

29. Campos JR, Werebe EC, Vargas FS, et al. Respiratory failure due to insufflated talc [letter]. *Lancet* 1997;349:251–252.

16

"Chest Pain" in Patients with Pulmonary Embolism

Nanette K. Wenger, MD

General Considerations

Pulmonary embolism is a common and often undiagnosed condition. Thrombotic pulmonary embolism occurs in patients with one or more of the components of Virchow's triad: venous stasis, endothelial damage, or a hypercoagulable state.

Clinical Setting

Venous stasis is an important common denominator and is characteristic of patients with prolonged immobilization due to bed rest, stroke, paralysis, heart failure, obesity, shock, hypovolemia, pregnancy, and the like. Endothelial damage is encountered with surgery and trauma. A hypercoagulable state is characterized by activated protein C resistance; deficiencies in protein C, protein S, antithrombin III; or by the presence of factor V Leiden; lupus anticoagulant/anticardiolipin antibodies; malignancies; oral contraceptive and estrogen use;[1] and pregnancy, among other things.

Characteristics of the "Pain"

In the International Cooperative Pulmonary Embolism Registry data base, 49% of patients had some "chest pain," not further specified, at the time of diagnosis of pulmonary embolism. Chest pain was inversely associated with 3-month mortality risk, possibly reflecting smaller, more distal

From: Hurst JW, Morris DC (eds): *"Chest Pain"* →. © Futura Publishing Co., Inc., Armonk, NY, 2001.

embolization.[2] In the PIOPED (Prospective Investigation of Pulmonary Embolism Diagnosis) study of 117 patients without pre-existing cardiac or pulmonary disease,[3] pleuritic pain was the second most common clinical symptom (66%) of pulmonary embolism. Angina-like chest pain occurred in only 4%.

Patient's characterization of the "chest pain"

A patient with a large *pulmonary embolism* usually complains of sudden difficulty in breathing. He or she may also complain of retrosternal pressure or tightness. An important point to remember is that elderly patients with acute myocardial ischemia due to coronary atherosclerotic heart disease commonly complain of dyspnea rather than chest pain, and patients with acute pulmonary embolism may experience chest pressure due to associated myocardial ischemia (see Chapter 39 for mechanism of "chest pain" due to pulmonary hypertension). Therefore, the separation of pulmonary embolism from myocardial ischemia due to coronary atherosclerotic heart disease is not always easy when the diagnosis is based on symptoms alone.

When *pulmonary infarction* develops as a consequence to pulmonary embolism the pain is pleuritic in nature and may be described as knife-like (see Chapter 14).

Common location of the "chest pain"

Dyspnea due to pulmonary embolism is a subjective feeling of being unable to breath properly or adequately. The chest pressure occasionally noted with acute massive pulmonary embolism is located in the retrosternal area (see Figure 16–1).

The "chest pain" of pulmonary infarction may be noted anywhere in the chest (see Figure 16–2). However, the "pain" is commonly located in the anterior or posterior portion of the left or right lower lung areas.

Uncommon locations of the "chest pain"

There are no uncommon locations of the chest pain.

Size of the painful "area"

When dyspnea due to pulmonary embolism dominates the clinical picture, the size of the distress area of cannot be determined. In the patients

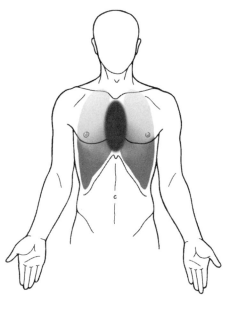

Figure 16–1. Frontal view. The location of "pain" in patients with pulmonary embolism and pulmonary infarction. The dark area in the center of the chest illustrates the location of chest pain that sometimes occurs with massive acute pulmonary embolism. The remainder of the figure shows the location of the lungs. Pleuritic chest pain is often associated with pulmonary infarction. This pain is located more often in the lower and lateral portions of the chest wall.

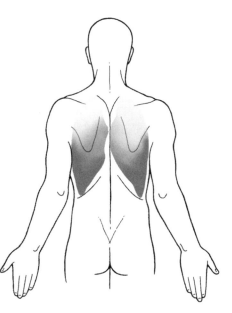

Figure 16–2. View from the back. The illustration shows the location of the pleuritic pain of pulmonary infarction. The pain is usually located in the lower and lateral portions of the chest wall.

with retrosternal pressure due to pulmonary embolism the size of the area of discomfort is larger than the fist.

The size of area of pleuritic pain due to pulmonary infarct varies, but is usually about the size of the hand.

Duration of the "chest pain"

Severe dyspnea due to acute pulmonary embolism may last a few minutes and be followed by less severe dyspnea that lasts for hours, or until appropriate treatment is initiated. The chest pressure due to acute pulmonary embolism usually lasts longer than angina pectoris, and for that reason may occasionally imitate the "chest pain" of myocardial infarction.

The knife-like pleuritic chest pain due to pulmonary infarct lasts for a brief moment each time an inspiratory breath is taken. This pain on inspiration continues for hours or days.

Tenderness of the chest wall

There is no tenderness of the chest wall.

Precipitating causes of the "chest pain"

The distress of pulmonary embolism and subsequent pleuritis due to pulmonary infarction may be a consequence of immobilization at bedrest, especially in patients with heart failure, and commonly follows a period of inactivity when the legs are not used, as when traveling for long periods in an airplane or automobile. Pulmonary embolism may occur in the post-partum period.

Straining at stool may also precipitate pulmonary embolism. The "pain" of pleuritis due to pulmonary infarction is, by definition, aggravated by inspiration.

The distress of pulmonary embolism is not precipitated by effort. The pain of pleuritis due to pulmonary infarction may be aggravated by exercise because it increases the frequency of the respiratory rate, which causes the accentuation of the pain.

Relief of the "chest pain"

The "chest pain" may gradually subside on its own, but as a rule, medical relief is sought and oxygen and narcotics are often needed.

Associated Symptoms

The acute onset of *dyspnea* is the most common presenting symptom of pulmonary embolism; hypotension may supervene. The occurrence of *syncope* is often associated with severe hemodynamic compromise and indicates life-threatening pulmonary embolism; *cardiac arrest* may follow. Less severe embolic obstruction of the pulmonary vascular bed is associated with less pronounced dyspnea as the typical presenting symptom. *Palpitations* may reflect the onset of atrial fibrillation or flutter or other supraventricular tachyarrhythmia. *Cough* may be prominent and acute anxiety is often evident, at times disproportionate to the apparent severity of the illness. *Hemoptysis* may occur. *Worsening symptoms in the patient with heart failure should also suggest pulmonary embolism.*

Although deep vein thrombosis of the leg is often clinically silent, symptoms of deep vein thrombosis, e.g., calf pain or tenderness, may be present.

Associated Signs

Physical examination

The signs vary with the severity of the pulmonary embolism. Acute right ventricular failure (cor pulmonale) is denoted by signs of pulmonary hypertension: a pulmonary artery impulse may be palpable, there is an accentuated pulmonic component of the second heart sound often with wide splitting, the jugular venous column is elevated with a prominent "a" wave, and a right ventricular impulse is palpable along the left parasternal edge. Right-sided gallop sounds may be present. Tachypnea and tachycardia are characteristic; *cyanosis,* when present, indicates a life-threatening pulmonary embolus.

With less severe obstruction of the pulmonary vascular bed, tachypnea is the most frequent sign, with tachycardia also common. Anxiety may be evident. Typically the cardiopulmonary examination is unremarkable and right ventricular function is normal. Evidence of worsening heart failure should raise suspicion of pulmonary embolism.

When pulmonary infarction occurs, there is often a pleural and, far less commonly, a pericardial friction rub. Râles and wheezes may be audible in the lung fields, and signs of pleural effusion may be present. Hemoptysis may be evident.

Signs of deep vein thrombosis include calf tenderness, palpable chords, swelling and warmth of one or both lower extremities, with skin discoloration and superficial venous distension. A Homan's sign may be present.

Rarely, there may be evidence of paradoxical embolism.

"Routine" laboratory tests

The *electrocardiographic abnormalities* are often transient and are most common with acute cor pulmonale.[2] They include the de novo appearance of complete or incomplete right bundle branch block, a right atrial abnormality, and rightward shift of the QRS vector with an S1 Q3 pattern, while the T wave vector is shifted to the left and posteriorly producing inverted T waves in leads II, III, and AVF, and the right precordial leads. Occasionally there is left axis deviation of the QRS vector. Atrial flutter or atrial fibrillation may be present. Rarely, changes of right ventricular infarction may be seen as a complication of massive pulmonary embolism.

With less extensive pulmonary vascular obstruction, sinus tachycardia and nonspecific ST and T wave changes are often the only electrocardiographic abnormalities. The electrocrdiogram is often normal in patients with small pulmonary emboli.

In the International Cooperative Pulmonary Embolism Registry data base,[3] cardiac enlargement was the most common *chest radiographic abnormality* in patients with all presentations of pulmonary embolism, likely reflecting the underlying cardiovascular disease in many instances. However, in this data base, neither pulmonary artery enlargement nor cardiomegaly were sensitive or specific predictors for the echocardiographic finding of right ventricular hypokinesis, an important predictor of mortality with acute pulmonary embolism.

There is often a pulmonary infiltrate or atelectasis on the chest radiograph when pulmonary infarction is present. This is encountered in about two-thirds of such patients; fewer have an elevated hemidiaphragm and/or evidence of unilateral pleural effusion. However, these findings are not specific for pulmonary infarction.

The chest x-ray film may be entirely normal in up to 25% of patients with pulmonary embolism following genitourinary, gynecologic, or orthopedic surgery; a pleural effusion appears more common after abdominal surgery. Focal oligemia has been described with massive central pulmonary artery occlusion, but is rare. A peripheral wedge-shaped density (Hampton's hump) indicates pulmonary infarction.

Exceptions to the
Usual Manifestations

Massive pulmonary embolism with resulting acute cor pulmonale is not characterized by chest pain but rather by severe dyspnea, often with concomitant hypotension. Sudden dyspnea is the presentation of submassive pulmonary embolism, with or without arterial hypoxemia and often without other laboratory test abnormalities. Some patients complain only of syncope.

Chest pain is characteristic for pulmonary infarction. Pleuritic pain occurs more commonly with small peripheral pulmonary emboli that result in pulmonary infarction.

Differential Diagnosis

Sudden unexplained dyspnea, the most common presentation of pulmonary embolism, is also common both with left ventricular failure and with chronic pulmonary disease; with both of these problems, worsening dyspnea may reflect superimposed pulmonary embolism. Sudden unexplained dyspnea may also be caused by pneumonia. Also included in the differential diagnosis are unstable angina or myocardial infarction, cardiomyopathy, primary pulmonary hypertension, asthma, costochondritis, and anxiety.

There is overlap between the pleuritic pain of pulmonary infarction and that of pericarditis and pleuritis, and less commonly with the nonpleuritic pain of angina. The nonpleuritic pain of esophageal spasm may also be confused with pulmonary embolism. Palpitations and/or syncope may reflect a primary cardiac arrhythmia; palpitations may likewise reflect an arrhythmia secondary to the pulmonary embolism or syncope may result from massive acute cor pulmonale.

Pneumonitis and pleuritis are included in the differential diagnosis of pulmonary infarction. Hemoptysis may be due to primary lung disease, but is far less common with heart failure than with pulmonary infarction.

Chronic thromboembolic disease must be differentiated from primary pulmonary hypertension (see Chapter 39).

It is important to recognize deep vein thrombosis as the potential source for pulmonary embolism.

Other Diagnostic Testing

Hypoxemia is a nonspecific finding and often is not present with submassive pulmonary embolism or pulmonary infarction. Normal arterial blood gases do not exclude the occurrence of pulmonary embolism. Neither does a normal alveolar-arterial oxygen gradient exclude pulmonary embolism.[4] Hypocapnia and respiratory alkalosis are nonspecific findings related to tachypnea.

Ventilation perfusion radionuclide pulmonary scanning is the initial diagnostic test.[5] A normal ventilation perfusion scan makes the diagnosis of pulmonary embolism highly unlikely. However, an abnormal scan is nonspecific, but its specificity is increased when there is laboratory documentation of deep vein thrombosis. Multiple areas of ventilation perfusion mismatch are virtually diagnostic for pulmonary embolism.

Spiral computed tomography[6] provides data essentially comparable to that for pulmonary ventilation perfusion scanning. The gold standard, pulmonary angiography, is not always needed for diagnosis.

The two-dimensional *transthoracic echocardiogram*[7] is valuable both for the diagnosis of pulmonary embolism and for the assessment of its hemodynamic significance. Acute cor pulmonale is characterized by enlargement of the right ventricle with a leftward septal shift and resultant decrease in left ventricular end systolic volume. The best clue to right ventricular hemodynamic compromise is flattening of the interventricular septum at end diastole as evidence of a reduced transseptal pressure gradient (RVEDP > LVEDP). This evidence of right ventricular systolic dysfunction is associated with an adverse prognosis.[8] The tricuspid valve gradient by Doppler echocardiography estimates the peak pulmonary artery pressure and the severity of obstruction of the pulmonary vascular bed. There may be pulmonary artery dilatation and lack of decreased inspiratory collapse of the inferior vena cava. Right ventricular hypokinesis at echocardiography doubled the risk of 3-month mortality in the International Cooperative Pulmonary Embolism Registry data base.[9]

Less commonly, a right atrial, right ventricular, or inferior vena caval thrombus is seen on transthoracic echocardiogram and even more rarely there is evidence of thrombus in the foramen ovale. Occasionally, a long thrombus may be coiled in the right atrium. It may dart in and out of the right ventricle with resultant emboli to the lung.

In the patient with septic emboli, tricuspid valve vegetations may be present.

When adequate views are not obtained with transthoracic echocardiogram, transesophageal echocardiography can provide the above information. Additionally, a clot in the central pulmonary arteries not seen with transthoracic echocardiogram may be evident with transesophageal echocardiography.

Venous ultrasonography of the lower extremities is recommended to evaluate for deep vein thrombosis, with use of contrast venography if the results of ultrasonography are inconclusive.[3,10]

Hemodynamic monitoring is usually unnecessary. Pulmonary capillary wedge pressure is not a good index of left ventricular preload; a normal or increased pulmonary wedge pressure can be present with left ventricular underfilling if there is external constraint to left ventricular filling as occurs with right ventricular dilatation. Pulmonary hypertension disproportionate to the severity of left-sided cardiac disease or pulmonary disease may be a clue to pulmonary embolism.

Etiology and Basic Mechanisms Responsible for the "Pain"

The pleuritic chest pain of pulmonary infarction is due to intra-alveolar hemorrhage. There is hemorrhage from the bronchial collateral circulation into the obstructed areas of the distal pulmonary circulation. Pulmonary infarction is more likely to occur when there is pre-existing cardiac or pulmonary disease; most episodes of pulmonary embolism are not associated with infarction of the lung owing to multiple sources of oxygen supply to the lung: this occurs predominantly from the pulmonary artery and the bronchial arterial circulation, and to a lesser extent from the airways, and from back diffusion from the pulmonary veins.

The mechanism of the retrosternal pressure with massive pulmonary embolism is uncertain but may reflect pulmonary artery dilatation or right ventricular subendocardial ischemia (see Chapter 39). The latter may result from increased wall tension due to acute pressure overload, and concomitant decreased coronary perfusion with massive pulmonary embolism.

Pleuritic pain suggests submassive pulmonary embolism occurring in the smaller distal pulmonary arteries in approximation to a pleural surface.

Treatment[8,9]

No specific therapy is indicated for hemodynamically well-tolerated pulmonary embolism other than oxygen for hypoxemia and morphine to relieve the respiratory distress. Therapy is directed to prevent recurrent pulmonary embolism.

In the patient with acute right ventricular failure and hemodynamic compromise, positive inotropic agents such as dobutamine (which is also a pulmonary artery vasodilator) or norepinephrine may be indicated. Evidence of proximal obstruction of the central pulmonary arteries, hemodynamic compromise, and echocardiographic evidence of right ventricular dysfunction are commonly considered indications for thrombolytic therapy. Thrombolytic agents accelerate hemodynamic improvement, but do not alter mortality. However, thrombolysis has been demonstrated to improve right ventricular dysfunction,[12] even in normotensive patients, suggesting that transthoracic echocardiography may be the appropriate approach to risk stratification. Thrombolysis reduces recurrent pulmonary embolism by lysis of the clot of origin. There are no studies comparing dosage regimens and durations of thrombolytic agents, and it is not clear whether one preparation is superior to another. Catheter-based embolectomy may be considered when thrombolysis is contraindicated or fails.

In the patient with cardiac arrest, prolonged cardiopulmonary resuscitation on occasion has been successful, likely because a central clot is fragmented and moves distally. Surgical embolectomy is rarely undertaken in patients with massive pulmonary embolism with contraindications to thrombolysis, as the operative mortality approximates 40%.

Rapid supraventricular tachyarrhythmias can be treated with atrioventricular nodal blocking drugs or electrical cardioversion if there is hemodynamic compromise.

Unfractionated heparin has been the traditional initial approach to the prevention of recurrent pulmonary embolism, but low molecular weight heparin has been recently studied extensively, although predominantly in the setting of deep vein thrombosis. Either full dose unfractionated heparin or low molecular weight heparin is recommended until warfarin anticoagulation reaches the therapeutic range, an International Normalized Ratio (INR) of 2–3.

Inferior vena caval interruption by filter or ligation is appropriate for patients with contraindications to anticoagulation, or for those who have failed anticoagulant therapy.

Often nonsteroidal antiinflammatory agents relieve the pleuritic pain of pulmonary infarction better than narcotic drugs. Patients receiving these drugs must be monitored for warfarin interaction.

References

1. Grady D, Wenger NK, Herrington D, et al, for the Heart and Estrogen/progestin Replacement Study Research Group. Postmenopausal hormone therapy increases risk for venous thromboembolic disease. The Heart and Estrogen/progestin Replacement Study. *Ann Intern Med* 2000;132:689–696.
2. Elliott CG, Goldhaber SZ, Visani L, et al. Chest radiographs in acute pulmonary embolism. Results from the International Cooperative Pulmonary Embolism Registry. *Chest* 2000;118:33–38.
3. Stein PD, Terrin ML, Hales CA, et al. Clinical, laboratory, roentgenographic, and electrocardiographic findings in patients with acute pulmonary embolism and no pre-existing cardiac or pulmonary disease. *Chest* 1991;100:598–603.
4. ACCP Consensus Committee on Pulmonary Embolism. Opinions regarding the diagnosis and management of venous thromboembolic disease. *Chest* 1996;109:233–237.
5. The PIOPED Investigators. Value of the ventilation/perfusion scan in acute pulmonary embolism: Results of the prospective investigation of pulmonary embolism diagnosis (PIOPED). *JAMA* 1990;263:2753–2759.
6. Remy-Jardin M, Remy J, Wattinne L, et al. Central pulmonary thromboembolism: Diagnosis with spiral volumetric CT with the single-breath-hold technique—comparison with pulmonary angiography. *Radiology* 1992;185:381–387.
7. Nazeyrollas P, Metz D, Jolly D, et al. Use of transthoracic Doppler echocardio-

graphy combined with clinical and electrocardiographic data to predict acute pulmonary embolism. *Eur Heart J* 1996;17:779–786.

8. Lualdi JC, Goldhaber SZ. Right ventricular dysfunction after acute pulmonary embolism: Pathophysiologic factors, detection, and therapeutic implications. *Am Heart J* 1995;130:1276–1282.

9. Goldhaber SZ, Visani L, DeRosa M. Acute pulmonary embolism: Clinical outcomes in the International Cooperative Pulmonary Embolism Registry (ICOPER). *Lancet* 1999;353:1386–1389.

10. Hirsh J, Hoak J. Management of deep vein thrombosis and pulmonary embolism: A statement for health care professionals from the Council on Thrombosis (in consultation with the Council on Cardiovascular Radiology), American Heart Association. *Circulation* 1996;93:2212–2245.

11. Goldhaber SZ, Morpurgo M, for the WHO/ISFC Task Force on Pulmonary Embolism: Diagnosis, treatment, and prevention of pulmonary embolism: Report of the WHO/International Society and Federation of Cardiology Task Force. *JAMA* 1992;268:1727–1733.

12. Goldhaber SZ, Haire WD, Feldstein ML, et al. Alteplase versus heparin in acute pulmonary embolism: Randomized trial assessing right-ventricular function and pulmonary perfusion. *Lancet* 1993;341:507–511.

17

"Chest Pain" in Patients with 'Café' Coronary

Stephen D. Clements, Jr., MD

General Considerations

Haugen, in 1963, coined the term café coronary to describe the obstructive asphyxia that occurred following aspiration of a large bolus of food into the hypopharynx.[1]

Clinical Setting

The age range of those affected with café coronary is broad (3–83 years) with the highest frequency in the 50–70 year range.[2] The overall male-to-female ratio of this syndrome is about 1:6, and it is distributed through all walks of life and professions. Although some café coronary events occur at home, mental institutions, nursing homes and hospitals, a large number occur in restaurants.[3]

Characteristics of the "Pain"

Patient's characterization of the "chest pain"

While eating, the subject may suddenly grasp the throat or point to the throat being unable to breathe, speak, or cough. Grasping the throat is the universal distress signal. Cyanosis and dyspnea are sometimes observed by bystanders.

From: Hurst JW, Morris DC (eds): *"Chest Pain"* →. © Futura Publishing Co., Inc., Armonk, NY, 2001.

Common locations of the "chest pain"

The patient grasps or points to the throat unable to speak, breathe or cough (see Figure 17–1).

Uncommon location of the "chest pain"

None.

Size of the pain "area"

The discomfort is limited to the neck area.

Duration of the "chest pain"

Total obstruction of the airway results in total collapse in a few minutes. Lack of oxygen to the brain can result in irreversible changes beyond 6 minutes. Partial obstruction can be more prolonged, but still lasting only minutes. Reflex reactions to include massive vasovagal responses may occur and hasten loss of circulation as food boluses come into contact with the inner surfaces of the hypopharynx and larynx.

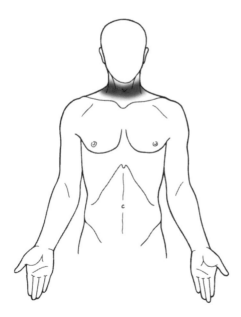

Figure 17–1. This figure illustrates the distress felt by a patient who has acute obstruction of the trachea (as occurs with café coronary). The patient points to his or her throat, unable to speak, breathe, or cough.

Tenderness of the chest wall

There is no tenderness of the chest wall.

Precipitating causes of the "chest pain"

The clinical setting in which café coronary occurs has been well defined. Restaurants or bars, in addition to lodgings, are the locations for the majority of deaths from foreign body airway obstruction.[3] Reports of these happenings also mention excessive alcohol intake and the instance of feeding periods for handicapped persons. Individuals with neurologic syndromes such as Parkinson's disease, Huntington's chorea, bulbar palsy, dementia, and stroke have been reported to have succumbed from café coronary events. Patients with psychiatric illnesses such as schizophrenia and those receiving drugs with strong anticholinergic effects are more prone to foreign-body airway obstruction.[4]

Suspicion should also be directed to the setting of older individuals talking while eating, occasions of hurried swallowing, presence of upper and lower dentures (a denture has been found in the hypopharynx in a fatal case of café coronary, and even a collar button in a child) and elevated blood alcohol levels. Any condition that alters the gag reflex will predispose the patient to café coronary.

The types of substances associated with choking varies, including pieces of poorly masticated meat, hot dogs, fish, vegetables, dentures, bananas, chewing tobacco, peanut butter and various other foods.[3]

Relief of the "chest pain"

The relief of choking of airway obstruction consists of removing the obstruction by coughing, Heimlich maneuver or tracheostomy (see treatment).

Associated Symptoms

See precipitating causes.

Associated Signs

Physical examination

In the predisposing clinical setting such as a restaurant, eating meat and drinking alcohol, the signs of grasping the neck, cyanosis, and inability to speak, breathe, or cough suggest that action must be taken immediately. Stridor with partial airway obstruction allows slightly more time for intervention. See below.

"Routine" laboratory tests

None.

Exceptions to the Usual Manifestations

Generally none.

Differential Diagnosis

Myocardial infarction or pulmonary embolus could be implicated in individuals found with circulatory collapse and sudden death. Clues to café coronary come when the setting is that of a restaurant, an indication of choking, pointing to the throat or neck, the lack of the ability to move air through the larynx, coughing, or cyanosis.

Other Diagnostic Testing

None.

Etiology and Basic Mechanisms Responsible for the "Pain"

Obstruction of the trachea or hypopharynx creates an acute sensation of suffocation and distress.

Treatment

Once the diagnosis of airway obstruction by a food bolus is made, immediate action should then be taken.[5] In 1974, Henry J. Heimlich described the abdominal thrust that bears his name. The maneuver consists of placing the fists one on top of the other between the naval and the xiphoid process (see Table 17–1).

Table 17–1.

Summary for Treatment of Complete Airway Obstruction.

1) The victim should be shaken so as to arouse him or her
2) If the victim is unresponsive, onlookers should be directed to bring about the necessary assistance such as emergency care if not already available.
3) An airway must be established. This is done by first checking for breathing by placing the ear over the mouth and listening and looking for rising of the chest. If not breathing, the rescuer should attempt to ventilate.
4) Ventilation begins by tilting the head and pinching the nostrils shut. However, if a neck injury is suspected, such as after a fall, then the airway is opened by the modified jaw thrust or chin lift method.
5) If the first ventilation is unsuccessful, then the head should be repositioned and ventilation attempted once again.
6) If still unsuccessful, one should now go through the procedure for relief of airway obstruction beginning with subdiaphragmatic abdominal thrusts.
7) If the foreign body is still lodged in the throat, the sequence of abdominal thrusts, finger sweeps and attempt to ventilate should be repeated.

(Source: Used with permission from *Nurse Practitioner* 1989 June 14 (6): 35–36 passim, ©Springhouse Corporation/www.springnet.com).

For the individual who is standing, the rescuer should stand behind the victim or, if the individual is sitting, the rescuer should be situated behind the chair. The rescuer should wrap both arms around the victim with one hand made into a fist, the thumb being located just above the umbilicus and the other hand grasping the fist. A quick, upward thrust should be given toward the diaphragm watching the mouth for evidence of the foreign body. Multiple attempts should be made, if necessary.

For victims lying down, the rescuer should straddle the victim with the knees of the rescuer at the victim's pelvis. The hand is then placed in the midline just above the umbilicus below the xiphoid and the second hand palm down placed upon the first. A quick, upward thrust toward the diaphragm should be made and repeated until the airway is opened. Exceptions in adults are individuals who are markedly obese or an advanced stage of pregnancy. In these situations, the arms should be higher under the armpits and the fist on the lower half of the sternum.

Children less than 1 year of age are exceptions to the usual abnormal thrust technique. It is recommended that a combination of back blows and chest thrusts be used. With the child draped over the rescuer's leg and head down, a blow is delivered to the infant's back in combination with chest thrusts.[6]

A finger sweep should be made by grasping the lower mandible and tongue with one hand and lifting forward, while the index finger of the other hand sweeps through the posterior pharynx searching for the foreign body.[7] If vomiting occurs, then the head and sometimes the trunk need to be turned to the side, the pharynx cleared, and the Heimlich maneuver repeated. If success is not obtained after a few attempts, emergency medical service should be called.

If the Heimlich maneuver is unsuccessful, then cricothyrotomy or tracheostomy should be performed by trained rescuers.

References

1. Haugen RK. The café coronary: Sudden deaths in restaurants. *JAMA* 1963;186: 142–143.
2. Jacob B, Weidbrauck C, Lamprecht J, et al. Dysphagia. 1992;7:31–35.
3. Mittleman RE, Wetli CV. The fatal café coronary. *JAMA* 1982;247:1285–1288.
4. Hsish HH, Bhatia SC, Andersen JM, et al. Psychotropic medication and nonfatal café coronary. *J Clin Psychopharmacol* 1986;6(2):101–102.
5. 1985 National Conference on Standards and Guidelines for Cardiopulmonary Resuscitation and Emergency Cardiac Care. Adult basic life support. *JAMA* 1986;255:2915–2932.
6. Heimlich HJ. Back blows and choking. *Pediatrics* 1983;71(6):983–984.
7. Kitay G, Shafer N. Café coronary: Recognition, treatment and prevention. *Nurse Practitioner* 1989;14(6):35–46.

Part VII

Diseases of the Gastrointestinal Tract as a Cause for "Chest Pain"

Although the definition of "chest pain"→ is discussed in Chapter 1, the definition is repeated here so that communication is clear.

The quotation marks around "chest" imply that different patients have different definitions of the word "chest." Here we use the word to indicate pain located above the waist. Then, too, *angina pectoris* is not always located in the pectoral region—it may be felt only in the jaw, neck, shoulder, elbow, or wrist. Therefore, the word "chest" implies that other parts of the upper body may also be involved with painful syndromes.

The quotation marks around "pain" imply that patients may assign other terms to their discomfort, such as indigestion, burning, ache, etc.

The arrow after "chest pain" implies that the physician initially may not know the cause of the symptom, so a differential diagnosis must be established that fits the available information.

18

"Chest Pain" in Patients with Esophageal Motility Disorders

J. Patrick Waring, MD

General Considerations

There are two important types of esophageal motility disorders: diffuse esophageal spasm and achalasia.[1,2] *Diffuse esophageal spasm* is commonly diagnosed but is actually quite rare; it is considered to be a disorder of esophageal peristalsis. *Achalasia* is also a rare disorder, manifested by poor relaxation of the lower esophageal sphincter and the absence of esophageal peristalsis.

The nutcracker esophagus is not discussed here because it is a controversial entity characterized by an increase in esophageal body pressure. Lowering the esophageal body pressure does not relieve the patient's chest pain.[3] Most patients with the nutcracker esophagus have other causes of chest pain.[4,5]

Clinical Setting

There is no particular clinical setting in which esophageal motility disorders are likely to occur. Adult males and females may have the condition.

Characteristics of the "Pain"

Patient's characterization of the "chest pain"

The patient with an esophageal motility disorder may complain of "chest pain" that is indistinguishable from angina pectoris or myocardial infarction (see Chapters 29 and 30).

From: Hurst JW, Morris DC (eds): *"Chest Pain"* →. © Futura Publishing Co., Inc., Armonk, NY, 2001.

Common location of the "chest pain"

The pain is centrally located, often at the subxiphoid level. It may be located in the area where angina pectoris is commonly detected (see Figure 18–1). The pain may radiate throughout the chest up to the jaw (see Figure 18–2).

Uncommon locations of the "chest pain"

The pain may radiate straight through to the back (see Figure 18–3).

Size of the painful "area"

The approximate size of the painful area is shown in Figures 18–1 and 18–2.

Duration of the "chest pain"

The pain can last for minutes, hours, or days. "Pain" lasting for days is rarely due to myocardial ischemia, but pain lasting for minutes to hours may simulate the pain of angina pectoris or myocardial infarction.

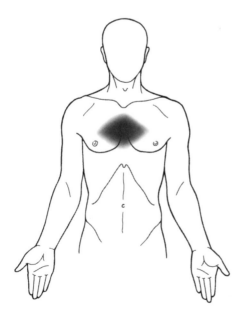

Figure 18–1. The "chest pain" related to esophageal motility disorders may be similar to that of angina pectoris, and is often located in the same general area where angina pectoris is usually identified.

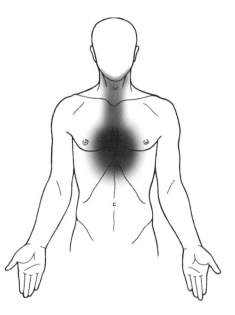

Figure 18–2. The "chest pain" of esophageal motility disorders may be located in the retrosternal area and radiate to the neck and jaw. This radiation is also often observed in patients with angina pectoris.

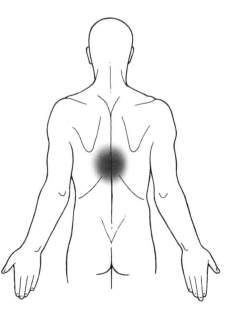

Figure 18–3. The "chest pain" of esophageal motility disorders may radiate through to the back. In virtually all cases the discomfort occurs in the anterior portion of the chest, and occasionally radiates to the back.

Tenderness of the chest wall

The epigastric area may or may not be tender.

Precipitating causes of the "chest pain"

The "chest pain" usually occurs without an obvious precipitating cause and is not necessarily related to eating. The "chest pain" is not precipitated by effort or detectable emotional turmoil.

Should eating precipitate the episode of pain, one should be reminded that angina pectoris can be precipitated by eating a full meal.

Relief of the "chest pain"

Esophageal pain from diffuse esophageal spasm or achalasia may or may not respond to antacid medication or sublingual nitroglycerin. Neither a rapid response or the lack of a response to symptomatic therapy is a reliable indicator of the cause of chest pain in these patients.

Associated Symptoms

These patients commonly describe dysphagia. Some patients use the word "spasm" to describe their discomfort. Most of these patients are describing pain, but occasionally they are describing dysphagia. The use of the word "spasm" by the patient may mislead the physician to believe the patient has an esophageal motility disorder. However, it must be emphasized that most patients who use the word "spasm" have gastroesophageal reflux. Patients with chest pain from diffuse esophageal spasm frequently have typical reflux symptoms as well. Some experts theorize that reflux can precipitate esophageal spasm. Regurgitation occurs in patients with diffuse esophageal spasm as well as gastroesophageal reflux.

Patients with *achalasia* almost always present with dysphagia or regurgitation. It is thought that fermentation of undigested food in the distal esophagus can lead to a burning sensation in patients with achalasia.

Associated Signs

The physical examination

The physical examination in patients with diffuse esophageal spasm or achalasia is usually normal. There may be slight tenderness in the epigastric area. Should other abnormalities be found, they are unrelated to either diffuse esophageal spasm or achalasia.

"Routine" laboratory tests

The "routine" laboratory tests are normal in patients with diffuse esophageal spasm or achalasia. The electrocardiogram may be normal or abnormal. If it is abnormal, the abnormalities are not related to the esophageal disease. The chest x-ray film is usually not helpful in establishing a diagnosis.

Exceptions to the Usual Manifestations

There are no exceptions to the description of the clinical findings that are described above.

Differential Diagnosis

Obviously, coronary atherosclerotic heart disease must be considered in patients with chest pain. The pain from gastroesophageal reflux can mimic angina. Additionally, it may be impossible to distinguish the pain of diffuse esophageal spasm from other esophageal causes; such as gastroesophageal reflux, based on the characteristic of the chest pain itself. *The best clue that you are dealing with diffuse esophageal spams or achalasia is the associated symptom of dysphagia.*

Other Diagnostic Testing

The symptoms of many of these patients mimic angina or myocardial infarction so closely that appropriate studies are often indicated to rule out coronary atherosclerotic heart disease before performing any tests to identify esophageal motility disorder.

A barium swallow can be a helpful diagnostic test in patients with dysphagia. It can distinguish achalasia from esophageal stricture quite nicely. A barium swallow is virtually diagnostic when it confirms the classic features of absent esophageal peristalsis, tapered narrowing at the lower esophageal sphincter (referred to as a bird-beaked appearance), and dilation of the esophageal body.[6] It is of benefit in the evaluation of esophageal spasm in patients whose prominent symptom is dysphagia. A rare patient will have the characteristic corkscrew appearance of tertiary contractions in the esophagus on barium swallow.

Esophageal manometry testing has been thought to be very helpful in the evaluation of unexplained chest pain. In truth, it is of little benefit given the rarity that esophageal motility disorders actually are responsible for the chest pain.[7] If diffuse esophageal spasm is suspected, esophageal manometry will have classic features, namely spontaneous, simultaneous esophageal contractions, mixed in with normal esophageal peristalsis. Esophageal manometry testing can confirm achalasia in patients with clinical and radiographic features of the disease. Findings of absent esophageal peristalsis and poor relaxation of the lower esophageal sphincter (with or without elevated pressure) are characteristic of achalasia.

Patients most likely to benefit from endoscopy are those with long-standing heartburn or odynphagia (painful swallowing). Patients with bothersome symptoms other than chest pain—such as weight loss, intestinal bleeding, nausea, vomiting, or dysphagia—should also have an endoscopy early on, to rule out more serious causes for their problems. Upper endoscopy is indicated in patients with achalasia to exclude a neoplastic cause for the radiographic and manometric findings.

Etiology and Basic Mechanisms Responsible for the "Pain"

The precise mechanism of pain sensation in the esophagus is not known.[8] The major pathways are along spinal and vagal afferent nerve fibers. The intraepithelial nerve endings, which are sensitive to acid exposure, are involved in the spinal pathways. Mechanosensitive spinal afferents are thought to be located in the esophageal muscle and serosa. Spinal pathways are largely responsible for the perception of pain and discomfort. The vagal afferents are sensitive to esophageal distension and appear to be important in pain modulation. Patients with chest pain appear to have a lower threshold to painful stimuli in the esophagus.[9,10] Balloon distension in the esophagus of chest pain patients prompts pain at lower volumes than in healthy controls.[11,12] The role of stress and psychological factors cannot be underestimated.

Treatment

The treatment of esophageal spasm is rather difficult. Historically, nitrates and calcium channel blockers have been used although with very little success. There are no data from objective testing suggesting that these drugs are useful.

Botulinim toxin injection into the lower esophageal sphincter has been used with modest success in patients with nonspecific esophageal motility disorders and chest pain or dysphagia.[13] One must remember that even in patients suspected of having diffuse esophageal spasm, there may be gastroesophageal reflux. The reflux may precipitate the motility disorder that causes the "chest pain." The most simple, and preferred, diagnostic test for gastroesophageal reflux-related chest pain is to offer the patient an empiric trial of the antireflux therapy.

The treatment of *achalasia* is to virtually obliterate the lower esophageal sphincter. This may be done by surgical, endoscopic, or pharmacological means.[14] Heller myotomy is the preferred surgical approach. The surgical results are comparable to those seen with pneumatic dilation. Injection of botulinum toxin into the lower esophageal sphincter is a safe, but less effective treatment for achalasia. Medical therapy with calcium channel blockers or nitrates provides limited benefit. The chest pain in achalasia does not respond as well to balloon dilation or dysphagia.[15]

References

1. Achem SR, Kolts BE. Current medical therapy for esophageal motility disorders. *Am J Med* 1992;92:98S–105S.
2. Langevin S, Castell DO. Esophageal motility disorders and chest pain. *Med Clin NA* 1991;75:1045–1063.
3. Richter JE, Dalton CB, Bradley LA, et al. Oral nifedipine in the treatment of noncardiac chest pain in patients with the nutcracker esophagus. *Gastroenterology* 1987;93:21–28.
4. Achem SR, Kolts BE, Wears R, et al. Chest pain associated with nutcracker esophagus: A preliminary study of the role of gastroesophageal reflux. *Am J Gastroenterol* 1993;88:187–192.
5. Kahrilas PJ. Nutcracker esophagus: An idea whose time has gone? *Am J Gastroenterol* 1993;88:167–169.
6. Vaezi MF, Richter JE. Diagnosis and management of achalasia. American College of Gastroenterology Practice Parameter Committee. *Am J Gastroenterol* 1999;94:3406–3412.
7. DiMarino AJ Jr, Allen ML, Lynn RB, et al. Clinical value of esophageal motility testing. *Dig Dis Sci* 1998;16:198–204.
8. Fass R, Fennerty MB, Vakil N. Non-erosive reflux disease (NERD) – current concepts and dilemmas. *Am J Gastroenterol* (in press).
9. Pasricha PJ. Noncardiac chest pain: From nutcrackers to nociceptors. *Gastroenterology* 1997;112:309–310.
10. Castell DO. Chest pain of undetermined origin: Overview of pathophysiology. *Am J Med* 1992;92:2S–4S.
11. DeVault KR, Castell DO. Esophageal balloon distention and cerebral evoked potential recording in the evaluation of unexplained chest pain. *Am J Med* 1992;92:20S–26S.
12. Paterson WG, Wang H, Vanner SJ. Increasing pain sensation to repeated

esophageal balloon distension in patients with chest pain of undetermined etiology. *Dig Dis Sci* 1995;40:1325–1331.

13. Miller LS, Parkman HP, Schiano TD, et al. Treatment of symptomatic nonachalasia esophageal motor disorders with botulinum toxin injection at the lower esophageal sphincter. *Dig Dis Sci* 1996;41:2025–2031.

14. Vaezi MF, Richter JE. Current therapies for achalasia: Comparison and efficacy. *J Clin Gastroenterol* 1998;27:21–35.

15. Eckardt VF, Stauf B, Bernhard G. Chest pain in achalasia: Patient characteristics and clinical course *Gastroenterology* 1999;116:1300–1304.

19

"Chest Pain" in Patients with Gastroesophageal Reflux

J. Patrick Waring, MD

General Considerations

Gastroesophageal reflux can cause "chest pain" that closely mimics the "pain" of angina pectoris and myocardial infarction. In fact, the pain of esophageal origin is the most common imitator of the "pain" of myocardial ischemia.

During the first 30–40 years of the 20th century, patients who died from unrecognized cardiac arrhythmias due to acute myocardial ischemia were said to have died from "acute indigestion." Today it is alarming to see the media hype designed to sell drugs to relieve "indigestion" when they show a patient in obvious "pain" with his fist placed in the mid-sternal area of the chest just as they do with the "pain" of angina pectoris. In fact, even expert cardiologists, such as Paul Wood, may misdiagnose their own "chest pain" due to angina pectoris or infarct as "indigestion" (see Chapter 1).

Gastroesophageal reflux is the most common treatable cause of "chest pain" due to esophageal disease.[1]

Clinical Setting

The patients with gastroesophageal reflux are usually adults and are commonly obese. Males and females are affected with this common disorder.

From: Hurst JW, Morris DC (eds): *"Chest Pain"* →. © Futura Publishing Co., Inc., Armonk, NY, 2001.

Characteristics of the "Pain"

Patient's characterization of the "chest pain"

The patient describes the "pain" as indigestion, burning (heartburn), tightness, pressure, or any of the other adjectives used by patients with angina pectoris (see Chapter 29). Occasionally the "pain" is described as a dull sensation.

Common location of the "chest pain"

The "pain" may be located in the retrosternal area as it is with angina pectoris (see Figure 19–1). It is usually located in the sub-xiphoid area and may radiate to the neck and jaw (see Figure 19–2).

Uncommon locations of the "chest pain"

The "pain" may radiate straight through to the back (see Figure 19–3).

Size of the painful "area"

The painful area is about the size of the fist or larger.

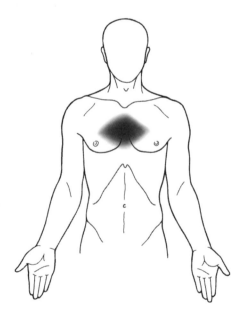

Figure 19–1. This figure illustrates the location of the "chest pain" caused by gastroesophageal reflux. Note the location of the "pain" is similar to the location of the "pain" due to myocardial ischemia (angina pectoris or myocardial infarction).

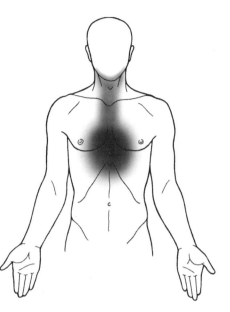

Figure 19–2. This figure illustrates that the "pain" of gastroesophageal reflux may be felt in the sub-xiphoid area, retrosternal area, neck, and jaw.

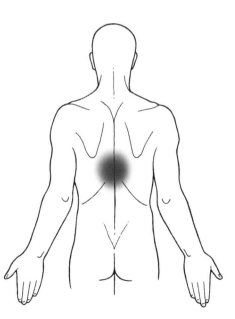

Figure 19–3. The "pain" of gastro-esophageal reflux may radiate to the back.

Duration of the "chest pain"

The "pain" may last minutes, hours, or days. The pain lasting minutes to hours may mimic the pain of angina pectoris or infarction. However, pain lasting for days is not characteristic of angina or infarct.

Tenderness of the chest wall

There is no tenderness of the chest wall. There may be slight tenderness in the sub-xiphoid area.

Precipitating causes of the "chest pain"

The pain may be precipitated when the patient assumes the recumbent position after a large meal. This is especially likely to occur in obese patients. The patient may identify certain foods, such as citrus fruit, that precipitate episodes of "indigestion" but this is not the case in most patients.

The "chest pain" associated with gastroesophageal reflux is not precipitated by effort. This point is useful when the person is active, but an individual who lives a sedentary life may not exert themselves so they cannot respond to an inquiry about exercise related "chest pain."

Relief of the "chest pain"

The use of antacids may or may not distinguish the difference between myocardial ischemia and gastroesophageal reflux. Should the patients obtain prompt relief of the "pain" after taking an antacid, we have to remember that untreated angina pectoris usually lasts only a few minutes. Also, should sublingual nitroglycerin be used, it is not always possible to deduce that the "pain" was due to angina pectoris because the pain of untreated gastroesophageal reflux may last only 2 or 3 minutes.

Still, in general, if the patient has had the "chest pain" for months and is an accurate observer, the apparent relief of the "pain" with antacids supports the idea that the "pain" was due to gastroesophageal reflux.

To confound the issue, some patients have angina pectoris *and* the pain of gastroesophageal reflux.

Associated Symptoms

The patient may notice slight regurgitation of gastric contents into his or her mouth. Belching may occur, but this is a nonspecific symptom.

Associated Signs

The physical examination

The physical examination is usually normal in patients with pain due to gastroesophageal reflux, as is the physical examination of patients with angina pectoris. Of course, the physical examination may be abnormal due to comorbid condition in both conditions.

The patient with pain due to gastroesophageal reflux may have tenderness to palpation in the sub-xiphoid area.

"Routine" laboratory tests

There are no abnormalities noted in the routine laboratory tests. The chest x-ray film and electrocardiogram are normal in patients with pain due to gastroesophageal reflux. Of course, the chest x-ray film and electrocardiogram may be abnormal due to a comorbid disease. The physician then must decide if the abnormalities seen in the electrocardiogram are caused by obstructive coronary disease or if the patient has both conditions—coronary disease and the pain of gastroesophageal reflux.

Exceptions to the Usual Manifestations

Gastroesophageal reflux can occur without symptoms, just as silent ischemia of the heart can occur without angina pectoris.

Differential Diagnosis

As stated earlier, angina pectoris must be differentiated from the "pain" of gastroesophageal reflux. Also, other types of esophageal disease must be identified because the "chest pain" itself does not differ sufficiently to make an accurate separation of the pain due to the other esophageal conditions.

Other Diagnostic Testing

The simplest, and preferred, diagnostic test is to offer the patient an empiric trial of the antireflux therapy.[2,3] It is more accurate than other traditional esophageal studies.[4] This is particularly true in patients who have other esophageal symptoms besides chest pain. A successful empiric trial prevents the need for further diagnostic testing, consequently decreasing the overall cost of health care for these patients.[5,6]

Ambulatory pH monitoring is probably the best test to establish a diagnosis of gastroesophageal reflux.[7] This involves placing a catheter transnasally into the esophagus. It is usually done for a 24-hour period to measure the amount of esophageal acid exposure. The test does have some shortcomings.[8] The patient may not have a typical day, if they don't eat or have the usual amount of activity during the study period. A good deal has been written about associating the symptoms of chest pain and reflux episodes during the pH test.[9] Unfortunately, this will not be helpful if the patient doesn't have chest pain during the study, or if the pain is constant.[10] The usual purpose of ambulatory pH monitoring in patients with "chest pain" is to make a diagnosis of gastroesophageal reflux.[11] Occasionally, however, ambulatory pH monitoring may be done to monitor the success of ongoing medical treatment. However, the data regarding the value of this approach are conflicting.[12,13]

Patients with bothersome symptoms besides chest pain—such as weight loss, intestinal bleeding, nausea, vomiting, dysphagia, or odynphagia—should have an endoscopy early on to rule out more serious causes for these problems. Otherwise, upper endoscopy is of limited benefit in patients with chest pain, as it is almost always normal.[1] Endoscopy is indicated for patients with long-standing reflux symptoms in order to exclude Barrett's esophagus.[14,15] Barium swallow is of limited value in diagnosing patients with gastroesophageal reflux, because of its poor sensitivity and specificity. Provocative tests, such as the acid-perfusion test or tensilon challenge, were popular in the 1980s.[16] However, they have been shown to be of little diagnostic value in the modern evaluation of unexplained chest pain.[17,18]

Etiology and Basic Mechanisms Responsible for the "Pain"

Gastroesophageal reflux is caused by a relaxed lower gastroesophageal sphincter. The chest pain associated with a hiatal hernia is rarely due to the hernia, but to associated gastroesophageal reflux.

The precise mechanism of pain sensation in the esophagus is not known.[19] The major pathways are along spinal and vagal afferent nerve fibers. The intraepithelial nerve endings, which are sensitive to acid exposure, are involved in the spinal pathways. Mechanosensitive spinal afferents are thought to be located in the esophageal muscle and serosa. Spinal pathways are largely responsible for the perception of pain and discomfort. The vagal afferents are sensitive to esophageal distension and appear to be important in pain modulation.

Patients with chest pain appear to have a lower threshold to painful stimuli in the esophagus.[20,21] Balloon distension in the esophagus of chest pain patients prompts pain at lower volumes than in healthy controls.[22,23] The role of stress and psychological factors cannot be underestimated. Numerous articles demonstrate a higher incidence of anxiety neurosis and panic disorder in patients with unexplained chest pain.[24–28]

Treatment

Nearly 60% of patients with unexplained "chest pain" have evidence of gastroesophageal reflux.[1,2,29] It would seem reasonable to consider antireflux therapy as the initial treatment approach. Accordingly, it would seem reasonable to consider antireflux treatment in patients who have normal coronary arteriograms and clinical symptoms consistent with those associated with gastroesophageal reflux. The optimum treatment for gastroesophageal reflux disease is with gastric acid suppression.[30] This admonition applies particularly to patients with recurring, troublesome chest pain.[9,31,32] In one study, double dose proton pump inhibitor therapy decreased chest pain symptoms in 81% of patients versus 6% in patients who were given a placebo.[33] There is probably no significant difference between the four available proton pump inhibitors. H2 blockers have been used, but in standard doses they usually fail and higher doses are required for relief.[9]

References

1. Richter JE. Chest pain and gastroesophageal reflux disease. *J Clin Gastroenterol* 2000;30:S39–41.
2. Fennerty MB. Extraesophageal gastroesophageal reflux disease. Presentations and approach to treatment. *Gastroenterol Clin NA* 1999;28:861–873.
3. Richter JE. Cost-effectiveness of testing for gastroesophageal reflux disease: What do patients, physicians, and health insurers want? *Am J Med* 1999;107:288–289.
4. Fass R, Fennerty MB, Ofman JJ, et al. The clinical and economic value of a short course of omeprazole in patients with noncardiac chest pain. *Gastroenterology* 1998;115:42–49.
5. Ofman JJ, Gralnek IM, Udani J, et al. The cost-effectiveness of the omeprazole test in patients with noncardiac chest pain. *Am J Med* 1999;107:219–227.
6. Borzecki AM, Pedrosa MC, Prashker MJ. Should noncardiac chest pain be treated empirically? A cost-effectiveness analysis. *Arch Int Med* 2000;160:844–852.
7. Kahrilas PJ, Quigley EM. Clinical esophageal pH recording: A technical review for practice guideline development. *Gastroenterology* 1996;110:1982–1988.
8. Singh S, Richter JE, Bradley LA, et al. The symptom index. Differential usefulness in suspected acid-related complaints of heartburn and chest pain. *Dig Dis Sci* 1993;38:1402–1408.

9. Stahl WG, Beton RR, Johnson CS, et al. Diagnosis and treatment of patients with gastroesophageal reflux and noncardiac chest pain. *South Med J* 1994;87:739–742.
10. Fass R, Fennerty MB, Johnson C, et al. Correlation of ambulatory 24-hour esophageal pH monitoring results with symptom improvement in patients with noncardiac chest pain due to gastroesophageal reflux disease. *J Clin Gastroenterol* 1999;28:36–39.
11. Wo JM, Hunter JG, Waring JP. Dual-channel ambulatory esophageal pH monitoring. A useful diagnostic tool? *Dig Dis Sci* 1997;42:2222–2226.
12. Katzka DA, Paoletti V, Leite L, et al Prolonged ambulatory pH monitoring in patients with persistent gastroesophageal reflux disease symptoms: Testing while on therapy identifies the need for more aggressive anti-reflux therapy. *Am J Gastroenterol* 1996;91:2110–2113.
13. Waring JP, Hunter JG. Patients failing moderately high doses of omeprazole. *Am J Gastroenterol* 1997;92:907–909.
14. DeVault KR, Castell DO. Updated guidelines for the diagnosis and treatment of gastroesophageal reflux disease. The Practice Parameters Committee of the American College of Gastroenterology. *Am J Gastroenterol* 1999;94:1434–1442.
15. Sampliner RE. Practice guidelines on the diagnosis, surveillance, and therapy of Barrett's esophagus. The Practice Parameters Committee of the American College of Gastroenterology. *Am J Gastroenterol* 1998;93:1028–1032.
16. Nostrant TT. Provocation testing in noncardiac chest pain. *Am J Med* 1992;92: 56S–64S.
17. Richter JE, Hewson EG, Sinclair JW, et al. Acid perfusion test and 24-hour esophageal pH monitoring with symptom index. Comparison of tests for esophageal acid sensitivity. *Dig Dis Sci* 1991;36:565–571.
18. Rose S, Achkar E, Falk GW, et al. Interaction between patient and test administrator may influence the results of edrophonium provocative testing in patients with noncardiac chest pain. *Am J Gastroenterol* 1993;88:20–24.
19. Fass R, Fennerty MB, Vakil N. Non-erosive reflux disease (NERD) – current concepts and dilemmas. *Am J Gastroenterol* (in press).
20. Pasricha PJ. Noncardiac chest pain: From nutcrackers to nociceptors. *Gastroenterology* 1997;112:309–310.
21. Castell DO. Chest pain of undetermined origin: Overview of pathophysiology. *Am J Med* 1992;92:2S–4S.
22. DeVault KR, Castell DO. Esophageal balloon distention and cerebral evoked potential recording in the evaluation of unexplained chest pain. *Am J Med* 1992;92:20S–26S.
23. Paterson WG, Wang H, Vanner SJ. Increasing pain sensation to repeated esophageal balloon distension in patients with chest pain of undetermined etiology. *Dig Dis Sci* 1995;40:1325–1331.
24. Ho KY, Kang JY, Yeo B, et al. Non-cardiac, non-oesophageal chest pain: The elevance of psychological factors. *Gut* 1998;43:105–110.
25. Ros E, Armengol X, Grande L, et al. Chest pain at rest in patients with coronary artery disease. Myocardial ischemia, esophageal dysfunction, or panic disorder? *Dig Dis Sci* 1997;42:1344–1353.
26. Mehta AJ, De Caestecker JS, Camm AJ, et al. Sensitization to painful distention and abnormal sensory perception in the esophagus. *Gastroenterology* 1995;108: 311–319.
27. Maunder RG. Panic disorder associated with gastrointestinal disease: Review and hypotheses. *J Psychosomatic Res* 1998;44:91–105.

28. Stollman NH, Bierman PS, Ribeiro A, et al. CO2 provocation of panic: Symptomatic and manometric evaluation in patients with noncardiac chest pain. *Am J Gastroenterol* 92:839–842.

29. DeMeester TR, O'Sullivan GC, Bermudez G, et al. Esophageal function in patients with angina-type chest pain and normal coronary angiograms. *Ann Surg* 1982;196:488–498.

30. Richter JE. Extraesophageal presentations of gastroesophageal reflux disease: The case for aggressive diagnosis and treatment. *Cleve Clin J Med* 1997;64:37–45.

31. Achem SR, Kolts BE, Wears R, et al. Chest pain associated with nutcracker esophagus: A preliminary study of the role of gastroesophageal reflux . *Am J Gastroenterol* 1993; 88:187–192.

32. Singh S, Richter JE, Hewson EG, et al. The contribution of gastroesophageal reflux to chest pain in patients with coronary artery disease. *Ann Int Med* 1992;117:824–830.

33. Achem SR, Kolts BE, MacMath T, et al. Effects of omeprazole versus placebo in treatment of noncardiac chest pain and gastroesophageal reflux. *Dig Dis Sci* 1997;42:2138–2145.

20

"Chest Pain" in Patients with Esophageal Rupture

J. Patrick Waring, MD

General Considerations

Rupture of the esophagus is a rare condition, but when it occurs it may produce "chest pain" that imitates acute myocardial infarction.

Clinical Setting

The "chest pain" of esophageal rupture usually occurs during or after an episodes of forceful vomiting.[1–3] In years past, the esophagus was occasionally ruptured during an endoscopic esophageal examination. This complication of endoscopy is currently almost nonexistent.

Characteristics of the "Pain"

Patient's characterization of the "chest pain"

The description of "pain" may simulate the "pain" of myocardial infarction (see Chapter 30). As associated inflammation develops, the pain may have a pleuritic component to it. The pain is usually classified by the patient as being severe, although occult rupture does occur.[4]

Common location of the "chest pain"

The pain is located in the epigastrium and anterior portion of the chest (see Figure 20–1). The "pain" may radiate to the neck and jaw.

From: Hurst JW, Morris DC (eds): *"Chest Pain"* →. © Futura Publishing Co., Inc., Armonk, NY, 2001.

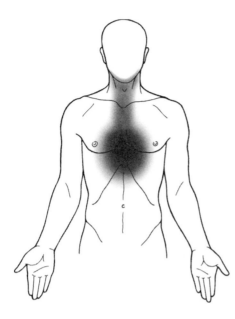

Figure 20–1. This figure illustrates the location of "chest pain" secondary to rupture of the esophagus. The "pain" may be located in the epigastric area; the lower retrosternal area, and may radiate to the neck and jaw.

Uncommon locations of the "chest pain"

The pain is usually located in the area shown in Figure 20–1; there are no unusual locations of the pain.

Size of the painful "area"

The approximate size of the painful area is shown in Figure 20–1.

Duration of the "chest pain"

The pain may last for hours unless it is relieved by appropriate medication.

Tenderness of the chest wall

Tenderness may be detected occasionally in the epigastric area.

Precipitating causes of the "chest pain"

Esophageal rupture almost always develops during or after episodes of severe vomiting. Inspiration may aggravate the pain as infection of adjacent structures develops.

Relief of the "chest pain"

There is nothing the patient can do to relieve the pain. Opiates are usually needed for relief.

Associated Symptoms

The patient with esophageal rupture usually presents with life threatening problems, including severe pain, a toxic appearance, hypotension, hypoxia, diaphoresis, or fever. Rarely, patients may present with occult injury.[4]

Associated Signs

The physical examination

Patients will have abnormal vital signs, such as hypotension, hypoxia, or fever. Patients may have subcutaneous emphysema. Many patients with esophageal rupture have a hydropneumothorax. Ninety percent of patients will develop a left-sided pleural effusion.

"Routine" laboratory tests

The chest x-ray film may reveal mediastinal emphysema and, at times, subcutaneous emphysema. Later in the course of the illness the x-ray film of the chest may reveal a left-sided pleural effusion or a hydropneumothorax.

The electrocardiogram reveals no abnormalities that are specific for esophageal rupture. These patients, however, may have hypotension and are desperately ill. Such patients may develop electrocardiograhic signs of subendocardial injury, or abnormal repolarization secondary to the hypotension and associated coronary atherosclerosis.

Exceptions to the Usual Manifestations

As a rule, the symptoms are quite severe. At times, however, the usual signs of esophageal rupture are not present and the symptoms may be mild.

Differential Diagnosis

The differential diagnosis includes any severe life-threatening event that can cause severe chest or upper abdominal pain, such as myocardial infarction, pneumonia or an intra-abdominal catastrophe.

Other Diagnostic Testing

The best diagnostic test is barium swallow. The contrast material may be seen flowing into the pleural space. The initial swallow may be done with gastrograffin, which is less injurious to bronchopulmonary tissues than barium. However, barium is a better contrast agent, and should be used if the gastrograffin swallow is normal.

Etiology and Basic Mechanisms Responsible for the "Pain"

Forceful vomiting can create sufficient intraesophageal pressure that the esophagus may rupture. This leads to mediastinal emphysema, subcutaneous emphysema, chemical irritation of adjacent structures which may be followed by infection, left pleural effusion, and hydropneumothorax.

Treatment

Prompt operative intervention is imperative. The mortality is high, occurring in at least one-quarter of patients even when the surgery is performed without delay. To delay surgery for a day or two increases the mortality more than two- to threefold.

References

1. Achem SR. Boerhaave's syndrome. *Dig Dis* 1999:17:256.
2. Brauer RB, Liebermann-Meffert D, Stein HJ, et al. Boerhaave's syndrome: Analysis of the literature and report of 18 new cases. *Dis Esophagus* 1997;10: 64–68.
3. Bjerke HS. Boerhaave's syndrome and barogenic injuries of the esophagus. *Chest Surg Clin NA* 1994;4:819–825.
4. Singh GS, Slovis CM. "Occult" Boerhaave's syndrome. *J Emergency Med* 1988;6: 13–16.

21

"Chest Pain" in Patients with Esophageal Stenosis

J. Patrick Waring, MD

General Consideration

Esophageal stenosis may be benign or malignant. This chapter deals with benign esophageal stenosis, which does not change greatly over a long period of time. A neoplastic cause should be considered in patients who have progressive worsening of dysphagia and weight loss.

Clinical Setting

Patients with symptoms of benign esophageal stenosis are usually adults, and can be males or females. The condition may follow the ingestion of caustic material in children. Occasionally, a patient with dysphagia related to an esophageal stricture may present with chest pain. However, it is usually fairly obvious that the patient has prominent dysphagia. The pain occurs at the time when *food impaction* is present. Once the food is dislodged, the pain subsides. This is different than odynophagia, which is pain during the act of swallowing. Odynophagia is usually related to an esophageal mucosal lesion, which becomes irritated when food passes by.

Charactreistics of the "Pain"

Patient's characterization of the "chest pain"

The patient notes that the "chest pain" is associated with eating. Patients describe the pain using many of the same adjectives they use to describe angina pectoris or myocardial infarction (see Chapters 29 and 30).

From: Hurst JW, Morris DC (eds): *"Chest Pain"* →. © Futura Publishing Co., Inc., Armonk, NY, 2001.

Common location of the "chest pain"

The "chest pain" is commonly located centrally as shown in Figure 21–1. The pain may be located in the sub-xiphoid region and radiate to the jaw (see Figure 21–2).

Uncommon locations of the "chest pain"

The pain may radiate straight through to the back (see Figure 21–3).

Size of the painful "area"

The size of the painful area is depicted in Figures 21–1, 21–2, and 21–3.

Duration of the "chest pain"

The "pain" is related to eating and occurs when food is stuck in the lower esophagus. Accordingly, the duration of the pain is determined by how long the food is stuck there. Therefore, the pain may last a few seconds, a few minutes, or an hour or more (esophageal impaction) until the food passes into the stomach, at which time the pain is instantly relieved. The brief episodes of pain may simulate unstable angina pectoris, while the long episodes of chest pain may simulate myocardial infarction.

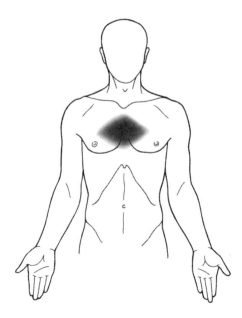

Figure 21–1. This figure illustrates the usual location of the "chest pain" caused by esophageal stenosis. The pain occurs when the lower esophagus is impacted with food.

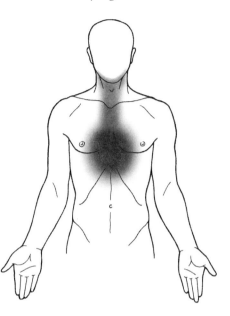

Figure 21–2. "Chest pain" due to esophageal impaction may be located in the sub-xiphoid and retrosternal area. The "pain" may radiate to the neck and jaw.

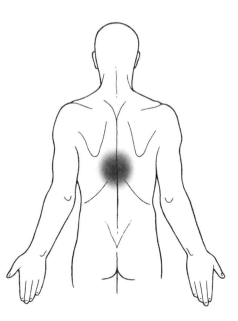

Figure 21–3. The "pain" of esophageal impaction may radiate to the back.

Tenderness of the chest wall

Occasionally there may be tenderness noted in the sub-xiphoid area of the abdomen.

Precipitating causes of the "chest pain"

The pain related to benign esophageal stenosis is produced by the failure of a bolus of food to pass from the lower esophagus into the stomach. The discomfort does not occur unless the food sticks in the esophagus for a varying length of time. The "chest pain" is not produced by effort.

Relief of the "chest pain"

The "chest pain" is relieved when the bolus of food passes from the lower esophagus into the stomach.

Associated Symptoms

When a patient presents with a history of chest pain that occurs during an episode of dysphagia, there are relatively few associated symptoms. Some patients may have a history of dysphagia or ingestion of pills known to cause esophageal stricture. If the patient presents with an esophageal impaction, then he or she appears extremely uncomfortable. Such a patient will not be able to drink water or swallow his or her own saliva.

When the symptoms of esophageal stenosis take place in a patient with known coronary atherosclerotic heart disease (especially when esophageal impaction has occurred), the physician is called upon to distinguish between myocardial infarction and esophageal impaction.

Associated Signs

The physical examination

The physical examination in patients with benign esophageal stenosis is almost always normal. Occasionally, patients may have some tenderness to palpation of the sub-xiphoid area. If other physical abnormalities are found they are unrelated to the esophageal problem.

"Routine" laboratory tests

The routine laboratory tests, including chest x-ray film and electrocardiogram, reveal no abnormalities that are related to esophageal stenosis. When the electrocardiogram is abnormal due to coronary atherosclerotic heart disease, the physician is called upon to distinguish myocardial infarction from esophageal impaction.

Exceptions to the Usual Manifestations

There are no exceptions to the symptoms and signs discussed above.

Differential Diagnosis

The finding of meal-related pain and dysphagia is characteristic of benign esophageal stenosis. As emphasized earlier, neoplastic cause for dysphagia should be considered in patients with progressively worsening dysphagia or weight loss. The symptoms of dysphagia, as occurs with benign esophageal stenosis, should be distinguished from odynophagia, which is pain while swallowing. Odynophagia is usually related to a mucosal lesion, which becomes irritated when food passes by the lesion.

Other Diagnostic Testing

Barium swallow can be helpful in patients with dysphagia. It will generally make the diagnosis of benign esophageal stricture very nicely. Upper endoscopy of the esophagus is of benefit in patients with dysphagia due to benign esophageal stenosis, because effective treatment can be offered to at the time of the procedure.

Etiology and Basic Mechanisms Responsible for the "Pain"

The cause most common of benign stenosis of the lower esophagus is gastroesophageal reflux disease. The cause of more serious esophageal stenosis is neoplasia and the ingestion of toxic material.

The symptoms of benign esophageal stenosis include dysphagia and pain. These symptoms result from the impaction of food in the lower esophagus and the subsequent increase in esophageal pressure.

Treatment

The treatment of benign esophageal stenosis is with esophageal dilation.[1] This is a safe, reliable treatment option. If the etiology of the stricture is identified, appropriate treatment may prevent a recurrence of the stricture.

References

1. Wo JM, Waring JP. Medical therapy of gastroesophageal reflux and management of esophageal strictures. *Surg Clin NA* 1997;77:1041–1062.

22

"Chest Pain" in Patients with Pill-Induced Esophagitis

J. Patrick Waring, MD

General Considerations

Americans are probably taking more pills now than ever before. Some of these pills can produce esophagitis which may cause chest pain and dysphagia.

Clinical Setting

These patients may present with dysphagia, odynophagia, or chest pain. Although any pill can theoretically lead to pill-induced esophagitis, most prominent are: non-steroidals; antibiotics such as tetracycline; alendronate; quinidine; and potassium. Often, the patient will be unaware of difficulty swallowing the pill. Patients may have been taking the medication at bedtime, which increases the likelihood of a problem.[1]

Characteristics of the "Pain"

Patient's characterization of the "chest pain"

Most patients experience odynophagia. Here, the pain is associated with swallowing. It is associated with mucosal injury to the esophageal lining as a result of direct injury caused by the pill. This should not be confused with dysphagia, which occurs when food is stuck in the esophagus. The sensation of odynophagia arises when the pain occurs as the food goes

From: Hurst JW, Morris DC (eds): *"Chest Pain"* →. © Futura Publishing Co., Inc., Armonk, NY, 2001.

past the esophageal lesion. The pain vanishes after the food is passed into the stomach.

Less commonly, patients may present with chest pain. There is no typical description of the chest pain associated with pill-induced esophagitis. Most esophageal causes for chest pain, including this one, can mimic angina perfectly, or it may be described as a dull sensation.

Common location of the "chest pain"

The "pain" is usually located centrally, as illustrated in Figure 22–1. It is often felt at the sub-xiphoid level. The "pain" may be felt in the anterior portion of the thorax and radiate to the neck and jaw (see Figure 22–2).

Uncommon locations of the "chest pain"

The pain may radiate straight through to the back (see Figure 22–3).

Size of the painful "area"

Figures 22–1, 22–2, and 22–3 illustrate the approximate size of the painful area.

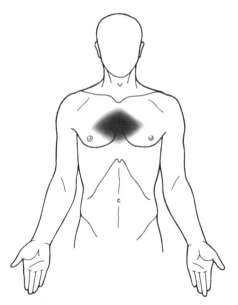

Figure 22–1. The location of "chest pain" produced by pill-induced esophagitis. The pain is worse with swallowing.

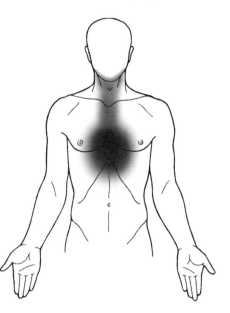

Figure 22–2. The "chest pain" of pill-induced esophagitis may be located in the sub-xiphoid and retrosternal area. The "pain" may radiate to the neck and jaw.

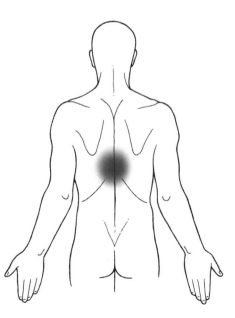

Figure 22–3. The pain of pill-induced esophagitis may radiate to the back.

Duration of the "chest pain"

The "pain" may last from minutes to hours, even days, but it is usually accentuated by swallowing. It may occur only when the patient swallows.

Tenderness of the chest wall

The sub-xiphoid area of the abdomen may be tender to palpation.

Precipitating causes of the "chest pain"

The "chest pain" is not produced by effort. There may be mild chest discomfort that is aggravated by the swallowing of food.

Relief of the "chest pain"

Neither a rapid response, nor the lack of a response to the use of antacids or sublingual nitroglycerin is a reliable indicator of the cause of the chest pain. Relief comes by discontinuing the drug if possible or altering the way it is taken.

Associated Symptoms

The major associated symptoms are dysphagia and odynophagia. The patient may or may not be aware of difficulty swallowing the pill.

Associated Signs

The physical examination

The physical examination in patients with pill-induced esophagitis is almost always normal. Occasionally, patients may have some tenderness to palpation of the sub-xiphoid area.

"Routine" laboratory tests

The routine laboratory tests, electrocardiogram, and chest x-ray film reveal no diagnostic information.

Exceptions to the Usual Manifestations

There are no exceptions to the manifestations discussed above.

Differential Diagnosis

The best clues to the diagnosis of pill-induced esophagitis are the associated symptom of odynophagia, and the patient's history of taking medications that can injure the esophagus.

Other Diagnostic Testing

Endoscopy is particularly helpful in patients who have odynophagia because the symptom is suggestive of esophageal mucosal injury. Barium swallow is of limited benefit in patients with odynophagia.

Etiology and Basic Mechanisms Responsible for the "Pain"

The mucosal erosion and esophagitis is caused by the direct action of the pill on the esophageal mucosa.

Treatment

The treatment of pill-induced lesions of the esophagus is to discontinue or change the drug if possible. Generally, esophageal lesions will heal within 4 to 7 days. If the drug cannot be safely discontinued, the patient should alter the manner in which he or she takes the drug. The pills should not be taken shortly before lying down, and the patient should drink a full glass of water to be certain the pill has moved from the esophagus into the stomach.

References

1. Kikendall JW. Pill esophagitis. *J Clin Gastroenterol* 1999;28:298–305.

"Chest Pain" of Esophageal Origin in Patients with HIV

J. Patrick Waring, MD

General Considerations

Human Immunodeficiency Virus (HIV) infection is a common condition, and some HIV patients have chest pain due to esophageal disease. HIV infection is more commonly seen in sexually active males and less often in females. The virus can also be transmitted through contaminated needles and transfusions.

Clinical Setting

Patients with HIV infection can present with dysphagia, odynophagia, or less commonly chest pain.[1]

Characteristics of the "Pain"

Patient's characterization of the "chest pain"

The "pain" may be described as especially painful when the patient swallows.

Common location of the "chest pain"

The "pain" is usually centrally located, often in the sub-xiphoid area (see Figure 23–1).

From: Hurst JW, Morris DC (eds): *"Chest Pain"* →. © Futura Publishing Co., Inc., Armonk, NY, 2001.

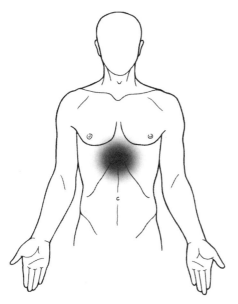

Figure 23–1. Esophageal pain in patients with HIV infection is commonly located in the epigastric area.

Uncommon locations of the "chest pain"

The "pain" may radiate throughout the anterior portion of the chest, to the jaw, and straight through to the back (see Figures 23–2 and 22–3).

Size of the painful "area"

The approximate size of the painful area is depicted in Figures 23–1, 23–2, and 23–3.

Duration of the "chest pain"

The pain may last until the infection is managed with antifungal drugs. There may be mild, steady pain that is made worse by swallowing (odynphagia).

Tenderness of the chest wall

The sub-xiphoid area may be tender to palpation.

Precipitating causes of the "chest pain"

The pain is made worse by swallowing. Pain due to esophagitis is not produced by effort and inspiration does not enhance the pain.

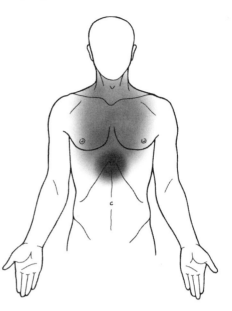

Figure 23–2. Esophageal pain in patients with HIV infection may be felt in the epigastric area, throughout the anterior portion of the chest, neck, and jaw.

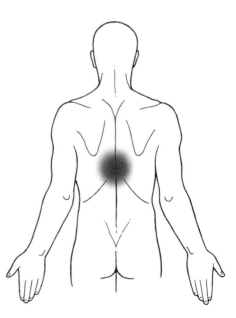

Figure 23–3. Esophageal pain in patients with HIV injection may radiate to the back.

Relief of the "chest pain"

Relief comes when the infection, which is usually due to Candida, is treated with antifungal drugs.

Associated Symptoms

The patient may have a history of symptoms that can be attributed to HIV infection or its sequelae.

Associated Signs

The physical examination

Occasionally, patients may have some tenderness to palpation of the sub-xiphoid area. There may be evidence of thrush on physical examination.

"Routine" laboratory tests

Routine laboratory tests are not helpful.

Exceptions to the Usual Manifestations

There are no exceptions to the description discussed above.

Differential Diagnosis

Patients with HIV infection should be asked about other esophageal symptoms because they can develop reflux strictures, pill-induced esophagitis, or esophageal motility disorders. It is well to remember that patients with HIV infection can have pericarditis and myocarditis that must be considered in the differential diagnosis.

Other Diagnostic Testing

Candida is the most common cause of esophageal disease in HIV patients. If empiric therapy fails to improve symptoms, an endoscopy should be done. Endoscopy is particularly valuable in patients who have odynophagia who may have esophageal mucosal injury.

Barium swallow is of limited value in patients with HIV infections, because of its poor sensitivity and specificity.

Etiology and Basic Mechanisms Responsible for the "Pain"

The cause of esophagitis in immunologically compromised patients is usually a Candida infection.

Treatment

The most efficient treatment is an empiric trail of an antifungal agent. As stated earlier, Candida is the most common cause of esophageal disease in HIV patients. If the diagnosis is made at the time of endoscopy, specific treatment for Candida infections, cytomegalic viral infections, or herpes infections can be offered. Esophageal ulcers may occur in an HIV infected patient with no evidence of infection. These patients often respond to a brief course of prednisone.

References

1. Dieterich DT, Wilcox CM. Diagnosis and treatment of esophageal diseases associated with HIV infection. Practice Parameters Committee of the American College of Gastroenterology. *Am J Gastroenterol* 1996;91:2265–2269.

24

"Chest Pain" in Patients with Peptic Ulcer Disease

Steve Goldschmid, MD

General Considerations

Peptic ulcer disease is a chronic inflammatory condition of the stomach or duodenum caused by the Helicobacter pylori, an infectious agent.

Clinical Setting

Peptic ulcer disease effects up to 10 percent of the U.S. population; however, there is no predisposition to peptic ulcer disease based on age, sex, or profession.

Characteristics of the "Pain"

Patient's characterization of the "chest pain"

Classically, the pain associated with peptic ulcer disease is described as a gnawing, burning, or aching pain. Some patients with peptic ulcer disease have no pain.

Common location of the "chest pain"

The pain associated with peptic ulcer disease is usually discreet and well localized to the epigastrium (see Figure 24–1). It is not unusual for the pain to radiate to the lower sternum.

From: Hurst JW, Morris DC (eds): *"Chest Pain"* →. © Futura Publishing Co., Inc., Armonk, NY, 2001.

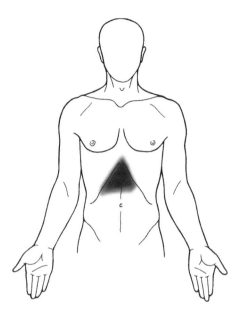

Figure 24–1. The "chest pain" due to peptic ulcer disease is located in the epigastric region. It may radiate to the lower retrosternal area.

Uncommon locations of the "chest pain"

At times, duodenal ulcers cause pain in the right upper quadrant and gastric ulcers cause pain in the left upper quadrant. It is unusual for ulcers to cause pain in the back, unless they are penetrating and associated with pancreatitis (see Figure 24–2). Pain in the upper chest can also occur, but this is very unusual and perforation should be considered if this pain is severe.

Size of the painful "area"

The size of the painful area is usually about the size of the fist.

Duration of the "chest pain"

Typically, the pain associated with peptic ulcer disease is constant, often waxing and waning in severity in relation to meals. The pain can be intermittent and infrequent, with pain-free intervals lasting for months or even years. When pain persists for months, other diagnoses should be considered.

Tenderness of the chest wall

The epigastric area may or may not be tender.

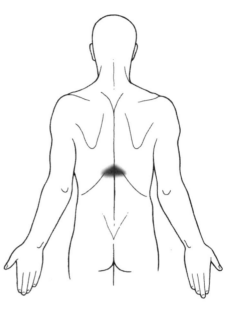

Figure 24–2. The "pain" of peptic ulcer may be located in the back if the ulcer is penetrating. Duodenal ulcers may cause pain in the right upper quadrant of the abdomen and gastric ulcers may cause pain in the left upper quadrant. On rare occasions the pain from a perforated ulcer may be located in the upper retrosternal area.

Precipitating causes of the "chest pain"

Two patterns of pain have been described that seem to relate to the location of the ulcer. Patients with duodenal ulcer often complain of pain when the stomach is empty, and they frequently have a constant feeling described as "hunger pains." This pain tends to occur before meals, and also very early in the morning, such as 1:00 AM or 2:00 AM, times when there is little food in the stomach to buffer acid and acid production is high.

Patients with gastric ulcers, in contrast, often complain of pain associated with meals. Either pattern can be seen in gastric or duodenal ulcers, however, so symptoms do not reliably distinguish ulcer location. There are three known causes of ulcers. Over 90% of duodenal ulcers and the vast majority of gastric ulcers are caused by Helicobacter pylori (H. pylori). Aspirin and non-steroidal anti-inflammatory drugs (NSAIDs) are the cause in most of the cases that remain. A minority of ulcers are secondary to Zollinger-Ellison syndrome. Patients infected with H. pylori that use aspirin or NSAIDs are most likely to develop complications related to their ulcer. As stated earlier, some patients experience pain in the absence of food, while others report that food precipitates the pain.

Relief of the "chest pain"

In patients who report pain in the absence of food, relief is fairly rapid and consistent with the ingestion of food or antacids. Over-the-counter H_2

blockers, antacids, and medical therapy almost always bring relief to patients with peptic ulcer disease. Eradication of H. pylori will prevent the recurrence of peptic ulcer disease. Cessation of aspirin and NSAID use will produce relief where they are precipitating factors.

Associated Symptoms

Ulcers are often associated with nausea and vomiting, whether or not gastric outlet obstruction or perforation has occurred. Nausea and vomiting can occur regardless of the location of the ulcer.

If the pain is severe, radiates to the shoulder, or is generalized over the entire abdomen, perforation should be considered. Ulcer penetration of the pancreas may lead to pain and symptoms associated with pancreatitis. Severe bleeding associated with ulcers may lead to melena or hematemesis. Occult bleeding can also occur and this may lead to symptoms associated with iron deficiency anemia. Patients with peptic ulcer disease can become anorectic, and the finding of significant weight loss does not necessarily signify the presence of a malignant ulcer.

Associated Signs

Physical examination

Very few physical findings are present in routine peptic ulcer disease. Epigastric tenderness to deep palpation is often found. Signs and symptoms of anemia may be present if there has been chronic occult bleeding.

"Routine" laboratory tests

There are also very few abnormal laboratory tests in patients with peptic ulcer disease. Radiographs of the chest and electrocardiograms are normal unless perforation of the ulcer has occurred. There may be occult blood in the stool.

Exceptions to the
Usual Manifestations

Remember that many patients have no symptoms suggestive of peptic ulcer disease until complications develop. The same is true of patients that do not have intact sensory systems such as quadriplegics, patients that are sedated, and patients with altered mental status.

Differential Diagnosis

There are typically two other diagnoses that should be considered in the differential diagnosis of peptic ulcer disease. These include pancreatitis and gallbladder disease. Pancreatitis can usually be distinguished from ulcer disease by the radiation of the pain from the epigastrium straight through to the back and an elevated serum amylase or lipase. Pain related to gallstones is typically located in the right upper quadrant and culminates to a peak over 1–2 hours, plateaus, and then resolves, unless acute cholecystitis occurs.

Other Diagnostic Testing

Esophagogastroduodenoscopy (EGD) is the diagnostic test of choice when considering peptic ulcer disease as the etiology of a patient's chest pain. The ulcer can be visualized over 95% of the time, malignancy can be excluded, and a sample for H. pylori can be obtained. Although not as sensitive or specific, contrast radiographs can be used as an alternative to EGD when diagnostic EGD is thought to be too invasive or the patient cannot tolerate the procedure.

Etiology and Basic Mechanisms Responsible for the "Pain"

Peptic ulcer disease is a chronic inflammatory condition creating the usual immunologic response with disruption of the involved mucosa. The true cause of the pain is uncertain. The cause of the ulcer itself is H. pylori, aspirin, or NSAIDs; in a small minority of patients the ulcer is part of the Zollinger-Ellison syndrome.[1,2]

Treatment

Treatment of peptic ulcer disease almost always involves the eradication of H. pylori.[3–5] The most effective regimens are the use of two or three antibiotics plus a proton pump inhibitor (PPI). The PPI almost always alleviates the pain in 1 to 3 days. The most common antibiotics include clarithromycin, amoxicillin, and metronidazole. When NSAIDs are the presumed precipitator of ulcer disease, the ulcer can be treated with a PPI alone and cessation of the offending agent. There are multitudes of regimens available for the treatment of H. pylori induced ulcer disease described in the literature.

References

1. Laine L, Cominelli F, Sloane R, et al. Interaction of NSAIDs and Helicobacter pylori on gastrointestinal injury and prostaglandin production: A controlled double-blind trial. *Aliment Pharmacol Ther* 1995;9:127–135.
2. William ME, Pounder RE. Helicobacter pylori: From the benign to the malignant. *Am J Gastroenterol* 1999;94(11 Suppl):S11–16.
3. Earnest DL, Robinson M. Treatment advances in acid secretory disorders: The promise of rapid symptom relief with disease resolution. *Am J Gastroenterol* 1999;94(11 Suppl):S17–24.
4. Quereshi WA, Graham DY. Diagnosis and management of Helicobacter pylori infection. *Clin Cornerstone* 1999;1(5):18–28.
5. Peterson WL, Fendrick AM, Cave DR, et al. Helicobacter pylori-related disease: Guidelines for testing and treatment. *Arch Intern Med* 2000;160(9):1285–1291.

Part VIII

Diseases of the Gallbladder as a Cause of "Chest Pain"

Although the definition of "chest pain" → is discussed in Chapter 1, the definition is repeated here so that communication is clear.

The quotation marks around "chest" imply that different patients have different definitions of the word "chest." Here we use the word to indicate pain located above the waist. Then, too, *angina pectoris* is not always located in the pectoral region—it may be felt only in the jaw, neck, shoulder, elbow, or wrist. Therefore, the word "chest" implies that other parts of the upper body may also be involved with painful syndromes.

The quotation marks around "pain" imply that patients may assign other terms to their discomfort, such as indigestion, burning, ache, etc.

The arrow after "chest pain" implies that the physician initially may not know the cause of the symptom, so a differential diagnosis must be established that fits the available information.

25

"Chest Pain" in Patients with Biliary Colic

Steve Goldschmid, MD

General Considerations

Gallstones continue to constitute a major medical problem in the United States. In developed countries, gallstones occur in 10% to 20% of the population. Fortunately, the majority of patients remain asymptomatic.

Clinical Setting

This common condition occurs in males and females who are usually beyond the age of 40 years.[1]

Characteristics of the "Pain"

Patient's characterization of the "chest pain"

The term "biliary colic" is a misnomer. Colic suggests intermittent pain, but biliary colic is characterized by a steady, unremitting pain, rather than intermittent as suggested by the term. Typically, the pain begins gradually, and reaches a peak over 1 to 2 hours. In approximately 30% of patients, it begins suddenly. It then plateaus for several hours and subsides rather slowly. The pain is deep, often described as a visceral type of pain. Because of its severity, medical attention is frequently sought as the pain worsens.

From: Hurst JW, Morris DC (eds): *"Chest Pain"* →. © Futura Publishing Co., Inc., Armonk, NY, 2001.

Common location of the "chest pain"

Most commonly, the pain of biliary colic occurs in the right upper quadrant or epigastrium (see Figure 25–1). The "pain" radiates to the back between the shoulder blades (see Figure 25–2). It is not unusual for the pain to be felt in other locations; however, the severity tends to be less in areas other than the epigastrium and right upper quadrant.

Uncommon locations of the "chest pain"

Although rare, the pain can occur in the left upper quadrant, the lower abdomen, and the precordium.

The pain associated with biliary colic can occasionally occur anywhere in the chest or abdomen. This is usually related to the location of the gallbladder. Pain that radiates straight through to the back should lead one to suspect gallstone-induced pancreatitis.

Size of the painful "area"

The area of pain may be about the size of the fist.

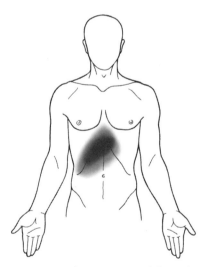

Figure 25–1. The location of the pain due to biliary colic is illustrated in this figure. The pain is almost always felt in the right upper quadrant of the abdomen and epigastrium.

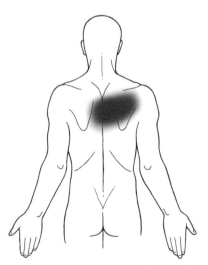

Figure 25–2. The pain of biliary colic is commonly felt in the back between the shoulder blades.

Duration of the "chest pain"

As noted previously, the pain of biliary colic lasts hours from onset to resolution. The interval between attacks is very unpredictable, and may last days, weeks, or months. However, the clinical activity of the disease tends to be constant, so that patients experiencing pain with a particular frequency tend to continue to experience pain in that same pattern. The pain rarely decreases in frequency or severity, but it can increase in severity.

Tenderness of the chest wall

The area of the gallbladder may be tender to deep palpation.

Precipitating causes of the "chest pain"

The classic case of biliary colic is right upper quadrant pain occurring after a fatty meal. In fact, biliary pain may occur in response to any meal, even the ingestion of water, or may even occur spontaneously. Although the clinical characteristics of the pain rarely change, factors that precipitate pain may be unpredictable.

Relief of the "chest pain"

The pain of biliary colic usually remits spontaneously, albeit rather slowly. Unfortunately, besides cholecystectomy, narcotic analgesics are the only agents that will relieve this discomfort. Any parenteral analgesic should be safe to use for relief of pain.

Associated Symptoms

Most patients with gallbladder colic experience nausea and vomiting. There are other associated symptoms that are often referred to as dyspepsia. In the absence of pain, these symptoms should not be associated with gallbladder colic. These symptoms include food intolerance, epigastric burning, abdominal bloating, early satiety, gas, pyrosis, nausea, and vomiting.

Associated Signs

Physical examination

Very few physical findings are present in patients with biliary colic. Right upper quadrant or epigastric tenderness to deep palpation may be present if the patient is examined before the symptoms begin to resolve.

"Routine" laboratory tests

There are no abnormal laboratory tests in patients with biliary colic. If a stone passes through the cystic duct, very mild and transient elevations of the alkaline phosphatase and bilirubin can be seen. Radiographs of the chest and electrocardiograms are normal or, if abnormalities are found, they are unrelated to the biliary colic.

Exceptions to the Usual Manifestations

On occasion, the most severe sensation of the pain may be in the chest, where it may be confused with the pain of myocardial infarction, or in the lower abdomen where it may be confused with some other cause of abdominal pains. This is likely related to the position of the gallbladder in the abdominal cavity.

Differential Diagnosis

The most common disorders in the differential diagnosis of biliary colic include peptic ulcer disease, pancreatitis, reflux esophagitis, gastroduodenitis, or myocardial infarction. At times, distinguishing between these different entities may be difficult. Endoscopy will confirm the absence of peptic ulcer disease, gastroduodenitis, or erosive esophagitis. The absence of radiation of the pain straight through to the back and normal serum amylase and lipase levels will eliminate pancreatitis. Stress testing or coronary angiography may be required to rule out cardiac ischemia as the cause of the pain.

Other Diagnostic Testing

Gallbladder ultrasonography is the test of choice when considering cholelithiasis as the cause of chest or abdominal pain. This will identify the location of the gallbladder, and gallstones can be seen in more than 95% of patients. Unless acute cholecystitis is suspected, there is no need to perform radionuclide studies such as a HIDA scan.

Etiology and Basic Mechanisms Responsible for the "Pain"

Intermittent obstruction of the gallbladder by a gallstone leads to the development of the pain referred to as biliary colic. Obstruction leads to distention, relative ischemia, and the possibility of infection within the gallbladder. An inflammatory response often follows which adds to the sensation of pain.

Treatment

Cholecystectomy is the only definitive treatment available for biliary colic.[2-5] In almost all instances, laparoscopic surgery can be performed. In patients unsuitable for open or laparoscopic surgery, lithotripsy and dissolution therapy can be attempted, but the success rate is low and the recurrence rate is high.

References

1. Caroli-Bosc FX, Deveau C, Harris A, et al. Prevalence of cholelithiasis: Results of an epidemiologic investigation in Vidauban, southeast France. General Practitioner's Group of Vidauban. *Dig Dis Sci* 1999;44(7):1322–1329.
2. Goldschmid S, Brady PG. Approaches to the management of cholelithiasis for the medical consultant. *Med Clin North Am* 1993;77(2):413–426.
3. Ahmed A, Cheung RC, Keeffe EB. Management of gallstones and their complications. *Amer Fam Physician* 2000;61(6):1673–1680.
4. Steinle EW, VanderMolen RL, Silbergleit A, et al. Impact of laparoscopic cholecystectomy on indications for surgical treatment of gallstones. *Surg Endosc* 1997;11(9):933–935.
5. Robertson GS, Wemyss-Holden SA, Maddern GJ. The best management for 'crescendo biliary colic' is urgent laparoscopic cholecystectomy. *Postgrad Med J* 1998;74(877):681–682.

26

"Chest Pain" in Patients with Acute Cholecystitis

Steve Goldschmid, MD

General Considerations

Abdominal pain, tenderness, and fever secondary to inflammation of the gallbladder wall constitute acute cholecystitis. Over 90% of patients with acute cholecystitis have gallstones, whereas the remainder develop cholecystitis in the absence of stones.

Clinical Setting

The patient with cholecystitis is usually above the age of 40. The disease occurs in males and females.[1]

Characteristics of the "Pain"

Patient's characterization of the "chest pain"

The pain of acute cholecystitis is very similar to that of biliary colic. As described in Chapter 25, biliary colic is characterized by a steady, unremitting pain rather than intermittent pain, as suggested by the term. Typically, the pain begins gradually, peaks over 1 to 2 hours, and then subsides. If acute cholecystitis ensues, the pain worsens and does not resolve. Because of its severity, medical attention is almost always sought.

From: Hurst JW, Morris DC (eds): *"Chest Pain"* →. © Futura Publishing Co., Inc., Armonk, NY, 2001.

Common location of the "chest pain"

Most commonly, the pain of acute cholecystitis occurs in the right upper quadrant. It may begin as biliary colic, producing pain as previously described. When it occurs in the chest, it usually localizes to the left lower portion of the chest (see Figure 26–1). The pain can also occur in the left upper quadrant and the lower abdomen. The pain commonly radiates around to the back and is often felt in the right shoulder (see Figure 26–2).

Uncommon locations of the "chest pain"

The pain associated with acute cholecystitis can be sensed anywhere in the chest or abdomen, but there is always pain in the region of the gallbladder since, as acute cholecystitis implies, the gallbladder wall is acutely inflamed.

Size of the painful "area"

The size of the painful area is about the size of the hand.

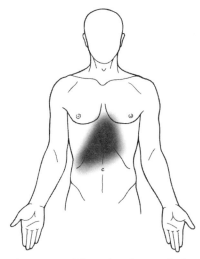 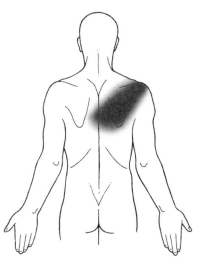

Figure 26–1. The pain of acute cholecystitis commonly occurs in the right upper quadrant of the abdomen. The pain may be felt in the left lower portion of the chest.

Figure 26–2. The pain of acute cholecystitis commonly radiates to the back and may be felt in the right shoulder.

Duration of the "chest pain"

Acute cholecystitis lasts for hours. Once the pain plateaus, it will continue to be severe until the patient receives appropriate medical attention.

Tenderness of the chest wall

The right upper quadrant of the abdomen is almost always tender in patients with acute cholecystitis.

Precipitating causes of the "chest pain"

The classic case of acute cholecystitis occurs most often in patients who have a history of biliary colic. It is not unusual for the episode to be precipitated by a meal.

Relief of the "chest pain"

Certain relief can only be obtained with urgent cholecystectomy, narcotics or less likely, non-narcotic analgesics.

Associated Symptoms

The majority of patients with acute cholecystitis experience fever, nausea and vomiting. The fever tends to be modest and the nausea and vomiting are usually not severe. Right-sided costal pain can be present and it can be pleuritic.

Associated Signs

Physical examination

The classic physical finding in acute cholecystitis is known as Murphy's sign. This is the abrupt cessation of inspiration upon palpation of the gallbladder. It is caused by the precipitation of pain when the gallbladder bed is thrust down against the palpating hand by the diaphragm. In some patients, physical findings include localized guarding or rebound, and the lower rib margin may be tender to palpation. The chest wall is usually not tender to palpation. The gallbladder may be palpable, especially if the patient has not had previous bouts of biliary colic.

"Routine" laboratory tests

Jaundice is present in approximately 20% of patients. The bilirubin may be mildly elevated with levels rarely surpassing 5 mg/dL. Mild elevations of the alkaline phosphatase and transaminases are also common. Liver tests that are more than two times normal should raise the suspicion of a common bile duct stone.

The white blood cell count is often modestly elevated in the range of 12,000 to 15,000 per cubic milliliter. The serum amylase may be slightly elevated, even in the absence of a common bile duct stone or pancreatitis. Radiographs of the chest and electrocardiograms are normal unless they are abnormal from other causes.

Exceptions to the Usual Manifestations

On occasion, the patient may have very little pain and minimal physical abnormalities. On the other hand, if the gallbladder is gangrenous or infected, fever and all the laboratory abnormalities may be exaggerated.

Differential Diagnosis

There are a variety of conditions that need to be considered in the differential diagnosis of acute cholecystitis. The principal conditions are pancreatitis, appendicitis, peptic ulcer disease, pyelonephritis, and nephrolithiasis. The most common diagnostic error occurring in the emergency room is misdiagnosis because of the misinterpretation of the laboratory abnormalities.

Other Diagnostic Testing

In about 15% of patients with suspected acute cholecystitis, gallstones can be seen on routine abdominal radiographs. Nuclear imaging studies such as the HIDA scan, are reasonably specific for acute cholecystitis.[2,3] Transcutaneous ultrasonography can also be very helpful in cases of suspected acute cholecystitis. Often, there is fluid surrounding the gallbladder, the gallbladder wall is thickened, and gallstones are visualized. If there is pain upon palpation of the gallbladder with the sonographic probe, this is another helpful sign in confirming the diagnosis. Radiologists refer to this as the sonographic Murphy's sign.

Etiology and Basic Mechanisms Responsible for the "Pain"

Over 90% of cases of patients with acute cholecystitis are due to complete obstruction of the gallbladder by a gallstone. Stasis without obstruction occurs in the remainder of cases. Stasis, ischemia, or infection leads to the inflammatory process within the gallbladder, but the true pathogenesis is unclear.

Treatment

Hospitalization for observation and treatment is necessary for acute cholecystitis. Intravenous fluids and analgesics should be given. Unless there are complications or infection, antibiotics are of no additional value. The patient should be assessed in anticipation of surgery, which should be performed early in the course if the patient's condition is suitable.[4–6]

References

1. Tyor MP. Acute Cholecystitis. In Hurst JW (ed). *Medicine for the Practicing Physician, 3rd ed.* Stoneham, MA, Butterworth-Heinemann Publishing, 1992, pp.1612–1613.
2. Simeone JF, Brink JA, Mueller PR, et al. The sonographic diagnosis of acute gangrenous cholecystitis: Importance of the Murphy sign. *Am J Roentgenol* 1989; 152(2):289–290.
3. Rall PW, Colletti PM, Halls JM, et al. Prospective evaluation of 99mTc-IDA cholescintigraphy and gray-scale ultrasound in the diagnosis of acute cholecystitis. 1982;144(2):369–371.
4. Eldar S, Eitan A, Bickel A, et al. The impact of patient delay and physician delay on the outcome of laparoscopic cholecystectomy for acute cholecystitis. *Am J Surg* 1999;178(4):303–307.
5. Wilsher PC, Sanabria JR, Gallinger S, et al. Early laparoscopic cholecystectomy for acute cholecystitis: A safe procedure. *J Gastrointest Surg* 1999;3(1):50–53
6. Eikman A, Cameron JL, Coleman M, et al. A test for patency of the cystic duct in acute cholecystitis. *Ann Intern Med* 1975:82(3):318–322.

Part IX

Pericardial Disease as a Cause for "Chest Pain"

Although the definition of "chest pain" → is discussed in Chapter 1, the definition is repeated here so that communication is clear.

The quotation marks around "chest" imply that different patients have different definitions of the word "chest." Here we use the word to indicate pain located above the waist. Then, too, *angina pectoris* is not always located in the pectoral region—it may be felt only in the jaw, neck, shoulder, elbow, or wrist. Therefore, the word "chest" implies that other parts of the upper body may also be involved with painful syndromes.

The quotation marks around "pain" imply that patients may assign other terms to their discomfort, such as indigestion, burning, ache, etc.

The arrow after "chest pain" implies that the physician initially may not know the cause of the symptom, so a differential diagnosis must be established that fits the available information.

27

"Chest Pain" in Patients with Acute Pericarditis

David H. Spodick, MD, DSc

General Considerations

Over the very large range of etiologies of acute pericarditis, pain is the most common single symptom, although it is frequently absent. For example, rheumatoid pericarditis is nearly always silent, while most acute infectious pericarditis rarely lacks some kind of pain. Pain can be due to potentiation of the algesic properties of bradykinin by pericardial prostacyclin[1] and inflammation of the pericardium, the phrenic nerves, the adjacent pleura and, probably, sympathetic nerves accompanying the coronary vessels in the epicardium.[2] Although the main coronary arteries run immediately under the visceral pericardium (epicardium), there is no evidence for coronary spasm despite the frequently striking electrocardiographic changes.

Clinical Setting

Pericarditis can occur in both sexes and at any age, but is more commonly seen in adults.

Characteristics of the "Pain"

Patients' characterization of the "chest pain"

Many varieties of pain—such as sharp, "sticking", dull, aching, and pressure-like—are described with intensities varying from 1–10 on a scale of 10, although commonly less than 5. The most characteristic pain of acute

From: Hurst JW, Morris DC (eds): *"Chest Pain"* →. © Futura Publishing Co., Inc., Armonk, NY, 2001.

pericarditis is sharp, precordial, and pleuritic. It is, as discussed under Precipitating Causes, made worse by recumbency, body movements and, especially, by inspiration. The onset is frequently perceived as sudden, particularly when it awakens patients from sleep. Once established, the pain may be worse with effort because of the greater excursion of the chest with deeper inspiratory effort. The discomfort is relieved by sitting up and leaning forward.[1] Rarely, the pain may be felt with each heartbeat, especially if the rate is slow. Some patients who have a large pericardial effusion may describe their pain as a dull, oppressive precordial sensation conjectured to arise from stretching of the pericardium. This type of pain is referred to as "protopathic."[2]

Common locations of the "chest pain"

Common locations of the "chest pain" are shown in Figure 27–1. Pain may radiate in all the distributions common to angina as well as to the epigastrium. This can create a problem in differential diagnosis when it has a pressing quality or is not pleuritic, particularly, when it radiates to the jaw or one or both shoulders. Pain in one or both trapezius ridges, usually the left, is practically pathognomonic and this history must be elicited by having the patient point to the pain zones (patients and even referring physicians usually refer to the trapezius ridges as either "shoulder" or "neck"). In some patients, pain is perceived only in a trapezius ridge.

Uncommon locations of the "chest pain"

The pain may be noted in the jaw (see Figure 27–1). This, of course, leads the physician to be concerned about myocardial infarction or angina pectoris. Other symptoms and signs are needed to determine if the jaw pain is due to myocardial ischemia, pericarditis, or esophageal disease.

The pain of pericarditis may be felt in the back (see Figure 27–2).

Size of the painful "area"

On the anterior chest, the painful area may be punctate, the size of a half-dollar or occupy practically the whole precordium.

With referral and radiation the painful zone tends to be small and vaguely delineated.

Duration of the "chest pain"

The pain associated with deep inspiration is brief. The dull pain related to distention of the pericardium from fluid may last for hours.

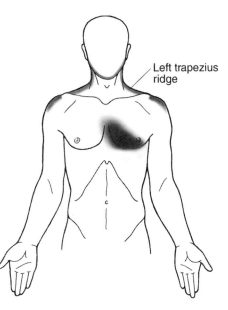

Figure 27–1. The chest pain associated with pericarditis is commonly located in the precordial area, along the left trapezius ridge, and occasionally in the shoulder and lower jaw (see text).

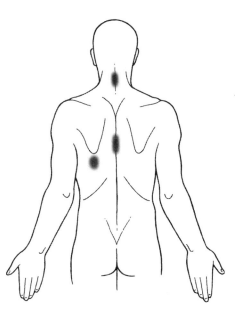

Figure 27–2. The pain associated with pericarditis may occasionally be located in the back.

The time from onset to the patient's first encounter with the physician is usually 30 minutes to a day. Because of the effectiveness of nonsteroidal antiinflammatory agents, depending on etiology, pain subsequently may last from minutes to an hour or two for most causes of acute pericarditis. Increasingly uncommon, excepting in immunocompromised patients and children, severe bacterial infection may prolong the duration of pain.

Tenderness of the chest wall

An occasional patient may have chest wall tenderness; however, the majority of these have costochondritis, Tietze's syndrome, or other chest wall syndromes (including rib fractures in patients with traumatic pericarditis).

Precipitating causes of "chest pain"

The pain of acute pericarditis is frequently aggravated when the patient is asked to take a deep breath. In fact, some patients will spontaneously breathe in a shallow fashion in order to avoid the pain.

The patient's "chest pain" of acute pericarditis is often precipitated by, or aggravated by, turning the trunk from side to side, swallowing, and assuming the recumbent position.

Relief of the "chest pain"

The patient often discovers that breathing in a shallow fashion may relieve the chest pain that is caused by pericarditis. The patient often finds relief by sitting and leaning forward.

Associated Symptoms

Patients usually adopt a rapid, *shallow breathing pattern* because of the pleuritic pain and its exacerbation by body movement, cough, and particularly inspiration. Any true dyspnea in patients with pericarditis is due to other disease such as transmural myocardial infarction.[3]

A nonproductive *cough* is common, while productive cough is due to associated illness as when pericarditis spreads from lung malignancy, pneumonia, or empyema.

Hiccough is relatively rare and probably due to inflammation of the diaphragmatic pleura and the phrenic nerves.

Odynophagia, rarely the only sign of pericarditis, occurs because the esophagus is applied to the posterior parietal pericardium.

Odynophagia and *dysphagia* also result from pericardial inflammation or effusion when pericardial disease is due to the spread of esophageal disease (inflammation, ulcer, malignancy, or trauma).

Significant arrhythmia (irrespective of whether symptomatic) may be due to anxiety since uncomplicated acute pericarditis does not cause arrhythmias. Here, if there is a large element of myocarditis (some is always present if the electrocardiogram has typical J(ST)-T abnormalities). It could qualify for an arrhythmogenic stimulus.

If the patient has a large pericardial effusion, especially with cardiac tamponade, there may be *faintness* and *dizziness,* especially on exertion; however, these also occur when there is considerable pain, tachycardia, or constitutional reaction.

Occasionally patients have *gastrointestinal symptoms* like nausea, anorexia, and even vomiting in the first few days but these are self-limited and tend to disappear with suppression of pain.

Low-grade *fever* is common and may precede the onset of chest pain. For example, pericarditis due to myocardial infarction (*epistenocardiac pericarditis*)[3] may appear mainly as a slight secondary temperature rise, whereas tuberculous pericarditis is frequently painless and may present as fever of unknown origin. Higher fevers may be accompanied by rigors (chills) especially in suppurative pericarditis.

Anxiety is common with a great deal of pain especially in patients with preexisting heart disease.

Any sustained *pallor* may be due to systemic illness like tuberculosis, uremia, or neoplasia.

In some individuals severely ill from antecedent or accompanying disease, symptoms and constitutional reaction provoked by acute pericarditis may be submerged in the total picture or suppressed by treatment already in progress.

Associated Signs

Physical examination

Physical examination may be unrevealing, however, the classic and quasi-diagnostic finding is the *pericardial rub*[4]—three or fewer friction sounds per cardiac cycle. The cardinal sign of pericarditis, rubs may be transient or intermittent; acute rubs can last from hours to 2 or more days (chronic rubs are usually permanent).[4] They tend to fluctuate so that their discovery may be due to a fortuitous timing of auscultation. Rubs may either be eliminated by or persist with even large pericardial effusions.

"Routine" laboratory tests

Unless there is pericardial effusion, a chest x-ray will show nothing alarming about the heart although adjacent disease in the mediastinum and lung may be demonstrable. *Electrocardiographic abnormalities*[5] occur in the majority of patients although atypical or absent in 40%–50% of mixed etiology.[6] Classic, quasi-diagnostic findings include Stage I: nearly ubiquitous J-point (ST-segment) elevation in most leads (depression always in aVR and usually in V1), usually accompanied by PR segment depressions which are approximately as widespread.[5] Stage I is quasi-diagnostic as is a typical evolution to Stage II—return to baseline of all J points; in Stage II T-waves invert where J points had been elevated; Stage III is inversion of all previously upright T waves; Stage IV is "resurrection" of the T-waves to their normal appearance. In modern times this sequence, except in some patients with suppurative pericarditis, is nearly always aborted by effective anti-inflammatory medications. The electrocardiographic abnormalities produced by pericarditis are compared with those of acute myocardial ischemia in Table 27–1.

Echocardiograms will demonstrate any fluid in "clinically dry" pericarditis but may also show fibrin either as epicardial masses within an effusion or if no effusion, a ragged "sunburst" appearance to the cardiac perimeter.

Leukocytosis is the rule, the dominant cell type being the result of the etiologic agent or of any primary illness accounting for pericarditis. Thus, bacterial pericarditis provokes higher neutrophil counts and tuberculous pericarditis usually a predominance of lymphocytes.

Table 27–1.

ECG: Acute Pericarditis Versus Acute Ischemia*

	Acute pericarditis	Acute ischemia (AP, MI)
J-ST	Diffuse elevation usually concave, without reciprocal depressions	Localized deviation usually convex (with reciprocals in infarct)
P-R segment Depression	Frequent	Almost never
Abnormal waves	None unless with infarction	Common with infarction ("Q wave" infarcts)
T waves	Inverted after J points return to baseline	Inverted while S-T still elevated (infarct)
Arrhythmia	None (in absence of heart disease)	Frequent
Conduction abnormalities	None (in absence of heart disease)	Frequent

*Source: Spodick DH. The Pericardium: A Comprehensive Textbook. New York, Marcel Dekker 1997. Used with permission.

Other acute phase reactants like the erythrocyte sedimentation rate (ESR) and C-reactive protein (CRP) are elevated.

Serum cardiac enzyme elevations and troponin elevations reflect the degree of myocardial[1] involvement by subepicardial myocarditis.

Exceptions to the Usual Manifestations

Any part of the syndrome, subjective or objective, may be missing and occasional patients have no detectable symptoms. Others lack electrocardiographic changes, notably with uremic pericarditis where the myocardium is not affected unless there is an intercurrent infection.[5] If there is pleuropericarditis, there will be both pleural and pericardial rubs, the independent pericardial rub being identified during suspended breathing.[4] Pericarditis of acute myocardial infarction will not have typical electrocardiographic changes unless due to an occasional "early" Dressler syndrome.

Differential Diagnosis

To recognize acute pericarditis and differentiate it from clinically and graphically similar syndromes requires realization that any pericarditis may be (1) part of a more generalized disease, (2) an apparently isolated illness or (3) part of a disorder affecting a neighboring organ like the heart or lung, and (4) occasionally the presenting syndrome of numerous disorders which only later declare themselves. Central pleuritic chest pain

Table 27–2.

Clinical Factors: Acute Pericarditis Versus Acute Ischemia*

	Acute pericarditis	*Acute ischemia (AP, MI)*
Myocardial enzymes	Normal or elevated	Elevated (infarct)
Pericardial friction	Rub (most cases)	Rub only if with Pericarditis
Abnormal S#	Absent unless preexisting	May be present
Abnormal S4	Absent unless preexisting	Nearly always present
SI	Intact	Often dull, mushy After first day
Pulmonary congestion	Absent	May be present
Murmurs	Absent unless preexisting	May be present

*Electrocardiographic differences in Table 27–4.
Source: Spodick DH. The Pericardium: A Comprehensive Textbook. New York, Marcel Dekker 1997. Used with permission.

Table 27–3.

Major Conditions That Can Simulate Pericarditis Without Effusion (Each may also occur with pericarditis).

Acute myocardial infarction
  Extension and/or reinfarction
Angina pectoris
Chest wall syndromes
Pulmonary embolism
Pneumonia and/or pleuritis
Chest pain in patients with early repolarization

Source: Spodick DH. The Pericardium: A Comprehensive Textbook. New York, Marcel Dekker 1997. Used with permission.

should always raise the question of acute pericarditis, especially if pleurisy can be ruled out, although both may occur simultaneously. Pain isolated to or referred to one or both trapezius ridges strongly compels consideration of pericarditis as long as it is not confused with shoulder or neck pain. Tables 27–1 through 27–5 capsulate the differential diagnosis.

Table 27–4.

Clinically "Dry" Acute Pericarditis: Principal Differential Diagnosis.

Manifestation	*To be differentiated*
Electrocardiogram	
Stage 1	Acute myocardial infarction
	Early repolarization
Stage 2	Ischemia/infarction
Stage 3	Ischemia/infarction/myocarditis
Pain	Myocardial ischemia
	Angina
	Infarction
	Pleuritis
	Pneumonia
	Chest wall pain
	Pulmonary embolus (usually small)
Tachypnea	Pleuropulmonary disease
	Cardiac failure
Pericardial rub	Murmurs
	Pleural rub
	Chest wall sounds
	"Conus rubs"
	Pulmonary embolism
	Acute hyperthyroidism (Means-Lerman "scratch")
	Pacemaker rub (endocardial)

Source: Spodick DH. The Pericardium: A Comprehensive Textbook. New York, Marcel Dekker 1997. Used with permission.

Table 27–5.

Ischemia/Infarction Versus Early/Late Pericarditis*[a,b]

	Pericarditis: Epistenocardiac or PMIS[b]	Ischemia: Angina or Infarction
Pain		
Usual quality	Sharp; waxes and wanes	"Pressure"; steady
Usual duration	Persistent: hours to days	Limited: minutes to hours
In trapezius ridge(s)	Yes: quasispecific	No
Respiratory variation	Pleuritic	No
Body position	Worse in recumbency	No effect
Nitroglycerin	No effect	Frequent relief
Significant pericardial Effusion	Common in PMIS and peri- cardial bleeding	Rare without heart failure
Fever	Low to moderate	Low
Cardiac signs	Pericardial rub (often faint, transient with episteno- cardiac pericarditis)	S4, S3 (heart failure)
		Mitral, tricuspid regurgita- tion
		Kussmaul's sign (RV Infarction)
Rales	Patchy when present (PMIS)	Diffuse when present
ECG	Rarely typical of pericar- ditis (Stage I) except "early" PMIS (Dressler)	Locates ischemia

[a]No findings obligatory. Symptoms and signs more intense with PMIS than epistenocardiac pericarditis. Ischemia/infarction signs often coexist with either kind of pericarditis.
[b]PMIS—post-myocardial infarction syndrome.
*Source: Spodick DH. The Pericardium: A Comprehensive Textbook. New York, Marcel Dekker 1997. Used with permission.

Other Diagnostic Testing

For acute, clinically "dry," pericarditis no special procedures are needed. For effusive pericarditis with or without cardiac tamponade, transthoracic Echo-Doppler echocardiography should suffice, but in case of confusion and particularly blood-containing effusions computed tomography (CT) or magnetic resonance imaging (MRI) may be necessary. Signs of cardiac tamponade will be found in respiratory effects on blood pressure and doppler flows, inspiratory fall in arterial blood pressure of over 10 mmHg, and increased velocity of flows in the right heart with decreased velocity in the left heart across all valves.

Etiology and Basic Mechanisms Responsible for the "Pain"[1,2]

With *trapezius ridge pain,* the mechanism is straightforward: irritation, i.e., inflammation, of one or both phrenic nerves which pass through the anterior parietal pericardium.[1] Since only the outer layer of the parietal pericardium below the sixth intercostal space is sensitive to direct noxious stimulation which produces sharp pain perceived in the nucha and trapezius ridge,[2] one can infer involvement of the phrenic nerve.

Pleuritic pain is considered to arise in the diaphragmatic or pulmonary pleura abutting the *pericardium.*

Simulation of angina may be a diagnostic problem, which may involve afferent pericoronary nerves or may arise from a superficial myocarditis, which is the origin of the electrocardiographic changes as well as diffuse or focal affection of the subepicardial fat and connective tissue within which ramify the larger coronary arteries.

Finally, with cardiac tamponade, engorgement of abdominal viscera, particularly the liver, may cause epigastric and abdominal pain.

Treatment

Treatment of all acute forms of pericarditis is aimed at relieving symptoms and eliminating etiological agents. Most patients are hospitalized, at least briefly, for complete diagnosis and observation for complications, particularly effusion and tamponade. Antiinflammatory and symptomatic treatments resemble those of other conditions producing comparable symptoms and thus are aimed at pain, fever, and malaise. Agents and dosage must be individualized commensurate with the degree of the patient's distress. Nonsteroidal antiinflammatory drugs (NSAIDs) are the main medications, possibly because many inhibit pericardial synthesis of prostaglandin I_2.[1] Any effective NSAIDs may be used (although indomethacin probably should be avoided in adults unless all else fails, since it reduces coronary flow, has deleterious effects on myocardial infarcts, has a strong side-effect profile, and has been implicated in coronary spasm). Ibuprofen has a good side-effect profile, may increase coronary flow and has the largest dose range. Cox2 inhibitors have not been used sufficiently to report, although their gastrointestinal side effects profile is excellent. Colchicine by itself or added to NSAIDs appears to be effective both for initial attacks and to prevent or treat recurrence in most patients. *Corticosteroid therapy should be avoided unless it is specific for an inciting illness like one of the connective tissue diseases or when all else fails.* If their use is unavoidable, corticosteroids should be used in minimally effective doses and slowly tapered on an individual basis. Opiates should be used only if there is severe pain at the onset of the illness. All patients should be monitored for side effects and, if they are on anticoagulants, monitored for bleeding (which can be significant, but appears to be infrequent).

References

1. Spodick DH. Physiology of the Normal Pericardium: Functions of the Pericardium. In: Spodick DH (ed). *The Pericardium: A comprehensive textbook.* New York, Marcel Dekker, 1997, pp. 15–26.
2. Spodick DH. Pain mechanisms in pericardial disease. *Bull Tufts-New England Medical Center* 1957;3:191–194.
3. Spodick DH. Epistenocardiac pericarditis: Atrial fibrillation is due to the infarct. *Euro Heart J* 1998;19:194–196.
4. Spodick DH. The pericardial rub: A prospective, multiple observer investigation of pericardial friction in 100 patients. *Am J Cardiol* 1975;35:375–362.
5. Spodick DH. Diagnostic electrocardiographic sequences in acute pericarditis: Significance of PR segment and PR vector changes. *Circulation* 1973;48:575–580.
6. Bruce MA, Spodick DH. Atypical electrocardiogram in acute pericarditis: Characteristics and prevalence. *J Electrocardiol* 1980;13:61–66.
7. Mewar SH, Shamsi SNH, Anjur-Kapali N, et al. Acute pericarditis. *Curr Treat Opt Cardio Med* 1993;1:73–77.
8. Adler Y, Finkelstein Y, Guindo J, et al. Colchicine treatment for recurrent pericarditis: A decade of experience. *Circulation* 1998;97:2183–2185.

Part X

Heart Disease as a Cause for "Chest Pain"

Although the definition of "chest pain" → is discussed in Chapter 1, the definition is repeated here so that communication is clear.

The quotation marks around "chest" imply that different patients have different definitions of the word "chest." Here we use the word to indicate pain located above the waist. Then, too, *angina pectoris* is not always located in the pectoral region—it may be felt only in the jaw, neck, shoulder, elbow, or wrist. Therefore, the word "chest" implies that other parts of the upper body may also be involved with painful syndromes.

The quotation marks around "pain" imply that patients may assign other terms to their discomfort, such as indigestion, burning, ache, etc.

The arrow after "chest pain" implies that the physician initially may not know the cause of the symptom, so a differential diagnosis must be established that fits the available information.

28

"Chest Pain" in Patients with Cardiac Arrhythmias

Paul F. Walter, MD and J. Willis Hurst, MD

General Considerations[1-3]

Cardiac arrhythmias are common. They may be associated with heart disease or may occur when there is no other evidence of heart disease. They may cause symptoms or they may not. They may be serious or benign.

Clinical Setting

Cardiac arrhythmias do not respect age or sex. They occur in subjects of all ages from youth to the elderly.

Characteristics of the "Pain"

Patient's characterization of the "chest pain"

Symptoms produced by cardiac arrhythmias vary with the nature of the arrhythmia. The sensations from premature beats differ from those generated by a tachyarrhythmia. Symptoms produced by premature beats from the atria or ventricles are similar and will be discussed as one subject. It should be emphasized that most patients with premature beats are unaware of their presence.

The sequence of a premature beat, a long pause and a subsequent strong contraction, produces an irregularity which may evoke a distressing heart consciousness or palpitation. Some patients feel the premature

From: Hurst JW, Morris DC (eds): *"Chest Pain"* →. © Futura Publishing Co., Inc., Armonk, NY, 2001.

beat as well as the stronger beat, which follows the pause that occurs after the early beat. The palpitation may be described as fluttering, thumping, skipping, or a sinking feeling. These sensations are generally felt in the left anterior precordium. Occasionally, the discomfort is localized in or radiates to the neck where the patient notes a fullness, tightness, pulsation, or a wave moving to the head. An urge to cough is sometimes noted. These sensations are attributed to contraction of the right atrium against a closed tricuspid valve, the pause that follows the premature beat, and the vigorous contraction that terminates the pause. The normal beat that follows the premature contraction may be felt as a strong thump against the chest wall. When runs of premature beats occur, there may be a pain simulating that of angina pectoris, especially in patients with symptomatic coronary atherosclerotic heart disease. Premature beats are especially annoying when patients are at rest and apparently relaxed. In some patients, premature beats are more apparent at slower heart rates, but the absence of other distractions may make the patient more aware of premature beating.

The uncomfortable sensation caused by premature contractions are more pronounced when they occur in patients with aortic valve regurgitation.

Tachycardias that may produce symptoms include: paroxysmal supraventricular tachycardia, atrial flutter, atrial fibrillation, and ventricular tachycardia. The onset of the tachycardia is sudden and without warning. Occasionally, a rapid change in position of the head or trunk or an unexpected emotional upset seems to trigger the attack. More commonly, there is no apparent precipitating cause. Tachycardia onset may be associated with a sudden thump against the chest wall, a seeming momentary heart stoppage followed by a continuous palpitation, fluttering, or racing of the heart. There may be a precordial discomfort or smothering sensation in the chest or throat, as well as a fullness and a sense of pulsation in the neck and head. Occasionally, the chest discomfort resembles the compressing retrosternal discomfort of angina pectoris. Slower tachycardia and tachycardias of brief duration produce milder symptoms or no symptoms at all. Symptoms of the tachycardia-bradycardia syndrome are dominated by the feelings of lightheadedness and near syncope. However, the sensation of heart racing or thumping may proceed the pause which is caused by the spontaneous termination of an atrial tachyarrhythmia.

Common location of the "chest pain"

The chest discomfort is usually located in the left precordium (see Figure 28–1).

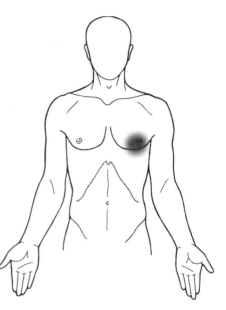

Figure 28–1. The common location of discomfort caused by premature contractions and supraventricular and ventricular tachycardia.

Uncommon locations of the "chest pain"

The discomfort may be located in the neck (see Figure 28–2). Occasionally the "pain" is characteristic of angina pectoris (see Associated Symptoms and Figures 28–3 and 28–4).

Size of the painful "area"

The size of the unpleasant pericardial sensation is shown in Figure 28–1. The size of the neck sensation is shown in Figure 28–2. The location of angina pectoris, which may be precipitated by tachyarrhythmias, is shown in Figures 28–3 and 28–4.

Duration of the "chest pain"

The duration of any arrhythmia is highly variable; it varies from seconds to hours to days. Premature beats may be felt at the precordium and neck by the patient the instant the abnormal beat occurs. The sensation produced by tachyarrhythmias usually lasts as long as the episode lasts.

Tenderness of the chest wall

There is no tenderness of the chest wall.

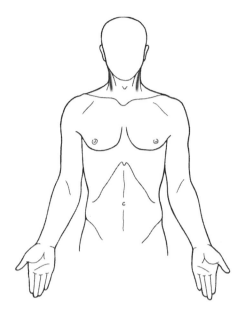

Figure 28–2. The "pain" of certain premature contractions and tachyarrhythmias may be felt in the neck. It is felt when the premature atrial contraction occurs during ventricular systole.

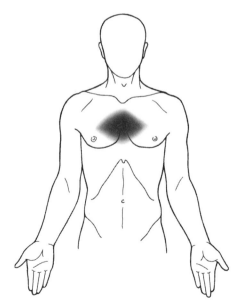

Figure 28–3. Angina pectoris may develop occasionally during tachyarrhythmias (see text). Angina occurring under these circumstances is referred to as secondary angina pectoris and may occur in patients with coronary atherosclerotic heart disease.

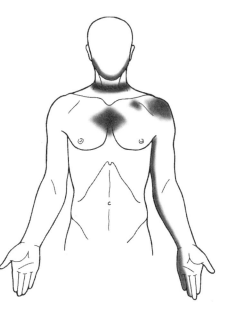

Figure 28–4. The radiation of the "chest pain" due to angina pectoris is shown in the illustration. This distribution of pain occurs occasionally during tachyarrhythmias (see text for discussion).

Precipitating causes of the "chest pain"

Cardiac arrhythmias often begin without an identifying cause. Occasionally a sudden change in body position, emotional upsetting events, excessive alcohol intake, fatigue, ingestion of caffeine-containing beverages, cigarette smoking, or exercise may serve as triggers. Various medical conditions that are conducive to the genesis of arrhythmias should be considered. These include hypokalemia, hyperchloremia, thyrotoxicosis, percarditis, and mitral valve proplapse.

Relief of the "chest pain"

The symptoms subside when the arrthymia, premature beats, or sustained tachyarrhythmia disappears.

Associated Symptoms

Any cardiac arrhythmia may generate a degree of anxiety. Premature beats appearing at bedtime delays the onset of sleep. A rapid, sustained, tachyarrhythmia produces fatigue and breathlessness, especially in patients with structural heart disease. A tachyarrhythmia may precipitate angina pectoris in patients with obstructive coronary artery disease. When this occurs the angina is labeled as *secondary unstable angina pectoris* (see Chapter 29). Polyuria often accompanies paroxysms of supraventricular tachycardia, atrial flutter, and atrial fibrillation.

Associated Signs

Physical examination

Cardiac auscultation should clarify whether premature beats are present or whether there is a sustained tachyarrhythmia. A tachycardia that is irregularly irregular strongly suggests the presence of atrial fibrillation. A venous pulsation in the neck that is coincident with the QRS complex offers a clue to the presence of typical atrioventricular node reentry. Atrioventricular dissociation occurs during certain ventricular tachycardias, and produces a variable peak systolic blood pressure, variable intensity of the first heart sound, intermittent cannon A waves in the jugular venous pulse, and intermittent gallop sounds. Reverse splitting of the second heart sounds is a clue to the presence of left bundle branch block. This may be due to ventricular tachycardia or a supraventricular tachycardia with left bundle branch block aberration. Similarly, a tachycardia with right bundle branch block QRS configuration is associated with wide splitting of the second heart sound.

"Routine" laboratory tests

The 12-lead electrocardiogram remains the most important and definitive diagnostic test. The response of a narrow QRS complex tachycardia to carotid sinus stimulation or to the administration of intravenous adenosine may help unravel the diagnosis. Carotid artery pressure, however, should not be used in elderly patients because of the possible presence of carotid artery atherosclerosis.

Exceptions to the Usual Manifestations

Many patients cannot describe the sensation they experience. They feel "something," but cannot describe it.

Differential Diagnosis

The major point concerns the patient with atrial or ventricular tachycardia who experiences anterior "chest pain" simulating angina pectoris during the episode of rapid heart action. Did myocardial ischemia precipitate the tachycardia, or did the abnormal tachycardia precipitate the angina pectoris? This question may be difficult to answer. When the electrocardiogram shows subendocardial injury *after* the tachycardia subsides, then the patient most likely has coronary atherosclerotic heart disease, but this does not answer the question as to which came first—the tachycardia or the myocardial ischemia. This difficult problem is more often raised in patients who are over the age of 40. When the patient is over 40 years of age and is being monitored with a Holter monitor he or she may be able to determine if the "chest pain" preceded the rapid heart action or followed it. Angina pectoris occurring before the tachycardia commences leads one to suspect that myocardial ischemia precipitated the tachycardia; when rapid heart action precedes development of angina pectoris one suspects that the episode of tachycardia precipitated the angina. Even when this information is available one senses the crudeness of the decision. Sustained monomorphic ventricular tachycardia associated with coronary atherosclerotic heart disease is usually due to scarring from a remote myocardial infarction. Myocardial ischemia is just one of many triggers that may initiate the ventricular tachycardia. Successful myocardial revascularization rarely eliminates this arrhythmia. On the other hand, ventricular fibrillation or ventricular flutter are frequently associated with myocardial ischemia, and restoration of coronary perfusion abolishes these malignant ventricular arrhythmias.

Other Diagnostic Testing

A Holter monitor may be required to clarify the problem in some patients. Electrophysiological studies may be indicated in some patients such as those with possible sick sinus syndrome or ventricular tachycardia.

Etiology and Basic Mechanisms Responsible for the "Pain"

Cardiac arrhythmias, perhaps more than any other condition, highlight the difference in sensitivity of individuals. Some individuals feel every ectopic beat and others do not feel ventricular tachycardia.

When the sensation is felt, it is caused by the movement of the heart itself or the abrupt distention of the neck veins.

Normally the moving heart stimulates the nerves of the adjacent structures, but because it occurs so frequently from the time of birth, the brain ignores the sensations. This is in contrast to the movement of the intestinal tract that occurs infrequently and is not always ignored by the brain. When the heart moves in a different manner than usual, the sensation is felt by the subject. The sensation is difficult to describe but, to some individuals, it is unpleasant and frightening. There is a "sinking feeling" as one feels when an elevator descends rapidly.

The discomfort in the neck occurs when the right atrium contracts against a closed tricuspid valve.

A discussion of the cause of arrhythmias is beyond the scope of the book (see references).

Treatment

The treatment of arrhythmias ranges from the reassurance offered the patient with benign rhythm problems to the use of modern drugs and electrical equipment such as the defibrillator, pacemakers, and procedures performed in the electrophysiological laboratory (see references).

References

1. Ruffy R, Roman-Smith P, Barkey JT. Palpitations: Evaluation and treatment. *Prog Cardiol* 1988;1/2:131.
2. Wood P. *Diseases of the Heart and Circulation, 2nd ed.* Philadelphia, J.B. Lippincott Company 1956:17–18.
3. Myerburg RJ, Kloosterman EM, Castellanos A. Recognition, clinical assessment, and management of arrhythmias and conduction disturbances. In: Fuster V, Alexander RW, O'Rourke RA, et al. (eds): *Hurst's The Heart, 10th ed*, New York, McGraw-Hill, 2001, pp. 797–873.

29

"Chest Pain" in Patients with Angina Pectoris

J. Willis Hurst, MD

General Considerations

Although some of the symptoms we now call angina pectoris were described by various individuals in different countries prior to the 18th century, credit for the classic description of the condition belongs to William Heberden. He first mentioned the condition and named it angina pectoris at a meeting of the Royal College of Physicians in London in 1768. The proceedings of the meeting were published in 1786 and his book, entitled *Commentaries on the History and Cure of Diseases,* was published in 1802.[1,2] Heberden did not know the etiology of the condition, but he did know it was a serious problem because some of his patients died and many others were seriously disabled.

We now know, as discussed in the section of this chapter labeled *Etiology and Basic Mechanisms Responsible for the "Pain,"* that the condition is usually caused by coronary atherosclerosis, but that there are many other less common causes of impaired oxygen delivery to the myocardium as well.

I wish to point out with great respect that those who discussed angina pectoris prior to 1968 had little collaborative information other than autopsy findings and, to some extent the electrocardiographic changes with exercise, to support their contentions. The discussion here is based on observations made during the last three decades when many helpful diagnostic methods have become available to assist in the total assessment of patients with "chest pain."

At the outset it must be realized that different patients may have different responses to similar stimuli. My former chief and teacher, Paul White, emphasized this point in the first edition of his book in 1931. He wrote:

From: Hurst JW, Morris DC (eds): *"Chest Pain"* →. © Futura Publishing Co., Inc., Armonk, NY, 2001.

249

"Symptoms are dependent on two primary factors: (1) stimulation of the sensory nerves, and (2) the sensitiveness of the nervous system. The percentage of the responsibility of each factor must be judged in every case; it is constantly varying, even in the same case at different times. . . ."[3]

His view was correct as proven by studies using devices that induce a measured amount of painful stimuli; different individuals respond differently at the same stimulus. This explains, to some degree at least, why mild "chest" discomfort in some patients may be serious and why severe "chest" discomfort in other patients may be less serious than the magnitude of the pain suggests. It is well known too, that myocardial ischemia can occur without chest "pain." This is especially common in patients with diabetes mellitus. The current belief is that patients with angina have more episodes of "painless" myocardial ischemia than they have episodes of angina. Elderly people commonly experience dyspnea as the symptom of myocardial ischemia rather than angina, and the severe coronary arteriopathy of transplanted hearts does not produce angina or pain with infarction.

Clinical Setting

It has not always been appreciated that coronary atherosclerotic heart disease is common in both sexes. Heberden reported on approximately 100 patients with the condition; there were only three females in the group.[2] This led to the view that the condition was rare in women. We now know that *one in two* males beyond the age of 40 will have angina pectoris, sudden death, or myocardial infarction during their lifetime due to coronary atherosclerotic heart disease.[4] We also know that *one in three* females beyond the age of 40 will have angina pectoris, sudden death, or myocardial infarction during their lifetime due to coronary atherosclerotic heart disease.[4] At age 70, with no prior symptoms of the disease, the lifetime risk of having angina pectoris, sudden death, or myocardial infarction due to coronary atherosclerotic heart disease is *one in three* in males and *one in four* in females.[4]

The explanation for the early misconception that the condition was a "male disease" is now explained by the fact that premenopausal women are protected against having atherosclerosis, but after menopause the condition gradually progresses in women to become almost as prevalent as it is in men. In Heberden's day, when the mean length of life was much shorter than it is today, women died of childbirth and infectious diseases before they developed coronary atherosclerotic heart disease. In addition, autopsy reports during the twentieth century on soldiers, who were all young men, swayed the profession toward believing that the condition was uncommon in women.[5,6] Now we know—angina pectoris due to coronary atherosclerosis is uncommon in women who are under 40 years of age, but is commonly observed in men who are less than 40 years of age. After age 50 angina pectoris is common in both sexes.

In industrialized countries, coronary atherosclerotic heart disease commonly occurs in patients who have a family history of the disease becoming manifest under the age of forty, who smoke tobacco, have hypertension, hyperlipidemia, diabetes, and are obese. The disease occurs less commonly in patients without these "risk factors," but it is sufficiently common to render it unwise to use the *absence* of "risk factors" to *exclude* the presence of the disease. To restate for emphasis—*despite their epidemiologic importance, the absence of risk factors must not be used to exclude the presence of coronary atherosclerotic heart disease.*

A normal aortic valve may become sclerotic by age 60 or 70 and a sclerotic aortic valve may become stenotic within one or more additional decades. The long-term follow-up of patients with aortic valve sclerosis revealed that they commonly develop coronary atherosclerotic heart disease and its complications.[7] In my opinion it seems likely that aortic valve sclerosis and stenosis are caused by certain aspects of the atherosclerotic process and mark the patient as already having coronary atherosclerosis. These conditions, as well as the signs of peripheral arterial disease due to atherosclerosis (such as a carotid bruit, an aortic aneurysm, and diminished pulsations of the arteries of the legs) may be regarded as coronary artery risk factors; but are, in fact, actually markers of existing coronary atherosclerosis that is likely to progress until the patient has angina pectoris, sudden death, or myocardial infarction.

Many individuals in all professions and all ethnic groups who eat and work like the average American are destined to have coronary atherosclerotic heart disease, and many of them will have sudden death, angina pectoris, or myocardial infarction.

Characteristics of the "Pain"

Patient's characterization of the "chest pain"[8]

Should the physician ask a patient, "Do you have chest pain?" the patient may answer, "Yes" and the physician then proceeds to ask other questions. However, this type of question is not a good one because many patients with angina pectoris do not describe it as being painful. Should this be the case, the diagnosis of angina pectoris may be missed. The physician should ask the patient, "Do you have any feeling, mild or severe, in the chest, arms, neck, or jaw that is unpleasant to you?" As the question is asked the physician should indicate the various anatomic parts just mentioned, by using his or her hand to point. The patient may respond by calling the unpleasant sensation any one of a number of common words such as indigestion, heartburn, a heavy feeling, burning, tightness, pressure, squeezing, ache, hurting, awful feeling, and strangling, but may deny the presence of "chest pain."[8] Older patients and diabetics may complain of shortness of breath with effort rather than chest pain. Less common complaints are "it feels like a weight on my chest or a tight rope around my chest."[8] Even more uncommon is for a patient to refer to the chest discomfort as *"it"* or to use strange descriptive words such as "I have a shoe box in my chest when I walk" or "I have a "wad" or "lump" in my chest" or "someone grabs my neck from behind" or "I have a toothache when I climb stairs," or a "hot flame hits my hard palate."[8] The patient's discomfort or feeling may be *severe* or it may be so *mild* that it is ignored until the patient is questioned by the physician. A patient may refer to his or her chest discomfort as a *terrible pain*, "like a car motor on my chest," whereas another patient may refer to his chest discomfort as a *"sternal whisper."*[8]

As discussed in Chapter 1, many patients, even doctors including the brilliant cardiologist, Paul Wood,[9] may self-diagnose their retrosternal "pain" that is actually due to myocardial ischemia as being due to indigestion. Emotionally stable patients often deny that they have a serious problem. On the other hand, patients who have anxiety only, are alarmed by benign "sticks" and "stabs" of pain located near the cardiac apex, and feel they undoubtedly have a serious disease.

The patient may respond to an inquiry about chest discomfort by saying nothing, but, as observed by Dr. Sam Levine, may place his or her clinched fist in the center of his or her sternum.[10]

Common location of the "chest pain"

The usual location of the chest discomfort called angina pectoris is retrosternal. The discomfort is usually located behind the mid or lower portion of the sternum often spreading upward, downward, and laterally from that area (see Figure 29–1).

It is helpful for the physician to ask the patient to "use your finger and draw a circle around the chest discomfort." When this is done the physician has a clear idea where the patient's discomfort is actually located as well as the size of the area.

The physician must also ask the patient, "Do you also feel the discomfort any place else, such as the lower jaw, neck, shoulder, inner surface of the left arm, little finger, or ring finger?" (See figure 29–2).

When the discomfort is located in the retrosternal area, or the other locations described above, it is interesting to inquire if the discomfort occurs in the little fingers, arm, neck, or jaw before it is felt in the retrosternal area or

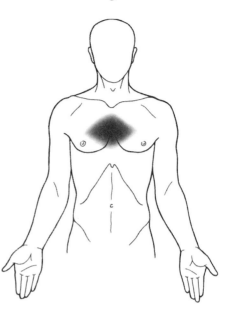

Figure 29–1. The usual location and size of the "chest pain" that is designated angina pectoris.

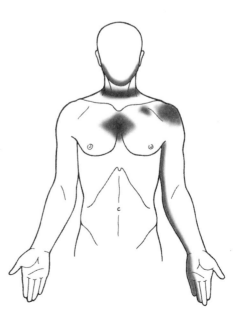

Figure 29–2. Common locations of the radiation of the "chest pain" that is designated angina pectoris. Note the radiation to the neck, jaw, left upper chest, left shoulder, inner surface of the left arm, left little finger, and left ring finger.

vice versa. Most often the discomfort begins in the retrosternal area and spreads to the neck, jaw, or arm but occasionally the discomfort is felt initially in the little finger, arms, neck or jaw before it is felt in the retrosternal area.

Uncommon locations of the "chest pain"

Whereas the discomfort of angina pectoris is usually located in the retrosternal area with or without radiation to the neck, jaw, shoulder, and inner surface of the left arm, the discomfort may, however, be felt *only* in the left precordial area, neck, lower or upper jaw, left or right shoulder, inner or outer surface of the left and right arms, epigastrium, left or right elbow, left or right wrist, and in the mid portion of the back (see Figures 29–3 and 29–4).

The most unusual patient I recall was a man who had angina in the lower jaw and teeth. He had three types of discomfort. He characterized a severe attack by placing his thumb under his mandible and pulling up "like a large hook under the jaw of a fish." He said a less severe attack was, "like catching a fish with a little hook." He said that the least severe attack was, "like pulling a needle and thread through the front lower teeth."[8]

Every physician has his or her own story of an unusual description of angina pectoris by a patient. *The discomfort is not atypical, it is simply less common than the usual retrosternal discomfort.* This is why the word atypical is avoided in this book. In fact, the more experience the physician has, the less often he or she uses the word atypical to describe chest discomfort. After all, the discomfort is typical of some condition.

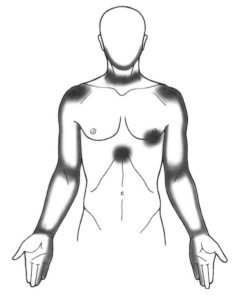

Figure 29–3. Unusual locations of the "pain" that is designated angina pectoris. The discomfort may be limited to the neck, jaw, right or left shoulder, left pectoral region, epigastrium, inner or outer surface of the right or left arms, elbows, wrists, ring, or little finger.

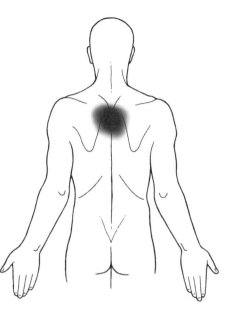

Figure 29–4. The location of the "chest pain" due to angina pectoris in the back. My estimate of the occurrence of angina pectoris in this location is about one percent.

Size of the "painful" area

As stated earlier, the physician should ask the patient with "chest" discomfort to, "use your finger and draw a circle around the area of discomfort." This important part of history taking is often overlooked and it is, in fact, one of the most useful diagnostic tools the physician has.

The area of discomfort located in the retrosternal area is about the size of a clinched fist, but may be larger. When the discomfort radiates to the neck, jaw, or shoulder, arm, elbow, wrist, finger, the size of the area is limited to the anatomic part. When the discomfort is located or radiates to the left or right arm, it is usually felt on the inner surface of the upper arm(s). Radiation of the "pain" to the left arm occurs more often than radiation to the right arm. The discomfort may be felt only in the inner aspect of the left or right arm but it is, on rare occasion, felt on the outer surface of the arms. When both arms are affected, the "pain" is usually more severe in the left arm. When the discomfort of angina is felt only in the back it is usually about the size of the open hand (see Figure 29–4).

The size of the area of "chest" discomfort of angina pectoris is never the size of a fingertip (see Figure 29–5).

Duration of the "chest pain"

The word *duration,* used in this chapter, has a dual meaning. The word is used in reference to the length of time an individual attack of angina pec-

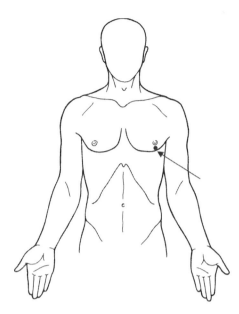

Figure 29–5. The "chest pain" located near the cardiac apex that is no larger than a fingertip is rarely due to angina pectoris.

toris lasts and is also used to designate how many hours, days, weeks or years a patient has had episodes of angina pectoris.

The duration of an episode of angina pectoris: The physician must always ask, "how long does the episode of discomfort last?" The patient usually responds, "not too long." This unsatisfactory answer should not be a surprise because patients have never heard of Lord Kelvin's admonition that science cannot be discussed without the ability to measure.[11] On the other hand, physicists and mathematicians, who know and live by the view of Kelvin, will give a similarly inadequate response to the question. Such scientists are laymen when a medical condition involves themselves. It is useful for the physician to ask a patient, as he or she squeezes the patient's hand, if the discomfort in the "chest" lasts the period of time he or she squeezes the hand. The physician should then squeeze the patient's hand for no longer than it takes to snap the fingers, again for 30 seconds, and again for a minute or longer. The physician should then ask the patient "which of the three squeezes matched the duration of the discomfort you feel in your "chest" or "elsewhere." Even this may not reveal the truth and it is bewildering that some patients cannot state precisely how long the discomfort lasts. It is useful to ask the patient if the "pain" feels like a brief "stick or stab"? Ask, "does the discomfort last about the time it takes to snap one's fingers?" This is important to know because "sticks" and "stabs" or sticks like "needles and pins" lasting no longer than it takes to snap the fingers are never angina pectoris.

The discomfort of angina pectoris that is precipitated by effort usually waxes gradually to its peak and then begins to wane promptly after the precipitating effort is discontinued. Heberden reported that, "the moment they stand still, all this uneasiness vanishes."[2] Paul White wrote that the . . . "attack may last only a few seconds to a half hour but, as a rule, it continues for about two to three minutes. . . ."[12] Paul Wood wrote that the attack lasts ". . . two to three minutes; occasionally five to ten minutes. . . ."[13] Angina pectoris precipitated by emotional reactions, such as anger, may occasionally last 10–20 minutes because it is more difficult for patients to dispel their emotional anguish than it is to discontinue exercise.

Nascent trainees and physicians have commonly labeled chest discomfort that is characteristic of myocardial ischemia that lasts 30 minutes or several hours as angina pectoris. *This is a grave error.* Chest discomfort lasting 30 minutes to several hours is either not due to myocardial ischemia, or is caused by myocardial infarction, or prolonged myocardial ischemia without electrocardiographic or cardiac enzyme changes of infarction.

The number of hours, days, weeks, or years the patient has had episodes of angina pectoris: The physician must never conclude that a patient has angina pectoris without specifying that it is *stable* or *unstable.* Just as the history is all-important in identifying angina pectoris in the first place, the history is also important in determining if the angina pectoris is *stable* or *unstable.* As will be discussed in the section on *Etiology and Basic Mechanisms Responsible for the "Pain,"* stable angina pectoris and unstable angina pectoris should be viewed as different subsets of the same disease because the molecular biology, pathophysiology, clinical manifestations, treatment, and prognosis of the two conditions are different. Only the difference in the clinical manifestations will be discussed in detail here.

Stable angina pectoris is defined as angina that has been present and unchanging for 60 days or more. These patients are the survivors of the unstable angina group of patients described below plus the group of patients who gradually develop atheromatous narrowing of one or more of the coronary arteries.

Unstable angina pectoris can be identified when angina pectoris has developed *during the last 60 days.* The discomfort may occur with effort, but commonly occurs de nova when the patient is at rest. Unstable angina pectoris should also be recognized in patients with a history of stable angina when the angina occurs with less effort, lasts longer than usual, or occurs at rest. Unstable angina is usually due to the abrupt rupture or a crack in an atheromatous plaque plus subsequent thrombosis and possibly coronary artery spasm. This is viewed as *primary* unstable angina pectoris. There are *secondary* causes of unstable angina pectoris such as the recent development of anemia or thyrotoxicosis in patients with obstructive coronary artery atherosclerotic lesions that have not ruptured.

Tenderness of the chest wall

The chest wall is not tender to touch during or after an episode of chest discomfort due to angina pectoris, although hypereresthesia may occasionally be present.

Precipitating causes of "chest pain" due to angina pectoris

Precipitating causes of stable angina pectoris: It is always necessary to identify the precipitating events that are responsible for the episodes of stable angina pectoris. Heberden's classic description of angina pectoris is reproduced at the end of this chapter and should be read by all students of medicine. The patient may volunteer that the chest discomfort is produced by effort such as climbing stairs, walking briskly up an incline, or rushing to catch a plane. Because the patient may have had 60 days to make observations, it is often possible for the physician to elicit many facets of the condition. For example, a patient noted no "chest" discomfort walking down a hill to his barn. In order to prevent the development of angina pectoris when he walked back, he learned to zig-zag. That is, he walked up one yard then walked sideways to the left and then stepped up another yard and walked sideways to the right until he reached his home. Such a story is virtually diagnostic of angina pectoris. Some patients may notice angina pectoris when they walk after eating large meals, or walk with cold wind blowing in their faces, or walk while smoking cigarettes. Walking and talking at the same time may precipitate stable angina in some patients. It is interesting to watch an individual who is so afflicted; he or she will stop walking to talk with his associates in order to make an important point in his or her conversation or stop to look in a store window. Rarely, smoking may precipitate angina when the patient is at rest.[14] Some patients notice their angina when they assume the recumbent position, while other patients notice their angina when they perform isometric exercise using their arms to raise a window. A patient may have an attack of angina pectoris precipitated by a nightmare. Circadian influence is obvious in some patients who develop angina pectoris when they arise in the morning and shave or bathe. This has been referred to as "getting-started" angina. They may have no more episodes during the day even though they lead active lives. An occasional patient will develop angina while walking and have it vanish even though he or she continues to walk. This has been called "walk-through" angina or "second-wind" angina. The patient may not spontaneously relate these situations to the physician and nascent history takers may not identify these variations of angina pectoris.

As discussed in Chapter 1, Paul Wood taught us to ask if arm pain tingled. If the patient answers yes, the pain is more likely caused by a neurologic problem than by coronary disease. Wood pointed out that patients rarely volunteer such information and that it is important to learn how to ask and interpret the answer to a leading question.[15]

As Dr. Sam Levine taught, it is sometimes useful to ask the following type of leading question.[16] If a patient responds negatively to such a question the response is likely to be true. For example, Levine would ask a patient whose history was vague, "I suppose your chest discomfort is less when you walk uphill, *isn't it?*" Should the patient disagree and say that the discomfort was worse under those circumstances, Dr. Levine believed he had a "true answer" to his question.

Patients may develop angina when singing, coughing, or during sexual intercourse, and during paroxysmal tachycardia.

Patients with stable angina may experience episodes secondary to an *emotional stimulus*. When angina is precipitated by anger or some other emotion it may last longer than it does when it is precipitated by effort. It is simply easier to discontinue effort than it is to abruptly decrease the catecholamine rush associated with emotional stimuli. Even so, the discomfort rarely lasts longer than 20 minutes.

The startle reaction must be recognized. A hunter may walk for hours and experience no angina, but may develop angina pectoris when he hears the rush and rustle of a frightened covey of birds or watches a frightened deer rushing to escape. Surely we can expect an article to appear soon that correlates road rage with the precipitation of angina pectoris and sudden death.

The startle reaction is usually obvious. But there are more subtle emotional stimuli that may precipitate angina pectoris (see description of John Hunter's angina reproduced at the end of the chapter). The grief of a man who has lost his wife may precipitate angina or even sudden death. The individual who holds a winning hand in the game of poker may have angina. On the other hand, a different poker player may have angina when he has a losing hand of cards. The individual who watches his or her favorite wrestler loose a rigged wrestling match may develop angina while another individual has angina pectoris watching his or her hero win a fake contest. Even more interesting is to discover that some patients develop angina while reading a passage in a book that strikes an emotional chord in their psychological makeup. John Hunter developed angina by the mere act of intense concentration (see the description of John Hunter's angina at the end of this chapter.) An ill Santa Claus may develop angina pectoris at Christmas when he views the television screen, and disagrees with the way his replacement "treats" children.[8] The point is, physicians must not use their own expected psychological response to situations to determine if various actions or statements are emotionally disturbing to a patient. Emotional responses are individualized reactions and an outsider should not make a judgment about them based on their own possible reactions.

The Canadian Cardiovascular Society classification should be used to classify stable angina pectoris (see Table 29–1).[17]

The television show Sanford and Son displayed the splendid talent of the actor Redd Fox who, in the show, had angina pectoris. When he did not get his way in a discussion he could easily fake his angina. This act weakened his sympathizing opponent and Fox won his point. This example is given to demonstrate that there are occasional patients who "use their angina" to live more happily; they often test the competence of their doctor and the patience of the family members.

Precipitating causes of unstable angina pectoris: Angina pectoris occurring for the first time, by definition, is labeled *unstable*. The first episode may appear *de novo*. Many times the chest discomfort has occurred

---

Table 29–1.
The Canadian Cardiovascular Society's Classification of Angina Pectoris.*

1. Ordinary physical activity does not cause . . . angina, such as walking and climbing stairs. Angina with strenuous or rapid or prolonged exertion at work or recreation.
2. Slight limitations of ordinary activity. Walking or climbing stairs rapidly, walking uphill, walking or stair climbing after meals, or in cold, or in wind, or under emotional stress, or only during the few hours after awakening. Walking more than two blocks on the level and climbing more than one flight of ordinary stairs at a normal pace and in normal conditions.
3. Marked limitation of ordinary physical activity. Walking one to two blocks on the level and climbing one flight of stairs in normal conditions and at normal pace.
4. Inability to carry on any physical activity without discomfort—anginal syndrome may be present at rest.

*This classification of angina pectoris has replaced the New York Heart Association classification, which was abandoned in 1973.
Source: Campeau L. Letter to the Editor, Circulation 1976;54:522. Reproduced with permission from the American Heart Association, Inc., and the author.

several times during the days preceding the patient's seeking the advice of a physician. The patient may or may not have observed the relationship of the chest discomfort to effort. This is why unstable angina pectoris is more difficult to diagnose than stable angina pectoris. As will be discussed later, the relationship of chest discomfort to effort is the most diagnostic feature of the symptom complex. When such a relationship cannot be established the predictive value of the history becomes less.

Unlike patients with stable angina pectoris, those with unstable angina pectoris may have angina pectoris at rest and it may last for 2 to 3 minutes to as long as 20 minutes. This is unlike effort produced stable angina that lasts 2 to 3 minutes if the patient discontinues the effort. Patients who have developed angina pectoris within the preceding 60 days are said to have unstable angina pectoris. Should a patient with stable angina pectoris begin to have episodes of angina during the preceding 60 days that lasts longer than unusual, occur at rest, or are precipitated by less effort, the changing angina is classified as being unstable. Noctural angina may be precipitated by nightmares or may occur without such an obvious stimulus. As a rule, noctural attacks of angina should be classified as being part of the unstable syndrome.

Unstable angina pectoris may be, and often is, precipitated by emotional events. The important point is that the chest discomfort has not occurred previously or has occurred only a few times during the recent past.

Braunwald's classification of unstable angina pectoris is recommended (see Table 29–2).[18] Note that Braunwald appropriately points out that there is a difference in those patients who have had episodes of angina for 48 hours compared to those who have episodes of angina pectoris for several weeks.

Relief of the "chest pain"

In years past it was customary for physicians to prescribe nitroglycerin so their patients could determine if the sublingual medication relieved their chest discomfort more quickly than occurred without the medication. While this so-called "diagnostic test" is used less often today than it was formerly there are situations where such an approach may be useful. Physicians also learned that sublingual nitroglycerin would precipitate an anginal episode in an occasional patient.

Angina pectoris can be relieved by slowing the heart rate. Some years ago this led to the use of carotid sinus pressure to slow the heart rate and possibly reduce the blood pressure, and patients were taught to perform the act. Even a carotid sinus nerve stimulator was introduced for such a purpose. Obviously, because of possible undesired complications of the proce-

---

Table 29–2.

Braunwald's Classification of Unstable Angina Severity.

Class I: New-onset, severe, or accelerated angina.
Patients with angina of less than 2 months' duration, severe or occurring three or more times per day, or angina that is distinctly more frequent and precipitated by distinctly less exertion; no rest pain in the last 2 months.

Class II: Angina at rest, subacute.
Patients with one or more episodes of angina at rest during the preceding month but not within the preceding 48 h.

Class III: Angina at rest; acute.
Patients with one or more episodes at rest within the preceding 48 h.

Clinical circumstances.

Class A: Secondary unstable angina.
A clearly identified condition extrinsic to the coronary vascular bed that has intensified myocardial ischemia, e.g., anemia, infection, fever, hypotension, tachyarrhythmia, thyrotoxicosis, hypoxemia secondary to respiratory failure.

Class B: Primary unstable angina.

Class C: Postinfarction unstable angina (within 2 weeks of documented myocardial infarction).

Intensity of treatment.

1. Absence of treatment or minimal treatment.
2. Occurring in presence of standard therapy for chronic stable angina (conventional doses of oral beta blockers, nitrates, and calcium antagonists).
3. Occurring despite maximally tolerated doses of all three categories of oral therapy, including intravenous nitroglycerin.

Source: Braunwald E. Heart Disease, 5th edition. Philadelphia: W. B. Saunders Company 1997;1332. Reproduced with permission of the publisher and author.

---

dure, the technique became contraindicated. William Dock relieved his own angina by performing a Valsalva maneuver on himself but even this safer method of slowing the heart rate is rarely prescribed.[19] The elimination of secondary causes of unstable angina pectoris may relieve the angina. For example, angina precipitated by any type of tachycardia may be relieved by the control of the rhythm. The method of controlling the rhythm, of course, is determined by nature of the rhythm. Also, angina that is aggravated by low hemoglobin may be relieved by a blood transfusion and the recognition and treatment of thyrotoxicosis is, of course, mandatory.

Associated Symptoms

In addition to the "chest pain" (with or without its associated neck, jaw, shoulder, elbow, wrist, little finger, and back pain) the patient may note shortness of breath. In fact, elderly patients commonly complain of dyspnea rather than angina as the symptom associated with myocardial ischemia. Also, the patient may feel a sense of impending doom or simply dislike what is happening to him or her, although for unexplained reasons, this symptom seems to be less common today than it was decades ago. Some patients who are experiencing an episode of angina pectoris may feel as though they may faint or recognize that they are not thinking clearly. This, and other symptoms, such as syncope and new dyspnea in the absence of lung disease are often referred to as angina equivalents when there is no "chest pain."

Associated Signs

Physical examination

Those individuals who witness a patient during an episode of angina may detect circumoral pallor or a gray color to the face. The blood pressure may be elevated, normal, or lower than usual during an episode. There is frequently an increase in heart rate and a left atrial gallop sound may be heard during the episode.

The physical examination is usually entirely normal before and after an attack of angina. The patient with a history of prior myocardial infarction may have a large heart, an abnormal precordial cardiac bulge, mitral regurgitation, and atrial and ventricular gallop sounds, the murmurs of aortic valve sclerosis or aortic valve stenosis, or a carotid bruit. There may be signs of peripheral arterial disease in the legs or an abdominal aneurysm. An occasional patient will exhibit xanthelasma, xanthoma, or an arcus senilis.

"Routine" laboratory tests

The electrocardiogram: The electrocardiogram made between episodes of angina pectoris is *usually normal* in patients with stable angina pectoris. An electrocardiogram made *during* an episode of angina pectoris may show S-T displacement due to subendocardial injury, but even when the tracing remains normal it does not exclude angina pectoris. When unstable angina is considered to be the diagnosis the tracing is usually normal, but may reveal the signs of myocardial infarction. This reminds the physician that the "pain" of myocardial infarction does not always last 30 minutes to several hours.

The tracing may reveal the signs of an old myocardial infarction. The following electrocardiographic abnormalities should stimulate a special type of thought process on the part of the physician. Coronary atherosclerotic heart disease does not usually produce the electrocardiographic signs of left ventricular hypertrophy just as intermittent claudication of the left calf does not make hypertrophy of the muscle of the left calf. Patients with an abnormal increase in QRS voltage who have angina pectoris may have coronary atherosclerosis *plus* systemic hypertension or aortic valve stenosis, or they may have idiopathic left ventricular hypertrophy with or without coronary atherosclerosis as a cause for the angina pectoris (see Chapter 38). Some patients with coronary atherosclerotic heart disease may occasionally exhibit low voltage of the QRS complexes when there have been multiple myocardial infarcts. However, when the QRS voltage is abnormally low it is wise to consider the possibility of dilated or restrictive cardiomyopathy, especially caused by amyloid infiltration of the myocardium as a cause for the angina pectoris (see Chapters 39 and 40).

The point is, increased or decreased QRS amplitude in the electrocardiogram should warn the physician to look carefully for conditions other than, or in addition to, coronary atherosclerosis.

The chest x-ray film: The chest x-ray film usually reveals no abnormality in patients with stable or unstable angina. Calcification of a short segment of a coronary artery is seen occasionally.

If there is radiographic evidence of an enlarged heart, it is usually caused by previous myocardial infarcts, hypertension, some type of cardiomyopathy, or valve disease.

If heart failure is present and the heart is normal size, the physician should search for evidence of recent myocardial infarction, because the heart does not become immediately larger following an infarction. Other causes for heart failure and normal heart size are rupture of a chordae tendineae of the mitral valve, or valve disease such as, mitral valve stenosis or aortic valve stenosis.

"Routine" Laboratory Tests

Routine laboratory tests are rarely directly useful in the diagnosis of angina pectoris. Occasionally, in a patient with unstable angina pectoris the physician is surprised that cardiac enzymes are elevated whereas the history revealed no episodes of prolonged "chest pain" suggesting myocardial infarction. A low hematocrit may suggest, but does not prove, that unstable angina may be due to a secondary cause in a patient with coronary atherosclerosis. An increase in the blood level of total cholesterol, low density cholesterol, and triglycerides increase the chances of coronary atherosclerosis but cannot be used to prove that the patient's "chest pain" is angina pectoris.

A high fasting blood sugar level indicating diabetes mellitus is very important. Coronary atherosclerotic heart disease is definitely more common in diabetics and diabetic cardiomyopathy is a real, but still ill-defined entity in the absence of occlusive coronary diseases. The value of the discovery is, however, quite different—patients with diabetes may not sense myocardial ischemia and the clinical syndrome of angina pectoris may not be present. Even large myocardial infarcts may not produce chest pain in diabetics.

Exceptions to the Usual Manifestations

Perhaps the most obvious exceptions to the general rules of diagnosis is that 10% to 20% of patients with episodes of "chest pain" for more than 60 days in whom the discomfort is definitely related to effort, is located in the retrosternal area, is relieved by discontinuing the effort, and lasts 1 to 3 minutes, do not have obstructive atheromatous lesions in the coronary arteries as determined by coronary arteriography. This, of course, does not eliminate other causes of myocardial ischemia such as cardiac syndrome X (see Chapter 50).

About 25% to 50% of patients who have what is thought to be unstable angina pectoris may not, on coronary arteriography, have obstructive atheromatous plaques in the coronary arteries. Some patients have coronary thrombosis without definite evidence of atherosclerosis and some patients have coronary artery spasm (see Chapters 31 and 32).

Another exception to the usual diagnostic criteria is that the discomfort called angina pectoris may not be located in the retrosternal area. Occasionally, the discomfort of angina pectoris is located near the cardiac apex rather than the retrosternal area but is unequivocally produced by effort and is definitely reproducible. Such symptoms should be considered to be angina pectoris. Earlier observers who did not have access to modern diagnostic equipment did not realize that this occurs in a small percentage of patients with angina. *It should not be called atypical—the angina is simply located in that area less often than it is located retrosternally.* The facts that 1) the discomfort is precipitated by effort and 2) has occurred often enough for the patient to recognize that it is reproducible are such powerful clues that they override the fact the discomfort is located near the cardiac apex rather than beneath the sternum which is more common. Pain in the lower jaw produced by effort is usually due to myocardial ischemia. It, too, should not be referred to as atypical pain. Angina pectoris may be felt in the back in about one percent of patients with transient myocardial ischemia, but should not be referred to as being atypical pain.

It should be emphasized that painless ischemia occurs commonly in patients with episodes of angina pectoris and, because of this, the number of episodes of myocardial ischemia is underestimated.

Finally, the symptom of dyspnea—"shortness of breath"—may be an angina equivalent. The dyspnea in such patients is due to acute left ventricular dysfunction and transient heart failure. This is commonly occurs in elderly patients who may already have diastolic dysfunction related to presbycardia, and in diabetics who may not sense the pain of myocardial ischemia but sense the dyspnea due to pulmonary congestion associated with transient left ventricular dysfunction.

Differential Diagnosis

The Predictive Value of the Symptom Complex in the Identifications of Angina Pectoris

The physician who examines the patient should, from the history alone, be able to weigh the value of the diagnostic clues he or she elicits, and determine the predictive value of the symptoms in the identification of angina pectoris. This cognitive skill is necessary and must be implemented in every patient with "chest pain."

The two aspects of the history that have the greatest diagnostic value are: the definite relationship of the "chest pain" to effort and its reproducibility by the patient. When all aspects of the history discussed above are present in patients with chest discomfort for more than 60 days, a diagnosis of stable angina pectoris can be made accurately in about 87% of men and 70% of women.[20-22] This concept is especially applicable in men who are older than 30 years and women who are beyond 45 years of age.

When the relationship of the chest discomfort to effort is not definite or its reproducibility by the patient is uncertain, but other features of the symptom complex are present, the predictive value of the history is about 50%. These limitations are common in patients with the recent onset of chest discomfort in whom unstable angina pectoris is considered to be possible. The problem here is that, on the one hand, the patient may not have unstable angina pectoris but, on the other hand, *if he or she does have unstable angina pectoris it is more serious* than stable angina or other causes of chest discomfort. Accordingly, the approach to further testing and treatment is different to that suggested for stable angina pectoris because the diagnosis is not certain.

When the components of the history include "sticks and stabs" like the sticks of "needles and pins" or chest discomfort that persists for hours or days and is located in a small spot near the cardiac apex, but is not related to effort, the likelihood that the discomfort is angina pectoris is almost nil.

When "pain" in the shoulder, elbow, or wrist is not related to effort produced by walking, climbing, or emotional stress, but is related to the movement of the part, the pain is likely to be due to disease of the part that hurts.

Gastrointestinal Disease

Gastroesophageal reflux and other esophageal conditions can produce chest discomfort that imitates the discomfort of myocardial ischemia (see Chapters 18 through 23). The discomfort is not produced by effort, but patients with unstable angina pectoris may not know if their chest discomfort is produced by effort or if it is reproducible because they have had too little time to make the observations. Also, many elderly patients with chest discomfort for more than 60 days may perform little exercise. Accordingly, they may not know if the chest discomfort is related to effort or not.

A common diagnostic trap is created should physicians forget that both angina pectoris and pain of esophageal origin occur commonly in the same patient.

As discussed in Chapters 24 through 26, the "pain" of peptic ulcer and gallstone colic, and cholecystitis may simulate the pain of myocardial ischemia.

Anxiety and Depression

The chest discomfort related to anxiety and depression are the most common causes of chest discomfort (see Chapters 45 and 46). The characteristic features of the chest discomfort are different to that described by patients with angina pectoris, but it is not always possible to obtain definite answers to carefully phrased questions. Also, because anxiety and depression are common, a patient may have both angina pectoris and anxiety or depression.

Dental Problems

Pain in the lower jaw produced by effort should be considered to be due to transient myocardial ischemia until proven otherwise. Teeth have been removed because the diagnosis of effort angina was not considered.[23]

"Pain" in Other Parts of the Upper Body

As pointed out earlier, transient myocardial ischemia may cause "pain" in many parts of the upper portion of the body. On the other hand, these same body parts can be intrinsically diseased and the pain may imitate the pain of myocardial ischemia. Accordingly, the symptoms caused by diseases of the skin, bone, nerves, pericardium, lung, gastrointestinal tract, and gall bladder that may be confused with myocardial ischemia are discussed in this book.

Other Diagnostic Testing

The history is the most important part of the examination because, even if coronary arteriography reveals objective evidence of obstructive coronary disease, the physician must be convinced that the symptoms are actually caused by what has been found. For example, the symptoms may be due to anxiety even though the coronary arteriogram reveals atheromatous lesions that cause a 50% narrowing of the diameter of one or more coronary arteries.

When the historical clues gleaned from the patient allow the physician to make a diagnosis of stable angina pectoris with almost 90% predictive value, it is not necessary to perform a stress exercise electrocardiogram, a stress echocardiogram, or a nuclear study. Such tests, when positive, will not increase the likelihood of the diagnosis sufficiently to justify the effort, and negative results do not exclude the diagnosis; such patients should usually undergo coronary arteriography.

Most patients whose differential diagnosis includes unstable angina pectoris, should undergo coronary arteriography. Electrocardiogram stress testing is generally contraindicated, and may be dangerous, in patients who *might* have unstable angina pectoris because such tests may precipitate cardiac arrhythmias, myocardial infarction, or sudden death and any other testing may delay obtaining a coronary arteriogram. If the arteriogram shows borderline obstructive lesions, a nuclear scan may then be indicated in an effort to determine if such lesions are indeed obstructive.

Stress tests are commonly performed on patients whose chest discomfort has been present for weeks and the highly diagnostic features of angina pectoris are not present while some of the less diagnostic features of angina pectoris are present.

Patients who have none of the diagnostic features of angina pectoris should not have a stress test or any additional tests. The usual patient is one who has a very small area of "sticks and stabs," or a larger area of persistent "dull ache" that has been present for days, or weeks, or months, that is located near the cardiac apex and has no relationship to effort. Should an exercise electrocardiogram be performed, hoping it will yield a negative result so the patient can be reassured, the physician must be prepared to manage the problem when a false positive response to the test is obtained. This is especially likely to occur in females under the age of 40. Should, under these circumstances, a positive response be obtained with an exercise electrocardiogram, some physicians attempt to clarify the problem by ordering a PET scan. Other physicians prefer to perform a dobutamine stress echocardiogram in such patients.

Physicians must not fall into the trap believing a normal stress test or even a normal coronary arteriogram will always be appreciated by a patient as "good news" and that the results of such testing will instantly reassure all patients. Many emotionally disturbed patients will simply believe the test results are not correct. Anxiety and depression must be attacked specifically.

Etiology and Basic Mechanisms Responsible for the "Pain"

The Etiology of Angina Pectoris

The most common cause of angina pectoris, myocardial infarction, or sudden death is coronary atherosclerotic heart disease. Less common causes include: coronary artery disease such as coronary artery spasm, coronary artery thrombosis without obstructive atheromatous lesions, cardiac syndrome X, coronary arteritis, the antiphospholipid antibody syndrome, anomalous coronary arteries, coronary ostial disease, and coronary embolism.[24] Angina pectoris may occur in patients with normal coronary arteriograms who have left ventricular hypertrophy due to hypertension or idiopathic hypertrophy, dilated or restrictive cardiomyopathy (see Chapters 42, 38, 39, and 40), and severe anemia.

Normal and Subnormal Myocardial Perfusion

Cardiac myocytes must have oxygen and other essential substances. The heart is designed so that the coronary arteries are able to transport sufficient oxygen and other essential substances to all of the cardiac myocytes when the heart is resting *and* when it is performing work. There is normally a perfect match—the amount of blood carrying oxygen and other substances matches the requirements of the ventricular and atrial myocytes.

A mismatch of the system described above occurs under three circumstances:

- First, when the coronary arteries are chronically narrowed by disease, they cannot deliver the amount of blood required for the cardiac muscle to perform the work associated with walking, climbing, or responding to an emotional stimulus such as anger. This is often referred to as an alteration in the demand portion of the supply-demand system. This type of system creates stable angina pectoris. At times the coronary obstructions occur so gradually that collateral circulation develops to partially make up for the diminished coronary artery blood flow created by the gradual narrowing of an artery. Therefore, some patients may have a totally occluded coronary artery and have no angina pectoris or infarction.

- Another mismatch occurs when an atheromatous plaque ruptures or a crack occurs on the surface of a plaque. This is more likely to occur when the roof of a plaque covers a large lipid core.[25] Low density lipoprotein (LDL) cholesterol becomes oxidized in the intima and the glutenous monocytes ingest it. This creates the soft lipid core. In addition, inflammatory cells soften the shoulders of the plaque causing it to rupture. Substances are then liberated from the plaque that initiate thrombosis and sometimes coronary artery spasm. When this happens the collateral vessels have no time to develop. This abrupt occlusion of a coronary artery alters the supply portion of the supply-demand system and leads to the unstable syndromes including unstable angina pectoris, sudden death, or infarction. Such a development causes primary unstable angina pectoris.

- The major function of the blood, lungs, and heart is to take in oxygen from the air and transport it to the cells of the body. When there is inadequate hemoglobin to transport the oxygen, then the poor quality of blood reaching the cardiac myocytes may contribute to the development of angina pectoris. This concept has practical value when assessing the cause of unstable angina pectoris. When a patient with stable angina pectoris begins to have more episodes of angina or has angina at rest, it is important to know if anemia, as from chronic blood loss, has contributed to a change in the angina. When this happens angina has been called secondary unstable angina (see Table 29–2).

    The cardiac myocytes require more oxygen than usual when the patient has thyrotoxicosis. Therefore, an increase in thyroid activity may precipitate angina pectoris or convert stable angina pectoris into unstable angina pectoris. Also, such a state may be produced by the over enthusiastic administration of thyroxin early in the therapy of myxedema. Here, again, is a secondary cause of unstable angina pectoris.

The Physiologic Events Associated with an Attack of Angina

The initial abnormality associated with myocardial ischemia is that the left ventricle, and occasionally the right ventricle, become stiff and noncompliant. This may produce a left atrial gallop sound and diastolic dysfunction. After that, left ventricular systolic dysfunction may develop producing a transient increase in left atrial pressure, pulmonary venous pressure, and even an increase in pulmonary artery pressure. The patient, especially elderly patients, who may have borderline diastolic and systolic dysfunction due to presbycardia, may develop transient dyspnea due to transient heart failure produced by transient myocardial ischemia. The electrocardiogram may, at about this time, show an S-T segment displacement due to subendocardial injury caused by the transient myocardial ischemia. "Chest pain" may, at times, be the last abnormality to appear in a patient with transient myocardial ischemia or infarction. The myocardium return to its previous non-ischemic state after the transient myocardial ischemia and "chest pain" vanishes.

The Nervous Pathway

The nervous pathway that enables an individual to sense the "pain" of myocardial ischemia is conceptually no different than the radiation pattern of other visercal pain. The autonomic nervous system from the heart is directly connected to major systems in the spinal cord and brain that enable a person to determine the actual location of the sensation of pain. The thoracic sympathetic cardiac nerves transmit impulses in their afferent fibers from the ischemic myocardium to the thoracic sympathetic ganglia and the middle and inferior cervical sympathetic afferent fibers transmit impulses from the ischemic myocardium to the cervical sympathetic ganglia. The impulses then travel in the rami communicantes into the upper four or five thoracic spinal nerves to the spinal cord where *fibers to and from the arms, neck, jaw and, most importantly, the brain are located.*

Treatment

The details of treatment are not discussed in this book on *"Chest Pain"*→. The reader is referred to reference 26 for the details of treatment.

It is sufficient to state here that: weight reduction in obese patients, a dietary and pharmacologic plan to reduce blood lipids and control diabetes; the exquisite control of hypertension; the discontinuation of smoking tobacco; the use of nitroglycerin, heparin, beta-blockers, calcium channel antagonists, coronary angioplasty, coronary bypass surgery, and properly prescribed exercise are all utilized in the management of stable and unstable angina pectoris.

Classic Descriptions

Knowledge of angina pectoris dates back over 200 years, but the classic description of angina pectoris due to effort is best revealed in William Heberden's 1802 text, a portion of which is reproduced below.

"But there is a disorder of the breast marked with strong and peculiar symptoms, considerable for the kind of danger belonging to it, and not extremely rare, which deserves to be mentioned more at length. The seat of it, and sense of strangling, and anxiety with which it is attended, may make it not improperly be called angina pectoris.

They who are afflicted with it, are seized while they are walking, (more especially if it be up hill, and soon after eating) with a painful and most disagreeable sensation in the breast, which seems as if it would extinguish life, if it were to increase or to continue; but the moment they stand still, all this uneasiness vanishes."

Source: Heberden W. Commentaries on the History and Cure of Diseases, Chapter 70. London: T. Payne, Mews-Gate, 1802.

The description of John Hunter's angina pectoris by his brother-in-law in 1796 in which he emphasizes the relationship of angina pectoris to various emotional events is reproduced below.

"Although evidently relieved from the violent attacks of spasm by the gout in his feet, yet he was far from being free from the disease, for he was still subject to the spasms, upon exercise or agitation of mind; the exercise that generally brought it on, was walking, especially on an ascent, either of stairs or rising ground, but never on going down either the one or the other; the affections of the mind that brought it on were principally anxiety or anger: it was not the cause of the anxiety, but the quantity that most affected him; the anxiety about the hiving of a swarm of bees brought it on; the anxiety lest an animal should make its escape before he could get a gun to shoot it, brought it on; even the hearing of a story in which the mind became so much engaged as to be interested in the event, although the particulars were of no consequence to him, would bring it on; anger brought on the same complaint and he could conceive it possible for that passion to be carried so far as totally to deprive him of life; but what was very extraordinary, the more tender passions of the mind did not produce it; he could relate a story which called up all the finer feelings, as compassion, admiration for the actions of gratitude in others, so as to make him shed tears, yet the spasm was not excited; it is extraordinary that he ate and slept as well as ever, and his mind was in no degree depressed; the want of exercise made him grow unusually fat.

In the autumn 1790, and in the spring and autumn 1791, he had more severe attacks than during the other periods of the year, but of not more than a few hours duration; in the beginning of October, 1792, one, at which I was present, was so violent that I thought he would have died. On October the 16th, 1793, when in his mind, and not being perfectly master of the circumstances, he withheld his sentiments, in which state of restraint he went into the next room, and turning around to Dr. Robertson, one of the physicians of the hospital, he gave a deep groan, and dropt down dead."

Source: Home E. A Treatise on the Blood, Inflammation, and Gun Shot Wounds by the Late John Hunter: To Which is Prefixed an Account of the Author's Life by His Brother-in-Law, Everard Home. Thomas Bradford, South Front Street, Philadelphia, 1796.

References

1. Heberden W. The first description of angina pectoris was made by Heberden at a meeting of the Royal College of physicians in London in 1768. His discussion, entitled *Some Account of Disorder of the Breast* was published in 1786 in their Medical Transactions (II 59).
2. Heberden W. Commentaries on the History and Cure of Diseases, Chapter 70. London: T. Payne, Mews-Gate, 1802.
3. White PD. *Heart Disease.* New York: The Macmillan Company, 1931, pp. 13.
4. Lloyd-Jones DM, Larson MG, Beiser A, et al. Lifetime risk of developing coronary heart disease. *Lancet* 1999;353:89–92.
5. Yater WM, Traum AH, Brown WG, et al. Coronary artery disease in men eighteen to thirty-nine years of age. *Am Heart J* 1948;36(4):481–526.
6. Enos WF, Beyer JC, Holmes RH. Pathogenesis of coronary disease in American soldiers killed in Korea. *JAMA* 1958;11:912–914.
7. Otto CM, Lind BK, Kitzman DW, et al. Association of aortic-valve sclerosis with cardiovascular mortality and morbidity in the elderly. *N Engl J Med* 1999;341:142–147.
8. Hurst JW, Logue RB. Angina pectoris: Words patients use and overlooked precipitating events. *Heart Disease and Stroke* 1993:2:89–91.
9. Silverman ME, Somerville W. To die in one's prime: The story of Paul Wood. *Am J Cardiol* 2000;85:75–88.
10. Levine S. Personal communication.
11. Thomson W, Lord Kelvin. Popular Lectures and Addresses, 1891–1894.
12. White PD. *Ischemic Heart Disease.* New York: The Macmillan Company, 1931, pp. 605.
13. Wood P. *Diseases of The Heart and Circulation, 2nd ed.* Philadelphia: JB Lippincott Company, 1956, pp. 711.
14. Hurst JW. Coronary spasm as viewed by Wilson and Johnston in 1941. *Am J Cardiol* 1986;57:1000–1002.
15. Wood P. *Diseases of The Heart and Circulation, 2nd ed.* Philadelphia: JB Lippincott Company, 1956, pp. 1–1005.
16. Levine S. Personal communication.
17. Campeau L. Letter to the editor. *Circulation* 1976;54:522.
18. Hurst JW, Morris DC, Alexander RW. The use of the New York Heart Association's classification of cardiovascular disease as part of the patient's complete problem list. *Clin Cardiol* 1999;22:385–390.

19. Dock W. Personal communication.
20. Douglas JS Jr, Hurst JW. Limitations of symptoms in the recognition of coronary atherosclerotic heart disease. In: Hurst JW (ed): *Update I: The Heart.* New York: McGraw-Hill 1979, pp. 3.
21. Proudfit WL, Shirey EK, Sones FM Jr. Selective cine coronary arteriography: Correlation with clinical findings in 1000 patients. *Circulation* 1966;33:901.
22. Welch CC, Proudfit WC, Sheldon WC. Coronary arteriographic findings in 1000 women under age 50. *Am J Cardiol* 1975;35:211.
23. Stribling WD, Hurst JW. Pain in the jaw due to heart disease. *J Am Dental Assoc* 1957;55:139.
24. Harrison DC, Baim DS. Nonatherosclerotic causes of coronary heart disease. In: Hurst JW (ed): *The Heart, 7th ed.* New York: McGraw-Hill 1990, pp 1130–1139.
25. Davies MJ. *Atlas of Coronary Artery Disease.* Philadelphia: Lippincott-Raven Publishers 1998.
26. Schlant RC, Alexander RW. Diagnosis and management of patients with chronic ischemic heart disease. In: Alexander RW, Schlant RC, Fuster V (eds): *Hurst's The Heart, 9th edition.* New York: McGraw-Hill 1998, pp 1275–1343.

30

"Chest Pain" in Patients with Myocardial Infarction

Douglas C. Morris, MD

General Considerations

Coronary heart disease is the leading cause of death in the United States and Western Europe. An estimated 1.5 million people in the US experience an acute myocardial infarction (MI) each year and one-third of these infarctions prove fatal.

Clinical Setting

While MIs occur most frequently in middle-aged males, it is also the leading cause of death in women. At the time of the occurrence of the infarction, women are, on the average, 5 to 8 years older than men. Women as compared to men are subject to having a worse outcome following their infarction. In the last decade, more than half of all patients experiencing an MI and approximately 80% of those patients suffering a fatal infarction were older than age 65 years. Women comprise a disproportionate majority of these elderly patients.[1]

Characteristics of the "Pain"

Patient's characterization of the "chest pain"

Most patients will describe an antecedent history of angina pectoris occurring days to weeks prior to their present pain. Patients with a prior history of angina pectoris usually describe their discomfort of infarction as

---

From: Hurst JW, Morris DC (eds): *"Chest Pain"* →. © Futura Publishing Co., Inc., Armonk, NY, 2001.

being similar in quality, but more severe (see Chapter 29). The "quality of pain" is often cited as critical in diagnosis. While the substernal 'pressure' sensation is unlikely to be of superficial origin, as discussed earlier, such descriptions as 'an elephant sitting on my chest' or the 'clenched fist sign' frequently reflect the level of patient sophistication and prior 'teaching' from other medical personnel or lay literature. Differentiation between burning and pressure, swelling and gnawing, commonly result from differing cultural backgrounds, for each of these descriptions applies to visceral pain. Once recognized as visceral, pain quality seldom provides further differentiation. . . ."[2] While the pain is characteristically quite severe, all gradations of intensity might be encountered, reflecting both different perceptions of the pain and different degrees of stoicism. The pain of an MI, as is the case with angina pectoris, is gradual in onset and the peak intensity is not reached for several minutes. While the intensity of the pain is usually steady following the initial crescendo, there is occasionally some waxing and waning in intensity.

Common location of the "chest pain"

The location of the "chest pain" is similar to that described for angina pectoris (see Chapter 29). The "pain" is usually located in the retrosternal area as shown in Figure 30–1. It often radiates to the neck, jaw, left shoulder, and inner aspect of the left arm (see Figure 30–2).

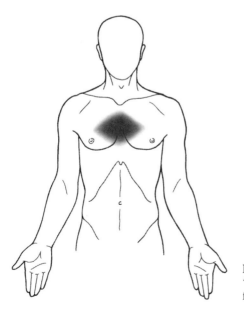

Figure 30–1. The common location of "chest pain" due to myocardial infarction.

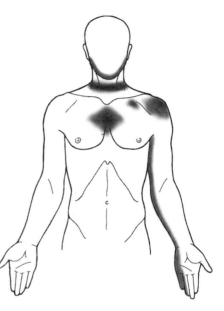

Figure 30–2. The "pain" of myocardial infarction may commonly radiate to the areas of the body shown in this illustration.

Uncommon locations of the "chest pain"

The uncommon locations of the "chest pain" are similar to that described for angina pectoris (see Chapter 29). The "pain" may be felt only in the lower jaw, left or right shoulder, inner or outer aspect of the left or right upper arm, left or right elbow, left or right wrist (see Figure 30–3). On rare occasion the pain is located in the upper portion of the back.

Size of the painful "area"

The painful area is the size of a clinched fist or larger (see Figure 30–1). When the "pain" is limited to the jaw, neck, shoulder, elbow, or wrist the size of the painful area is determined by the anatomy of the structure involved.

Duration of the "pain"

The "pain" of MI usually lasts longer than 30 minutes. After resolution of the most intense pain the patient may describe a less intense heaviness or ache that may last for 12 to 24 hours.[3] Angina pectoris produced by effort usually lasts 2 to 3 minutes after the effort is discontinued. Angina pectoris may last 10–20 minutes when it is precipitated by anger or some other emotional stimulus. It must be emphasized, however, that infarction

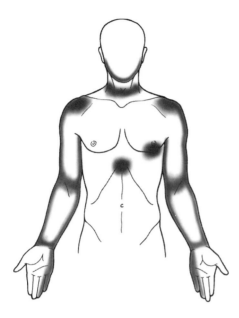

Figure 30–3. The "pain" of myocardial infarction may be limited to one or more areas shown in this illustration. For example, the pain may be located in the jaw, neck, shoulder, elbow, or wrist.

(proven by electrocardiographic changes and elevated cardiac enzymes) can follow an episode of "chest pain" that lasts no longer than the "pain" of angina pectoris.

Tenderness of the chest wall

There is no tenderness of the chest wall. The area of "pain" may occasionally be slightly hypersensitive, but steady pressure with the hand produces no exaggeration of the "pain" of infarction.

Precipitating causes of the "chest pain"

Myocardial infarction does not occur randomly throughout the day, but shows a marked circadian variation with a peak during the period from 6 AM to 12 noon.[4] While heavy physical exertion and emotionally upsetting events may serve as triggers for MIs, these factors are not so closely tied to the onset of an MI as exertion is to angina pectoris.

Relief of the "chest pain"

The patient with stable angina pectoris learns to stop his or her activities until the "pain" vanishes. Some patients who are experiencing their first MI may walk the floor in an attempt to relieve the chest pain while others with MI remain as still as possible.

The use of sublingual nitroglycerin commonly relieves angina pectoris, but fails to give satisfactory relief of the "pain" of MI. The "pain" of infarction continues as long as the ischemic process continues. Therefore, the "pain" of infarction gradually subsides as the ischemia wanes or is relieved by an injection of a narcotic such as morphine.

The "pain" of infarction compared to the "pain" of angina pectoris

If we were to refer back to Heberden's original description of angina pectoris,[5] we would note the following differences between the pain of angina pectoris and acute MI: "There is a disorder of the breast" (holds true for both disorders) . . . "they who are afflicted with it are seized while they are walking" (likely not the case with an acute infarction as the patient may be inactive or have just recently completed heavy exertion) . . . "with a painful and disagreeable sensation in the breast which seems as if it would extinguish life if it were to increase or continue" (the character of the pain is the same in the two disorders with the only possible difference being that the pain of infarction is even more painful or disagreeable) "but the moment they stand still all this uneasiness vanishes" (not the case with an acute infarction).

Associated Symptoms

The presence of associated symptoms is more commonly associated with an acute MI than with angina pectoris. Those symptoms most often associated with an acute MI include dyspnea, diaphoresis, nausea, and vomiting. Marked apprehension or restlessness is common. Inferior MIs are more often associated with gastrointestinal symptoms. The clinical presentations of an acute MI are more protean in the elderly patient. These patients may present with syncope or near-syncope, acute confusion, a stroke, appearance or worsening of heart failure, or profound weakness.

Associated Signs

Physicial examination

In reviewing the physical findings associated with an acute MI, it is important to emphasize that the findings will depend on both the size and location of the infarction and, secondly, they will vary according to the amount of time that has elapsed following the occlusion of the coronary artery.

The patient's general appearance will reflect the anxiety, sense of impending doom, pain, exhaustion, and nausea they may be experiencing. Pallor, restlessness, and diaphoresis are common sequelae.

The pulse will vary widely depending on the patient's degree of anxiety, the hemodynamic status, and the autonomic milieu. During the initial hours of an inferior infarction, the pulse rate will often be in the 50s or 60s. After the initial 12 hours, sinus tachycardia usually reflects significant left ventricular dysfunction.

The systemic arterial blood pressure will likewise show marked variation among patients with an acute MI. Mild hypotension is common in the early phase of an MI with a gradual return to normal levels over the ensuing two weeks. In patients with a larger infarction the blood pressure may never return to baseline levels. Other patients will experience an acute hypertensive reaction in the early hours of an infarction due to sympathetic overactivity.

The jugular venous pressure is usually low or normal. An elevated jugular venous pressure usually implies right ventricular infarction. In addition, an elevated "A" wave or Kussmaul's sign may be present in such patients. If atrioventricular dissociation due to high-grade heart block or ventricular tachycardia is present, "cannon" A waves may be noted.

Palpation of the precordium may reveal a "bulge" reflecting a regional wall abnormality. Frequently, there is a palpable presystolic impulse at the apex corresponding to an audible fourth heart sound.

Besides an atrial gallop, auscultation of the heart may reveal a ventricular gallop (reflecting severe left ventricular dysfunction) and a new systolic murmur at the apex. The likely explanation of a new murmur is papillary muscle dysfunction, although papillary muscle rupture or ventricular septal rupture should be considered if the murmur is accompanied by the development of heart failure. A pericardial friction rub may appear one to three days after the occurrence of the infarction.

Auscultation of the lungs should be aimed toward detecting the presence of inspiratory râles and establishing how much of the lung fields they involve. The presence of râles should be attributed to heart failure until proven otherwise.

The diagnostic *serial electrocardiographic* changes of an acute MI will vary according to the time that has elapsed since occlusion of the coronary artery, the size and location of the infarction, and the pre-existing electrocardiographic abnormalities. The hallmark of an acute MI is the development of abnormal Q waves. The Q waves develop because the infracted myocardium produces no electrical forces and, consequently, the electrical forces of the intact diametrically opposed myocardium dominate the electrical field. Actually, these abnormal Q waves appear in less than 50% of acute infarctions.[4] Furthermore, since they appear on the average of 8 to 12

hours after the onset of symptoms, they are not helpful in the initial therapeutic triage of these patients.[4] Epicardial injury creates the ST-segment elevation and the ST-segment vector points toward the region of injury. This
ST-segment elevation is generally the initial electrocardiograhic manifestation of a "Q wave" infarction. The ST-segment displacement decreases in
amplitude over the initial few days following the infarction. Persistence of
this ST-segment elevation for weeks and months after an infarction suggests a ventricular aneurysm. Following the appearance of the ST-segment
elevation is the development of a T wave vector, which is caused by epicardial ischemia and is directed away from this region of ischemia, which
surrounds the region of epicardial injury. The T wave abnormality will decrease in size and often disappear. The electrocardiographic manifestations
of a non-Q wave infarction include the T wave changes of epicardial ischemia, the T wave changes of endocardial ischemia (T wave vector directed toward the segment of ischemia, or the ST-segment changes of endocardial injury (ST vector directed away from the endocardial injury).

The *chest x-ray film* contributes little to the diagnosis of an acute MI, except to occasionally bring to the forefront another possible cause of the chest
pain such as dissection of the ascending aorta or pneumothorax. During the
course of the infarction the chest x-ray film can be helpful in diagnosing
complications of the infarction such as pulmonary edema or pleural effusion. The heart size remains normal early after MI even when there is pulmonary edema in patients who were normal prior to the infarction.

"Routine" laboratory tests

The routine laboratory tests are of no direct diagnostic value in the diagnosis of MI. Elevation of the levels of blood sugar and cholesterol are in-
directly helpful as risk factors for coronary atherosclerosis, but do not aid
in the diagnosis of infarction.

Differential Diagnosis

Myocardial infarction is customarily diagnosed on the basis of the
triad of prolonged chest pain, evolutionary electrocardiographic changes,
and characteristic plasma enzyme activity. While the absence of chest pain
(20% to 25% of patients with an acute MI will be pain-free) does not exclude an MI, this is usually the symptom that causes the patient to seek
medical attention. The differential diagnosis of prolonged chest pain is
listed in Table 30–1. Note that the etiologies of "chest pain" that should be
considered are listed in the table and the appropriate chapter numbers are

designated for easy reference. In addition to the entities listed, it is occasionally necessary to rule out *acute pancreatitis*.

The clinical features of acute pancreatitis may simulate those due to MI, aortic dissection, or rupture of an aortic aneurysm. Acute pancreatitis may be caused by viruses, drugs, neoplasia, penetrating duodenal ulcer, biliary obstruction, and for unknown or undetermined reasons.

Patients with acute pancreatitis complain of "pain" in the epigastric or periumbilical area. The "pain" commonly radiates to the back, and lower abdomen. Occasionally the "pain" may radiate superiorly and in such cases the "pain" may simulate that of MI.

The patient with acute pancreatitis may be febrile. Hypotension, tachycardia, and shock may develop as it may with MI. Nausea and vomiting may occur also as it may with MI. Tenderness of the painful area may be present. Some patients with acute pancreatitis develop râles and pleural fluid.

The white blood count is commonly elevated. The serum amylase and serum lipose are elevated. Ultrasonography may be useful in making the diagnosis. An argument surrounds the interpretation of the abnormal electrocardiogram that can be recorded occasionally in patients with acute pancreatitis. Some physicians contend that the electrocardiographic abnormalities are caused by the pancreatic enzymes on the heart while others believe the changes are due to associated myocardial ischemia.

Another distinction that should be immediately made is whether the patient has an ST-segment elevation infarction. ST-segment elevation infarctions, unlike other acute ischemic syndromes, should be considered for urgent thrombolytic therapy or mechanical reperfusion. The examining physician must distinguish the ST-segment elevation of an acute MI from: the more diffuse ST-segment elevation accompanying acute pericarditis;

Table 30–1.

Differential Diagnosis of Prolonged Chest Pain.

Acute myocardial infarction (see Chapter 30)
Aortic dissection (see Chapter 43)
Rupture of aortic aneurysm (see Chapter 44)
Pericarditis (see Chapter 27)
Anxiety disorders (see Chapter 45)
Chest wall pain (see Chapter 5)
Musculoskeletal (see Chapters 3 and 5, 7, 8, 9)
Neuropathic (see Chapters 4, 11, 12)
Pulmonary embolus (see Chapter 16)
Esophageal reflux with esophagitis (see Chapter 19)
Acute pancreatitis (see text of this chapter)
Cholecystitis and gallstones (see Chapters 25 and 26)
Mondor's syndrome (see Chapter 10)

the chronic ST-segment elevation of a ventricular aneurysm; and the ST-segment elevation of the "early repolarization" syndrome (these ST-segments maintain their normal concavity).

Abnormal Q waves mimicking those of an MI may be seen with the Wolff-Parkinson-White syndrome, with a dilated or restrictive cardiomyopathy, or with a diastolic overload of the left ventricle. The entire electrocardiographic complex of abnormal Q waves, ST-segment displacement, and T wave abnormalities may accompany myopericarditis and hypertrophic cardiomyopathy. The absence of R waves resulting in QS waves in leads V_1, V_2, and V_3 can be seen in systolic pressure overload of the left ventricle.

Other Diagnostic Testing

Serologic markers of myocardial necrosis are the third method used for the diagnosis of an acute MI. Measurement of the total creatine kinase (CK), CK-MB, and their relative index (CK-MB as a percentage of total CK) are the assays of choice for the detection of an acute MI. Skeletal muscle diseases such as rhabdomyolysis and Duchenne's muscular dystrophy may elevate the CK-MB in the absence of an acute MI. Hypothyroidism and renal failure may also falsely elevate the serum CK-MB levels. The myocardial-specific isoforms of troponin T and I are also sensitive serologic markers of an acute MI. Cardiac troponin T and I discriminate between cardiac and skeletal muscle damage in the setting of rhabdomyolysis and renal failure. Myoglobin is the serologic marker that rises the most rapidly following the onset of an infarction. Unlike the other two serologic markers, myoglobin is not cardiac specific.

Echocardiography can detect regional wall abnormalities associated with an acute MI. In the setting of ambiguous clinical and electrocardiographic findings, the echocardiogram may help to establish the diagnosis of infarction.

Perfusion imaging of *radioactively labeled substances* may help to establish the diagnosis of an MI. Uptake of the radioactive substances is dependent upon adequate regional perfusion and viable myocardium. Technetium-99m sestambi, because of its minimal redistribution, has become the radionuclide of choice to establish a perfusion defect in the early hours of an infarction.

Etiology and Basic Mechanisms
Responsible for the "Pain"

Myocardial infarction is defined as cardiac necrosis due to myocardial ischemia. The myocardial ischemia is secondary to the absence of coronary blood flow due to coronary artery occlusion. As the ischemia is sustained, the necrosis progresses from the subendocardium toward the epicardium. It takes several hours to complete the infarction of all the myocardium at risk.

Experience with patients undergoing successful reperfusion of an occluded coronary artery argues convincingly that the pain associated with an acute MI is secondary to myocardial ischemia. In such patients, the pain frequently disappears abruptly upon re-establishment of blood flow to the jeopardized myocardium. The mechanism of the pain in an acute MI is, consequently, that which was outlined for angina pectoris (Chapter 29). Furthermore, "what has previously been thought of as the 'pain of infarction' sometimes lasting for many hours, probably represents pain caused by ongoing ischemia."[6]

There are three components to myocardial ischemic pain: (1) a dull, poorly localized visceral component, (2) a much sharper somatic component with a well-defined dermatomeric distribution, and (3) an interpretative component of anguish and fear of imminent death (angor animi).[7]

Treatment

The initial management of the patient with an acute MI is the treatment of life-threatening arrhythmias, alleviation of pain and anxiety, and preservation of as much myocardium as possible. Narcotics remain the drugs of choice in the treatment of the pain and anxiety, which so often accompanies an acute MI. *Morphine* seems particularly well suited for this task as it provides adequate analgesia with little cardiac depression. Since it can produce respiratory depression and peripheral vasodilatation, morphine should be administered intravenously in doses of 2 to 4 mg every 15 to 30 minutes until the desired analgesia is obtained. Any tachyarrhythmia accompanied by hemodynamic compromise warrants immediate electrical cardioversion. Symptomatic bradyarrhythmias should be initially treated with intravenous *atropine*. The insertion of a *transvenous pacemaker* should be reserved for the bradyarrhythmias that are refractory to medical treatment.

Aspirin should be administered by mouth in all patients experiencing an acute MI unless the patient is allergic to the drug.

All patients with an ST-elevation infarction should be considered for reperfusion therapy either with *thrombolytic agents* or *angioplasty* or a combination of the two. It is imperative that this decision be made and enacted quickly in order to preserve as much myocardium as possible.

Other drugs, which seem to offer some myocardial protection, are *intravenous nitroglycerin* and *intravenous beta-blockers*. Beta-blockers also offer some benefit in reducing the frequency of arrhythmias such as ventricular ectopy and atrial fibrillation. These drugs are best avoided in patients with a systolic blood pressure level of 100 mmHg or less and beta-blockers should be avoided with a heart rate of less than 60 beats per minute.

References

1. Huggins GS, O'Hara PT. Clinical presentation and diagnostic evaluation. In Fuster V, Ross R, and Topol EJ (eds): *Atherosclerosis and Coronary Artery Disease.* Philadelphia, Lippincott-Raven Publishers, 1996, pp. 835–854.
2. Christie LG, Jr, Conti CR. Systematic approach to evaluation of angina-like chest pain: Pathophysiology and clinical testing with emphasis on objective documentation of myocardial ischemia. *Am Heart J* 1981;102:897–901.
3. Gersh BJ, Clements IP. Acute myocardial infarction: Diagnosis and prognosis. In Giuliani ER, Gersh BJ, McGoon MD, et al. (eds): *Mayo Clinic Practice of Cardiology.* St. Louis, Mosby,1996, pp. 1216–1256.
4. Alexander RW, Pratt CM, Roberts R. Diagnosis and management of patients with acute myocardial infarction. In Alexander RW, Schlant RC, and Fuster V (eds): *Hurst's The Heart, Arteries, and Veins.* McGraw-Hill, New York, 1998, pp. 1345–1433.
5. Heberden W. The first description of angina pectoris was made by Heberden at a meeting of the Royal College of physicians in London in 1768. His discussion, entitled *Some Account of Disorder of the Breast* was published in 1786 in their Medical Transactions (II 59).
6. Pasternak RC, Braunwald E, Sobel BE. Acute myocardial infarction. In Braunwald E (ed): *Heart Disease: A Textbook of Cardiovascular Medicine.* Philadelphia, W. B. Saunders Company, 1988, pp. 1222–1313.
7. Maseri A, Crea F, Kaski JC, et al. Mechanisms and significance of cardiac ischemic pain. *Prog Cardiovasc Dis* 1992;35:1–18.

31

"Chest Pain" in Patients with Prinzmetal's Angina

David Waters, MD and Rabih R. Azar, MD

General Considerations

In 1959, Prinzmetal et al. described a syndrome characterized by angina at rest with transient ST segment elevation.[1,2] With the advent of coronary arteriography a few years later, it soon became apparent that the syndrome was caused by coronary spasm, usually focal, and often at the site of a coronary stenosis.[3] The underlying coronary disease can vary from a subtotal occlusion to a very mild stenosis, and in some cases, the coronary arteries are angiographically normal.[3]

Diagnosing Prinzmetal's, or variant, angina is important because most patients with this syndrome respond very well to calcium channel blockers and very poorly to beta-blockers.[4] Myocardial infarction (MI) is a common complication within the first 3 months after diagnosis, particularly among patients with coronary diameter stenoses of greater than 50%.[5] Spontaneous remission occurs eventually in most patients with Prinzmetal's angina, leaving the residual underlying coronary atherosclerosis.[6]

Clinical Setting

Prinzmetal's angina is uncommon. Most patients are heavy cigarette smokers, but their age, sex, and risk factor profiles are otherwise similar to other coronary patients. Those with angiographically normal coronary arteries tend to be younger and more often women.

From: Hurst JW, Morris DC (eds): *"Chest Pain"* →. © Futura Publishing Co., Inc., Armonk, NY, 2001.

Characteristics of the "Pain"

Patient's characterization of the "chest pain"

In most patients with Prinzmetal's angina, the presenting symptoms are not specific enough to suggest the diagnosis. The description of the chest discomfort is similar to the description given by patients with myocardial ischemia due to other causes. Although the extent and severity of ischemia is more severe in Prinzmetal's compared to classic angina, the severity of the discomfort is usually not appreciably worse. Many or most patients describe the pain as increasing gradually in intensity and then gradually dissipating in a crescendo/decrescendo pattern. *Burning, squeezing, aching, pressure, heaviness* and *tightness* are commonly used words. Patients often seem to be groping for accurate terms to describe the symptom that they experience. As with other forms of chest pain, the description of the symptom is heavily colored by the patient's cultural background and fluency.

Common location of the "chest pain"

The usual location of the chest discomfort of Prinzmetal's angina corresponds to the usual location for other forms of angina; that is, retrosternal (see Figure 31–1). Chest pain that is described as being on or near the surface of the skin is unlikely to be caused by myocardial ischemia. The

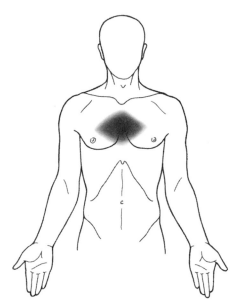

Figure 31–1. The usual location and size of the "chest pain" that is designated angina pectoris.

pattern of radiation for Prinzmetal's angina is also not different that that of classic angina. Radiation to the neck, jaw, shoulder(s), elbow(s) or inner aspects of the arm(s) are most common. If the discomfort radiates to one side, it is usually the left.

Uncommon locations of the "chest pain"

Discomfort may be limited to one or both shoulders, elbows or arms, or to the jaw, teeth, back, or epigastrium (see Figure 31–2). These atypical locations are similar to those of classic angina (see Figure 31–3). Transient ST segment elevation due to coronary spasm may occur with no symptoms at all, just as ST depression may reflect silent myocardial ischemia from other causes.

Size of the painful "area"

Most patients are not able to define precisely the size of the painful area. As with the more common type of angina, the patient might state that

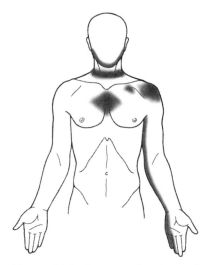

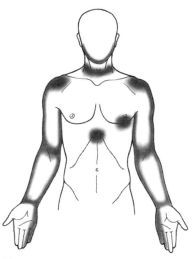

Figure 31–2. Common locations of the radiation of the "chest pain" that is designated angina pectoris. Note the radiation to the neck, jaw, left upper chest, left shoulder, inner surface of the left arm, left little finger, and left ring finger.

Figure 31–3. Unusual locations of the "pain" that is designated angina pectoris. The discomfort may be limited to the neck, jaw, right or left shoulder, left pectoral region, epigastrium, inner or outer surface of the right or left arms, elbows, wrists, little or ring finger.

the discomfort is the size of a baseball, a grapefruit or even a basketball (but almost never a golf ball).

Duration of the "chest pain"

The chest pain of Prinzmetal's angina usually lasts from 1 to 5 minutes, but may last for 10 or even 20 minutes. Most attacks exhibit a crescendo decrescendo pattern. Nitroglycerin relieves the pain promptly, as it does in classic angina.

Tenderness of the chest wall

The chest wall is almost never tender. This finding suggests a different diagnosis.

Precipitating causes of the "chest pain"

The underlying precipitating cause of the chest pain is coronary spasm, which can be initiated by a variety of physiologic and nonphysiologic mechanisms. Coronary arteries tend to be narrowest in the early morning hours. Episodes of Prinzmetal's angina are most common at this time because lesser degrees of spasm are required to produce ischemia. Many patients are awakened by attacks almost every morning, but are free from symptoms during the rest of the day. Exercise tolerance is often normal in Prinzmetal's angina; however, in approximately one-third of patients with active symptoms, exercise will precipitate an attack. Unlike classic angina, the threshold at which angina occurs is extremely variable.

Exposure to cold is a common trigger for attacks of Prinzmetal's angina. Attacks have also been reported to occur after alcohol ingestion, with ingestion of cold beverages, and with allergic reactions. Cocaine use can provoke coronary spasm, but the presenting picture is dissimilar to Prinzmetal's angina.

Relief of the "chest pain"

Nitroglycerin relieves attacks of Prinzmetal's angina as well as it relieves attacks of classic angina. Prolonged attacks of variant angina are dangerous because prolonged severe transmural myocardial ischemia can induce life-threatening ventricular arrhythmias and conduction disturbances. Sudden death is a real, potential complication of an attack of Prinzmetal's angina. Nitroglycerin should therefore be used promptly to abort an attack as early as possible.

Associated Symptoms

Raynaud's phenomenon and migraine headaches have been reported to occur in up to one-quarter of patients with Prinzmetal's angina, suggesting that a generalized vasospastic disorder may be present.[7] Esophageal and coronary spasm may coexist in the same patient. Syncope occurs in approximately one-quarter of variant angina patients during attacks, and provides a useful clue as to the diagnosis.

Associated Signs

Physical examination

The cardiovascular examination is usually entirely normal in patients with Prinzmetal's angina. During an attack, signs of left ventricular dysfunction may transiently appear, such as a ventricular gallop, a mitral regurgitation murmur, a palpable anterior dyskinetic movement, or basilar râles.

"Routine" laboratory tests

During a typical attack of Prinzmetal's angina, ST segment elevation develops in the territory of the artery undergoing spasm. Milder attacks may be associated with ST depression or pseudonormalization of a negative T wave. Other laboratory tests are unchanged.

Exceptions to the Usual Manifestations

As mentioned above, coronary spasm may produce transient ST elevation in the absence of angina. Many patients have both silent and symptomatic attacks, but in a few patients all attacks are silent. Coronary spasm after cardiac transplantation might be expected to be silent because the heart is denervated.

Coronary spasm can sometimes be documented at angiography in patients without episodes of transient ST elevation. ST depression or pseudonormalization of persistently negative T waves may be the only abnormality documented in some patients. A few patients have been described who present with syncope that has been attributed to ventricular arrhythmias or conduction disturbances secondary to spasm, but with no history of chest discomfort.

Differential Diagnosis

The combination of episodes of chest discomfort at rest associated with transient ST segment elevation relieved by nitroglycerin cinches the diagnosis of Prinzmetal's angina. If the ST segment and chest pain do not begin to resolve within 5 minutes after nitroglycerin administration, acute myocardial infarction becomes an increasingly likely diagnostic possibility.

Coronary spasm is often used as a convenient diagnosis of default when the coronary arteriogram is normal and no cause can be found for chest pain. The overwhelming majority of such patients have neither coronary spasm nor Prinzmetal's angina.

Chest discomfort at rest suggestive of myocardial ischemia should prompt consideration of unstable angina as the most likely diagnosis. Most patients with unstable angina will also have symptoms on exertion, but the absence of exertional symptoms does not exclude unstable angina. Gastro-esophageal reflux, others disorders of the esophagus, intermittent musculoskeletal pain, and psychogenic causes of chest pain should be considered in a differential diagnosis of patients who have chest pain typical of Prinzmetal's angina. Other cardiac conditions associated with chest pain, such as pulmonary hypertension, cardiomyopathy and mitral valve prolapse are usually easy to distinguish from Prinzmetal's angina.

Other Diagnostic Testing

Variant angina can be most easily diagnosed by recording an ECG during an episode of rest angina. When variant angina is suspected, ambulatory ECG monitoring or an event monitor can sometimes be useful to confirm the diagnosis. The development of transient ST elevation during an exercise test is often the first clue to diagnosis, although other conditions can cause this response.

Provocative testing has been used to confirm the diagnosis of Prinzmetal's angina when a spontaneous attack cannot be documented.[4] The cold pressor test, exercise, and hyperventilation are physiologic stimuli for coronary spasm, but each has a sensitivity that is too low to be useful clinically. Ergonovine and acetylcholine are much more potent stimuli to induce attacks; both agents combine high sensitivity and specificity for diagnosis. These drugs should only be used under controlled circumstances, such as during coronary arteriography, and in carefully selected patients.

All patients with Prinzmetal's angina should undergo coronary arteriography unless an absolute contraindication is present. Coronary arteriography is the only certain method to distinguish between patients who have severe multivessel organic stenoses and those who have only narrowings or angiographically normal coronary arteries.

Etiology and Basic Mechanisms Responsible for the "Pain"

Prinzmetal's angina is caused by episodic coronary spasm, but the cause of coronary spasm has remained elusive.[4] Evidence of parasympathetic nervous system overactivity and reduced sympathetic activity have both been presented; however, coronary spasm has been demonstrated in the transplanted denervated heart, making a central neural mechanism unlikely. Alpha-adrenergic blockade, blockade of serotonin receptors, inhibition of thromboxane A_2 production, and prostacyclin administration have each failed to prevent attacks. Magnesium deficiency, hyperinsulinemia and vitamin E deficiency have been reported to be present in patients with Prinzmetal's angina. Vitamin C has been reported to attenuate the abnormal coronary vasoconstriction in these patients by inhibiting oxygen free radical generation. A mutation in the endothelial nitric oxide synthase gene has recently been reported to be significantly more common in patients with coronary spasm compared to controls.

The pathophysiologic consequences of coronary spasm are better understood. Total coronary occlusion due to spasm induces transmural myocardial ischemia within a very few minutes, with ST elevation and segmental dyskinesis. If the territory is large, left ventricular filling pressure will rise and cardiac output and arterial pressure will fall. Ventricular arrhythmias and conduction disturbances will develop if the ischemia is severe, extensive and lasts for more than a few minutes.

Treatment

Nitroglycerin relieves attacks of Prinzmetal's angina within seconds to minutes. It should be used promptly at the onset of an attack both for relief and to prevent the complications that are more likely with prolonged episodes. Long-acting nitrates are effective in reducing the frequency of attacks, but the rapid development of nitrate tolerance limits their utility. Beta-blockers should be avoided in patients with Prinzmetal's angina because of their propensity to increase the frequency and duration of attacks.

Calcium channel blockers are very effective in preventing attacks of Prinzmetal's angina.[4-6] The response is better at higher doses and the relative efficacy of drugs within this class appears to be roughly equal. Patients who respond incompletely to one drug often become completely asymptomatic on a combination of either diltiazem or verapamil plus nifedipine or amlodipine.

Coronary bypass surgery should be considered for most patients with Prinzmetal's angina and multivessel organic coronary disease because of their high short-term risk of MI. The perioperative mortality rate and infarction rate are higher than for comparable patients without Prinzmetal's angina, but surgery almost always eliminates symptoms and the long-term prognosis is excellent.

Many patients with Prinzmetal's angina have coronary lesions that are ideal for angioplasty. When such patients are pretreated with calcium channel blockers and given intracoronary nitroglycerin during the procedure, the primary success rate is high. However, coronary spasm may persist or recur after successful angioplasty, and the restenosis rate is high.[8] Definitive evidence is lacking as to whether or not stenting yields better outcomes. Revascularization procedures are not indicated in the absence of organic stenosis.

Spontaneous remission has been reported to occur within 1 to 2 years in over half of patients with Prinzmetal's angina.[6] The long-term prognosis depends upon the severity of the underlying coronary atherosclerosis.[5]

Classic Description

"From a study of 35 patients with this variant form of angina, a typical composite picture emerges. All of these features are, or course, not seen in every case. The typical patient, while at rest or engaged in ordinary activity, develops pain in the same location as the patient with classic angina. There is a sense of oppression, and then the discomfort subsides. Several minutes go by, then often the uncomfortable substernal sensation recurs. Although mild and quite bearable at first, the distress mounts, the pain becomes intense, and there is apprehension and often a fear of death. These symptoms, fortunately, pass away quickly, and all seems well . . .

If a continuous electrocardiogram is recorded throughout an attack, a remarkable series of changes is observed. With the appearance of pain, the S-T segments become elevated. As the pain becomes more severe, the R waves may become taller in the leads showing S-T segment elevation. When the pain reaches its peak, arrhythmias may appear, most often ventricular. The pain then diminishes and the process is reversed. The arrhythmias disappear and the R waves and S-T segments revert to their appearance prior to the onset of the pain. As the cycles of pain and relief recur, this extraordinary sequence of electrocardiographic changes is repeated."

Source: Prinzmetal M, Ekmekei A, Kennamer R, Kwoczynski JK, Shubin H, Toyoshima H. Variant form of angina pectoris. Previously undelineated syndrome. *JAMA* 1960;174:1794–1800. (Used under the "fair use" rule.)

References

1. Prinzmetal M, Kennamer R, Merliss R, et al. Angina pectoris. I. A variant form of angina pectoris. *Am J Med* 1959;27:375–388.

2. Prinzmetal M, Ekmekei A, Kennamer R, et al. Variant form of angina pectoris. Previously undelineated syndrome. *JAMA* 1960;174:1794–1800.
3. Maseri A, Severi S, De Nes M, et al. "Variant" angina: One aspect of a continuous spectrum of vasospastic myocardial ischemia. *Am J Cardiol* 1978;42:1019–1035.
4. Waters DD. Diagnosis and management of patients with unstable angina. In *Hurst's The Heart, 10ᵗʰ ed.*, Alexander RW, Schlant RC, Fuster V, et al. (eds): McGraw-Hill (New York), 2001, pp. 1237–1274.
5. Walling A, Waters DD, Miller DD, et al. Long-term prognosis of patients with variant angina. *Circulation* 1987;76:990–997.
6. Waters DD, Bouchard A, Théroux P. Spontaneous remission is a frequent outcome of variant angina. *J Am Coll Cardiol* 1983;2:195–199.
7. Miller D, Waters DD, Warnica W, et al. Is variant angina the coronary manifestation of a generalized vasospastic disorder? *N Engl J Med* 1981;304:763–766.
8. Bertrand ME, Lablanche JM, Thieuleux FA, et al. Relation of restenosis after percutaneous transluminal coronary angioplasty to vasomotion of the dilated coronary arterial segment. *Am J Cardiol* 1989;63:277–281.

32

"Chest Pain" in Patients with Myocardial Infarction with Normal or Near-Normal Coronary Arteriograms

Rabih R. Azar, MD, MSc and David Waters, MD

General Considerations

Some patients have myocardial infarction (MI) with normal or near-normal coronary arteriograms. This condition and discussion should not be confused with patients who have symptoms suggesting myocardial ischemia only, who have normal coronary arteriograms.

Clinical Setting

The typical patient with MI with normal or near-normal coronary arteriograms is a young male smoker[1] or a young woman under the influence of pregnancy or oral contraceptives.[2] The prevalence is inversely related to the age of the patients and varies from 1% to 12%.[3] Typical patients are less than 35 years old but this syndrome can occur at any age.

Characteristics of the Pain

Patient's characterization of the "chest pain"

The description of the "chest pain" in patients with MI with normal or near-normal coronary arteriograms is similar to that given by patients

From: Hurst JW, Morris DC (eds): *"Chest Pain"* →. © Futura Publishing Co., Inc., Armonk, NY, 2001.

with MI secondary to coronary atherosclerotic heart disease. The terms of *pressure, squeezing, tightness, heaviness, burning* and *aching* are frequently use. The onset of the pain is usually sudden. The majority of these patients do not have prodromal attacks before the onset of the MI, such as a history of exertional angina or unstable angina.[4,5] Patients with coronary spasm as an etiology for their MI (see below) may give a prior history of chest pain at rest. The pain is usually severe in intensity, because it is caused by complete occlusion of an artery supplying a large amount of myocardium with no collateral circulation. In rare instances, MI may be silent.[4]

Common Location of the "chest pain"

The location of the pain is also similar to that of patients with MI and abnormal coronary arteries. In its typical location, the pain is retrosternal radiating to the left shoulder, inner aspect of the left upper extremity and sometimes to the neck, jaw, right side of the chest, and both upper extremities (see Figures 32–1 through 32–3). The pain may also begin in the epigastrium and simulate a variety of abdominal disorders.

Uncommon locations of the "chest pain"

In rare instances, the chest discomfort could be minor and the pain could be mainly localized to one of its areas of radiation such as the left

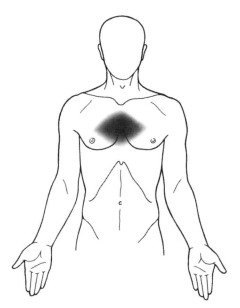

Figure 32–1. The usual location and size of the "chest pain" that is designated angina pectoris.

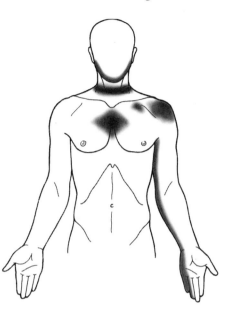

Figure 32–2. Common locations of the radiation of the "chest pain" that is designated angina pectoris. Note the radiation to the neck, jaw, left upper chest, left shoulder, inner surface of the left arm, left little finger, and left ring finger.

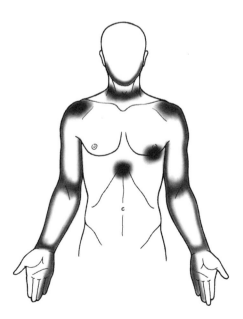

Figure 32–3. Unusual locations of the "pain" that is designated angina pectoris. The discomfort may be limited to the neck, jaw, right or left shoulder, left pectoral region, epigastrium, inner or outer surface of the right or left arms, elbows, wrists or little ring fingers.

arm, left shoulder, inner aspect of the left or both upper extremities, or the jaw (see Figure 32–3).

Size of the "painful" area

The size of the painful area is usually large and diffuse. Pain that occupies a small area that can be pinpointed by the patient's finger is almost never cardiac. The pain is usually deep. Chest pain that is described as being near the surface of the skin is unlikely to be caused by MI.

Duration of the "chest pain"

By definition, the pain of MI usually lasts more than 30 minutes. Pain lasting less than 30 minutes is usually classified as unstable angina. The physician will, however, be occasionally surprised to observe the changes of infarction in the electrocardiogram in patients who have only unstable angina. Typically, the pain of MI lasts several hours, and does not resolve until reperfusion or complete necrosis of the involved myocardium have occurred.

Tenderness of the chest wall

The chest wall is rarely, if ever, tender.

Precipitating causes of the "chest pain"

The most commonly reported triggers for MI with normal or near-normal coronary arteriograms are heavy physical exercise or a strong mental stress such as that caused by anger. Other potential triggers are atrial fibrillation which can rarely cause embolization into one of the coronary arteries, and pregnancy, especially during the puerperal period which predisposes to coronary dissection.[6] Cocaine use can also precipitate MI because it stimulates platelets, triggers coronary spasm and increases myocardial oxygen demand.[7] Binge alcohol drinking has also been reported as a trigger for acute MI with a normal coronary arteriogram.[8] However, in the majority of cases no precipitating factor can be identified. The onset of MI is acute and unheralded.

Relief of the "chest pain"

Myocardial infarction occurs when blood flow to a myocardial territory is completely interrupted. The pain is thus persistent and does not resolve until blood flow is re-established in the culprit vessel or until the whole myocardium supplied by the culprit vessel dies. The pain is usually not relieved with nitroglycerine. The pain resolves very quickly once flow is restored in the occluded vessel. This can happen spontaneously (spontaneous lysis of an intra-coronary clot) or following reperfusion therapy.

Associated Symptoms

Nausea, vomiting, weakness, fatigue, and diaphoresis are frequently associated with acute MI. All of these symptoms are nonspecific and do not allow differentiation between patients with and those without atherosclerotic coronary artery disease. Light-headedness and syncope may also occur and are commonly caused by ventricular tachycardia or by bradyarrhythmia. Symptoms of congestive heart failure (dyspnea, orthopnea) are less common in patients with normal or near-normal coronary arteries. This is because they are usually younger and have a better baseline cardiac function than patients with coronary atherosclerosis.

Other associated symptoms may be present and may orient the physician toward the etiology of the MI. For example, patients with coronary artery spasm may give a history of migraine headache or Raynaud's disease and patients with coronary embolization, may experience palpitations preceding the onset of the "chest pain".

Associated Signs

Physical examination

No specific signs allow differentiating patients with MI with normal or near-normal coronary arteriograms from those with abnormal coronary arteriograms. Patients in the former group are usually younger and have fewer risk factors. The patients often show signs of distress from pain and anxiety. Cardiac auscultation may reveal an S4 gallop or a murmur of mitral regurgitation. Signs of congestive heart failure such as hypotension, rales, and S3 gallop are rare.

"Routine" laboratory tests

The *electrocardiographic* abnormalities and *serum markers* such as creatine-kinase and its MB subfraction and the cardiac troponin T and I are useful in confirming the diagnosis. All these findings are similar to those of MI caused by coronary atherosclerotic heart disease.

The chest x-ray film is not useful for the diagnosis of MI, but is helpful to exclude other conditions that can simulate an MI. A fresh MI does not produce cardiac enlargement, but may reveal pulmonary congestion.

Exceptions to the Usual Manifestations

The clinical presentation may be very subtle and in some cases the infarct may be silent. Sudden death may be the first manifestation of the MI and was reported more frequently in cases of coronary dissection.

Differential Diagnosis

Coronary spasm can produce chest pain and ST-segment elevation. Coronary spasm however, resolves promptly after sub-lingual nitroglycerin and if the pain persists for more than 15 minutes, MI becomes a more likely diagnosis. Patients with cocaine use may present with a wide variety of chest complaints which may mimic myocardial ischemia and/or infarction and usually respond to benzodiazepines. However, because cocaine is associated with MI, these patients should be carefully monitored and treated.

Patients with focal myocarditis can sometimes be falsely diagnosed as having MI with normal or near normal coronary arteriograms. The exact differentiation between the two conditions may be difficult because both are associated with abnormal cardiac enzymes and wall motion abnormalities on imaging studies. The characteristics of the pain as well as the pattern of the cardiac enzymes elevation and subsequent normalization, allow the correct identification of patients with acute MI.

Overall, the differential diagnosis for patients with MI with normal or near-normal arteriograms is similar to that of patients with coronary atherosclerotic heart disease. Because the former patients are usually younger, have fewer risk factors and do not have a prior cardiac history, it is easier to attribute their complaints to noncardiac causes, such as pulmonary hypertension, gastroesophageal problems, pulmonary hypertension or embolism. The findings on the electrocardiogram and abnormal rise in cardiac enzymes are extremely useful in making the correct diagnosis. Sometimes a brief period of observation on a telemetry floor may be the only way to completely exclude an MI.

Other Diagnostic Tests

Acute rest myocardial perfusion imaging may be extremely useful in rapidly identifying patients with MI, especially those with nonspecific electrocardiographic findings who have not yet elevated their cardiac enzymes. Injection of these patients with Tc-99m sestamibi as soon as possible during or after the episode of pain, allows visualization of the infarct as an area with reduced (or absent) perfusion.

Coronary angiography allows visualization of the coronary arterial tree. If angiography is performed emergently during the acute phase of the infarction, occlusion of the coronary artery is the universal finding. The causes of the occlusion are however multiple (see next paragraph). If angiography is performed a few days or weeks after the infarct, these patients have normal coronary arteriograms or mild luminal irregularities. Coronary angiography however, depicts coronary anatomy from a planar 2-dimensional silhouette of the lumen and cannot detect early signs of atherosclerosis. Thus, many "normal" angiograms may be false normals. Intra-vascular ultra-sound is a new technique that allows a more accurate assessment of the coronary tree, and allows identification of early atherosclerosis, ruptured plaque and extra-luminal pathology, such as dissection or mural hematoma. These findings may be extremely important in determining the etiology of the infarction.

Etiology and Basic Mechanisms Responsible for the "Pain"

The mechanism of "chest pain" is similar to that of patients with MI due to atherosclerotic coronary artery disease. The syndrome is a consequence of an occlusion of a coronary artery, with complete interruption of the forward blood flow resulting in ischemia and necrosis of the myocardium supplied by that vessel. However, the causes of the occlusion are different from MI with abnormal coronary arteriograms where plaque rupture and formation of an occlusive intra-coronary thrombus are by far the most common mechanism of infarction. This mechanism remains possible, even if coronary angiography reveals normal looking arteries or mild coronary artery disease. This is because plaques that rupture are usually minimally stenotic and by the time patients are referred to coronary angiography, the occlusive clot might have lysed leaving only the nonocclusive plaque.

Other mechanisms may account for MI in patients with normal or near-normal arteries (see Table 32–1). Coronary artery spasm is one of the most popular etiologies and is supported by the finding that patients with Prinzmetal's angina can develop MI. In addition, angiographic observations in the early hours after the onset of acute MI thought to be secondary to intra-coronary thrombosis, have demonstrated severe coronary spasm which resolved after the administration of intra-coronary nitroglycerin.[9,10]

Table 32–1.

Causes of Myocardial Infarction in Patients with Normal or Near-Normal Coronary Arteriograms.

- Rupture of a non-obstructive coronary plaque
- Coronary spasm
- Emboli to the coronary arteries
- Coronary dissection
- Trauma to the coronary arteries
- Cocaine use
- Cardiac contusion
- Hematological causes: thrombocytosis, polycythemia vera
- Anomalous origin of the coronary arteries
- False negative coronary angiography

Spasm can lead to complete interruption of the blood flow and MI. Some patients may also develop coronary thrombosis at the site of spasm. High levels of fibrinopeptide A and of plasminogen inhibitor activator have been reported in patients with vasospastic angina.[11]

Embolization into the coronary artery is another cause of MI and is reported mainly in patients with atrial fibrillation or abnormalities of the mitral valve, such as endocarditis, a prosthetic mitral valve, or patients with left atrial or ventricular myxoma, or with a mural thrombus. Paradoxical embolization can also occur in patients with a patent foramen ovale.

Myocardial infarction can also result from coronary dissection. This condition is more common in women, especially during the puerperal period.[6,12] The dissection occurs in the outer media and causes luminal occlusion by pushing the inner media against the opposing wall. The hormonal and hemodynamic factors of pregnancy or contraceptive use may result in a weakening of the tunica media thereby explaining the higher incidence of female patients with spontaneous dissection. By the time angiography is performed, the dissection might have healed.

Myocardial bridging is another rare cause of MI with normal coronary arteriograms. In this condition, a portion of the coronary artery runs deep in the myocardial muscle and is subject to the trauma caused by repeated contractions which can predispose to thrombosis.

Finally, it should be remembered that angiography is an imperfect technique and may underestimate the degree of coronary atherosclerosis or may sometimes completely miss a "tight" coronary lesion or even a total occlusion of a small or medium caliber artery. Simply stated, a normal coronary arteriogram does not guarantee that the coronary arteries are normal.

Treatment

There are no clinical or electrocardiographic criteria that allow beforehand identification of patients with acute MI who have normal or near normal coronary arteriograms. As a result, the treatment of these patients is initially similar to that of patients with acute MI caused by coronary atherosclerosis: aspirin, heparin, sublingual and intravenous nitroglycerin, followed by prompt reperfusion therapy (thrombolytics or primary coronary angioplasty depending on institutional preferences). The diagnosis is made only retrospectively after coronary angiography has been performed. Further management depends on the suspected etiology. Patients with coronary spasm should be treated with calcium channel blockers and nitrates and the tobacco should be prohibited. Patients with suspected embolization should be carefully evaluated to determine the source of the embolism and decide about the use of long-term anticoagulation therapy. Substances that can enhance platelets activity or stimulate the coagulation system should be discontinued (estrogen and progesterone). Patients should be questioned about cocaine use. Risk factor modifications should always be a central part of the long-term plan of care, especially in patients with mild coronary atherosclerosis. The majority of patients will probably benefit from life-long aspirin therapy.

References

1. Khan AH, Haywood LJ. Myocardial infarction in nine patients with radiologically patent coronary arteries. *N Engl J Med* 1974;291:427–431.
2. Erlebacher JA. Transmural myocardial infarction with "normal" coronary arteries. *Am Heart J* 1979;98:421–430.
3. Alpert JS. Myocardial infarction with angiographically normal coronary arteries. *Arch Intern Med* 1994;154:265–269.
4. Rosenblatt A, Selzer A. The nature and clinical features of myocardial infarction with normal coronary arteriogram. *Circulation* 1977;55:578–580.
5. Raymond R, Lynch J, Underwood D, et al. Myocardial infarction and normal coronary arteriography: A 10 year clinical and risk analysis of 74 patients. *J Am Coll Cardiol* 1988;11:471–477.
6. Roth A, Elkayam U. Acute myocardial infarction associated with pregnancy. *Ann Intern Med* 1996;125:751–762.
7. Amin M, Gabelman G, Karpel J, et al. Acute myocardial infarction and chest pain syndromes after cocaine use. *Am J Cardiol* 1990;66:1434–1437.
8. Williams MJ, Restieaux NJ, Low CJ. Myocardial infarction in young people with normal coronary arteries. *Heart* 1998;79:191–194.
9. Vincent GM, Anderson JL, Marshall HW. Coronary spasm producing coronary thrombosis and myocardial infarction. *N Engl J Med* 1983;309:220–223.

10. Lindsay J, Jr., Pichard AD. Acute myocardial infarction with normal coronary arteries. *Am J Cardiol* 1984;54:902–904.
11. Irie T, Imaizumi T, Matuguchi T, et al. Increased fibrinopeptide A during anginal attacks in patients with variant angina. *J Am Coll Cardiol* 1989;14:589–594.
12. Basso C, Morgagni GL, Thiene G. Spontaneous coronary artery dissection: A neglected cause of acute myocardial ischaemia and sudden death. *Heart* 1996;75:451–454.

33

"Chest Pain" in Patients Who Use Cocaine

Jessica Haberer, MD and David Waters, MD

General Considerations

An estimated 25 to 30 million Americans have used cocaine, five to six million use it regularly and 5,000 use it for the first time daily.[1] Concern over cocaine-induced cardiac disease has grown in the last decade because of the increasing popularity of crack cocaine, a free base form of the drug that is smoked in a pipe. Crack is less expensive and more potent than intranasal cocaine. Chest pain is the most common cocaine-related medical problem and leads to the evaluation of more than 64,000 patients annually in the US.[2] Unfortunately, the actual incidence of cocaine-associated chest pain is not known, largely because patients are not asked about cocaine use. Cocaine is known to cause ischemia with or without myocardial necrosis via coronary vasospasm, fixed coronary atherosclerosis, increased demand or a combination of these mechanisms. Additionally, cocaine has been associated with myocarditis, cardiomyopathy, acute pulmonary edema, ventricular arrhythmias and aortic dissections. Although many cocaine users are young and otherwise healthy, many also have substantial risk factors for coronary artery disease, particularly tobacco use and hypertension. Cardiac evaluation must therefore be tailored to the individual patient.

---

[1]This chapter, written by two cardiologists, on *"chest pain" in adults who use cocaine* is somewhat similar to Chapter 48 that was written by a psychiatrist. Both chapters are included in an effort to characterize all aspects of patients with chest pain who are addicts.

From: Hurst JW, Morris DC (eds): *"Chest Pain"* →. © Futura Publishing Co., Inc., Armonk, NY, 2001.

Clinical Setting

Some patients admit to their cocaine use; many do not. A higher level of cocaine use is seen in urban areas; however, the use of cocaine should be screened in any patient presenting with chest pain. One study involving three urban and one suburban hospitals reported 17% cocaine use in patients under the age of 60 who were admitted for chest pain.[3] Suspicion of cocaine-associated chest pain should be higher in younger, otherwise healthy patients, as well as patients with a known history of cocaine use. Although any patient with chest pain can exhibit hypertension and tachycardia, other physical signs of adrenergic stimulation such as dilated pupils, agitation and psychosis should suggest recent cocaine use.

Characteristics of the "Pain"

Patient's characteristics of the "chest pain"

Chest pain in the setting of cocaine use can be caused by a variety of conditions and the characteristics of the pain vary accordingly. Patients typically describe a constant stabbing or crushing pain that does not vary with position or degree of exertion. A pleuritic component may be present as well. Cocaine users often have a low tolerance for pain and characterize it as quite severe. The pain is frequently associated with palpitations and diaphoresis and may radiate to the back, arms or jaw. Nausea is seen less frequently. Classic anginal pain (i.e., pain that lasts a few minutes, worsens with exertion and improves with rest) may also be seen and is more common in older patients. When these symptoms are present, suspicion for actual myocardial ischemia must be higher. Additionally, when the pain radiates to the back, aortic dissection must be considered.

Common location of the "chest pain"

The chest pain is usually located in the retrosternal area and may involve the entire chest (see Figure 33–1). The "pain" may radiate to the neck, shoulder and inner surface of the left arm (see Figure 33–2).

Uncommon locations of the "chest pain"

Cocaine-associated chest pain is rarely located outside the retrosternal area. It can, however, be experienced in the back, epigastrium and shoulders (see Figures 33–3 and 33–4).

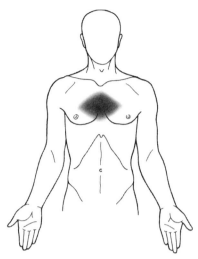

Figure 33–1. The "chest pain" due to cocaine usage is commonly located in the retrosternal area.

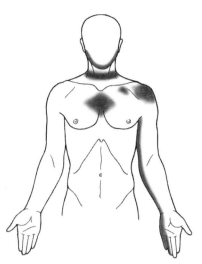

Figure 33–2. The "chest pain" due to cocaine usage may radiate to the neck, left shoulder, and inner surface of the left arm.

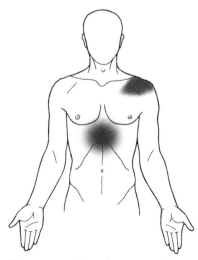

Figure 33–3. The "chest pain" due to cocaine usage may occasionally be located in the epigastric area.

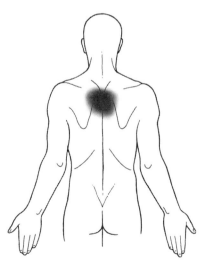

Figure 33–4. The "chest pain" due to cocaine usage may rarely radiate to the back.

Size of the painful *"area"*

Retrosternal chest pain is typically the size of a fist, but may involve the entire precordium.

Duration of the *"chest pain"*

Cocaine-associated chest pain can last for minutes to several hours. The pain may result from the effects of cocaine itself or its metabolites: benzoylecgonine and ethyl methyl ecgonine.[4] The onset of pain is often acute; however, cocaine's euphoric effects may mask the patient's ability to recognize the actual time onset. Medication is frequently needed to provide the patient with relief.

Tenderness of the chest wall

The chest wall may or may not be tender. Patients under the influence of cocaine and other "street drugs" are more likely to be involved in coincident trauma and consequently complain of musculoskeletal injury.

Precipitating causes of the *"chest pain"*

Cocaine can cause chest pain within minutes of use, but symptoms may not develop for hours or even weeks. In a study of 21 young men in a cocaine rehabilitation program, ST elevation was seen on ambulatory electrocardiographic monitoring in eight of the men up to 6 weeks after the last use.[5] Because only one patient was found to have myocardial infarction (MI), however, the changes were attributed to vasospasm similar to that seen in Prinzmetal's angina. Additionally, patients with underlying coronary disease may be more prone to chest pain with exercise or emotional stress.

Relief of the *"chest pain"*

The pain associated with cocaine use can be quite severe. As with classic angina, nitroglycerin and morphine are often effective. Higher doses of morphine may be needed, because cocaine users frequently take other "street drugs" and have a high tolerance for opiates. Calcium channel blockers help reverse the underlying coronary vasoconstriction and aid in relieving pain. Benzodiazepines can also be used to decrease the patient's overall agitation.

Associated Symptoms

Cocaine is a potent stimulator of the sympathetic nervous system. In addition to the cardiovascular effects described above, it initially induces euphoria, garrulousness, increased motor activity and occasionally seizures and hyperthermia. Excessive use can cause tremor, respiratory and vasomotor depression, and paranoia. These symptoms are almost indistinguishable from amphetamine use. Following the initial stimulant effects, the patient develops dysphoria and depression. The length of time between these feelings depends on the route of administration. Nasal inhalation produces a slower onset of euphoria, while oral inhalation and injection produce quite rapid onset and withdrawal. In addition, patients may complain of nausea, dyspnea, anxiety, palpitations, and dizziness.

Associated Signs

Physical examination

Given the adrenergic-stimulation of cocaine, patients typically have dilated pupils, tachycardia, and hypertension. Cocaine, however, is often mixed with other "street drugs" that may alter these findings. The cardiovascular exam frequently reveals hyperdynamic pulses and precordium. Decreased peripheral pulses are suggestive of aortic dissection, and the blood pressure should be measured in both arms to assess if a discrepancy exists. If MI is indeed present, other abnormalities, such as a ventricular gallop or mitral regurgitation murmur, may be heard. Cocaine has also been associated with flash pulmonary edema, and râles may be present.

"Routine" laboratory tests

The significance of electrocardiographic abnormalities is difficult to interpret in cocaine users. As many as 84% of electrocardiograms are abnormal in cocaine-associated chest pain.[6,7] In a study of young, male cocaine users, Chakko et. al. found that 54% had left ventricular hypertrophy, 23% had increased QRS voltage, 50% had ST-segment elevation (early repolarization) and 15% had non-specific ST-T changes.[1] These abnormalities may be due to hypertension, which often results from repeated cocaine use. Alternatively, they may simply reflect the youth of many cocaine users. Evidence of old MI was also seen in 4% of electrocardiograms.

The incidence of MI in cocaine users as determined by enzyme testing is not clear, and reports have ranged from 0% to 31% in retrospective stuides.[6,7] Of note, a prospective study reported a 6% incidence.[8] Because cocaine use is associated with musculoskeletal injury, troponin tends to be a more specific marker than CK/CK-MB.[9]

Exceptions to the Usual Manifestations

The vast majority of cocaine use is not associated with chest pain. Further, patients may experience cardiac complications of cocaine without noticing symptoms during the euphoric effects of the drug.

Differential Diagnosis

Given the hyperadrenergic state and paranoia induced by cocaine, some proportion of chest pain may reflect anxiety or panic attacks. More serious conditions, such as aortic dissection and ventricular arrhythmia, must also be considered in any cocaine user presenting with chest pain. The actual incidence of these conditions is not known, and the latter may be responsible for sudden death seen in cocaine users.[1] Pneumothorax, pneumomediastinum and pneumopericardium have been reported after inhalation or insufflation of cocaine.[10] Musculoskeletal injury is also common in hyperadrenergic states. Drug users are more susceptible to infections, such as pneumonia, endocarditis, sternal osteomyelitis/septic arthritis, which could present as chest pain. Esophageal spasm and gastroesophageal reflux disease should also be considered, as with any patient presenting with chest pain. Like cocaine, Prinzmetal's angina is due to vasospasm, although it presents quite differently (see Chapter 31).

Other Diagnostic Testing

The majority of cocaine-associated chest pain does not cause permanent cardiac injury and requires no further diagnostic testing. If the history, electrocardiographic changes and/or enzyme levels are consistent with MI, atherosclerotic coronary disease should be suspected and evaluated further. Suspicion for athersclerosis should be higher in patients with known cardiac risk factors such as older age, tobacco use, hypertension, high cholesterol, diabetes, and prior history of cardiac disease. Some data, however, suggest that cocaine use enhances atherogenesis, and risk factors do not necessarily predict with accuracy the amount of coronary artery disease seen on diagnostic testing.[11-13]

Echocardiography may be useful in detecting regional wall motion abnormalities and depressed ejection fractions (<50%) which suggest infarction. Dilated cardiomyopathy, however, is associated with cocaine use alone and may not indicate ischemic disease.[11,13] Additionally, alcohol abuse is common in cocaine users and may account for some of the dilated cardiomyopathy observed in this group.

Myocardial perfusion studies are frequently abnormal in cocaine users; however, electrocardiographic findings suggestive of ischemia do not necessarily correlate with reversible defects. In one study of cocaine users with chest pain and normal electrocardiograms, 71% had normal perfusion scans and 15% had fixed defects.[14] The other 14% of patients had abnormal stress scans, but did not return for resting images. The nature of those defects is therefore not known. Another study found perfusion defects in 34% of patients with normal electrocardiograms, 31% of which were reversible.[15] Cardiac catheterizations revealed significant coronary stenosis (>75%) in 89% of these patients.

When clinical suspicion for MI is high, cardiac catheterization studies indicate that 60 to 72% of cocaine users have abnormal arteries.[11,13] Om et al. found mild stenosis (<70%) in 21% of patients and moderate to severe stenosis (>70%) in 40% of patients. These results are supported by an autopsy study of young men with cocaine in the bloodstream at the time of death in which 47% were found to have greater than 75% stenosis of the coronary vessels.[12]

Etiology and Basic Mechanisms Responsible for the "Pain"

Cocaine blocks the reuptake of norepinephrine, epinephrine, and dopamine in the synapse and stimulates the presynaptic release of norepinephrine. It thus produces an excess of neurotransmitters in the central and peripheral nervous systems. The hyperadrenergic state results in tachycardia, vasoconstriction, hypertension, and potentially arrhythmia.[1] The tachycardia and hypertension induced by cocaine increases myocardial oxygen demand and may lead to demand ischemia in patients with underlying atherosclerotic disease.

Vasoconstriction produced by cocaine may cause temporary ischemia and thrombus formation due to sluggish blood flow. Infarction may occur if blood flow is obstructed for several hours. Cocaine also increases platelet aggregation, which may cause thrombus formation in the setting of vasoconstriction. The magnitude of effect is unrelated to the amount of cocaine used, the route of entry (i.e. nasal/oral inhalation versus injection) or underlying heart disease.[6,11]

The pro-arrhythmogenic effects of cocaine can be understood via its effect on electrical conduction within the heart. Cocaine blocks the fast sodium channels, which causes a depression of depolarization, slowing of conduction velocity and a prolonged QRS complex. It also depresses the calcium current responsible for A-V nodal conduction and prolongs the PR interval. Potassium currents are also depressed, which prolong repolarization and the QT interval. Early afterdepolarizations may occur and result in ventricular arrhythmia, including torsade de pointes. Reperfusion abnormalities may then occur and result in arrhythmia.

Treatment

The course of treatment depends on the individual and the probability that the patient may have underlying coronary disease. Unfortunately, there have been no well-designed, prospective clinical trials to determine the best means of therapy in this subset of patients. The patient's history is therefore vital in guiding choice of therapy. Because the incidence of ischemia is low in the majority of patients, most require only pain control with narcotics and blood pressure control as discussed below.

When ischemia is suspected, all patients without contraindication should be given aspirin and monitored on telemetry for arrhythmias. Benzodiazepines are useful as anxiolytics and provide some reduction of blood pressure and heart rate, thereby decreasing myocardial oxygen demand.

While beta-blockers are commonly used in the setting of ischemia, they should be avoided in cocaine users. Cocaine causes stimulation of both the alpha- and beta-adrenergic systems, and beta-blockade poses a theoretic risk of unopposed alpha-adrenergic stimulation.[2,16] In that setting, heart rate and blood pressure could rise dramatically. Labetalol is a beta-blocker that also has alpha inhibition properties, but has not been proven to be safe in cocaine-associated chest pain. The beta blockade effect appears to dominate, and animal studies have revealed increased rates of seizure and mortality. Further, labetalol has been studied in the treatment of pheochromocytoma, an adrenal tumor causing increased alpha and beta-receptor stimulation, and hypertension was found to worsen in those patients.[17] Labetalol should be used, however, in the setting of cocaine-induced aortic dissection in order to rapidly decrease the sheer forces of severe hypertension. Anti-hypertensive therapy should therefore consist of calcium channel blockers and nitrates. These agents also serve to decrease coronary vasospasm, which is commonly seen in cocaine-induced pain and ischemia. Phentolamine may be used in refractory hypertension and tachycardia.

If the clinical suspicion for coronary artery disease is high, heparin (or low molecular weight heparin) should be used for anti-coagulation. The use of thrombolytic therapy is controversial. Cocaine-induced MI often occurs in the absence of thrombus, and severe hypertension associated with increased adrenergic stimulation theorectically places this subset of patients at higher risk for bleeding. One case series, however, reported no complications and some evidence of reperfusion had been documented.[18]

As many as 60% of patients with cocaine-associated chest pain have a second such event within 1 year.[10] Long-term treatment is therefore best aimed at cessation of cocaine and tobacco use. Unfortunately, rehabilitation failure is common. One study found that 24% of cocaine users reported weekly cocaine use in the year following treatment, and an additional 18% returned to another drug treatment program during that time.[19] Recurrent chest pain is less common in patients who stop using cocaine, and fatal or non-fatal MI is rare.[2] Aspirin may have some benefit in preventing cocaine-induced platelet aggregation and should be given to all patients who do not have a contraindication. The benefits of long-acting nitrates and calcium channel blockers have not been proven; however, they are recommended in patients with recurrent pain and persistent cocaine use.

References

1. Chakko S, Myerburg RJ. Cardiac complications of cocaine abuse. *Clin Cardiol* 1995;18:67–72.
2. Hollander JE. The management of cocaine-associated myocardial ischemia. *NEJM* 1995;333(19):1267–1272.
3. Hollander JE, Todd KH, Green G, et al. Chest pain associated with cocaine: An assessment of prevalence in suburban and urban emergency departments. *Ann Emerg Med* 1995;26(6):671–676.
4. Brogan WC 3rd, Lange RA, Glamann DB, et al. Recurrent coronary vasoconstriction caused by intranasal cocaine: Possible role for metabolites. *Ann Int Med* 1992;116(7):556–561.
5. Nademanee K, Gorelick DA, Josephson MA, et al. Myocardial ischemia during cocaine withdrawal. *Ann Int Med* 1989;111:876–880.
6. Amin M, Gabelman G, Karpel J, et al. Acute myocardial infarction and chest pain syndromes after cocaine use. *Amer J Cardiol* 1990;66:1434–1437.
7. Gitter MJ, Goldsmith SR, Dunbar DN, et al. Cocaine and chest pain: Clinical features and outcome of patients hospitalized to rule out myocardial infarction. *Ann Int Med* 1991;115:277–282.
8. Tokarsi GF, Paganussi P, Urbanski R, et al. An evaluation of cocaine-induced chest pain. *Ann Emerg Med* 1990;19:1088–1092.
9. Hollander JE, Levitt MA, Young GP, et al. Effect of recent cocaine use on the specificity of cardiac markers for diagnosis of acute myocardial infarction. *Amer Heart J* 1998;135(2 pt 1):245–252.
10. Hoffman RA, Hollander JE. Medical toxicology: Evaluation of patients with chest pain after cocaine use. *Crit Care Clin* 1997;13(4):809–828.
11. Om A, Warner M, Sabri N, et al. Frequency of coronary artery disease and left ventricular dysfunction in cocaine users. *Am J Cardiol* 1992;69:1549–1552.

12. Dressler FA, Malekzadeh S, Roberts WC. Quantitative analysis of amounts of coronary artery narrowing in cocaine addicts. *Am J Cardiol* 1990;65:303–308.
13. Rezkalla SH, Hale S, Kloner RA. Cocaine induced heart diseases. *Am Heart J* 1990;120:1403–1408.
14. Feldman JA, Bui LD, Mitchell PM, et al. The evaluation of cocaine-induced chest pain with acute myocardial perfusion imaging. *Acad Emer Med* 1999;6(2):103–109.
15. Giola G, Manuel M, Russell J, et al. Myocardial perfusion pattern in patients with cocaine-induced chest pain. *Am J Cardiol* 1995;75:396–398.
16. Boehrer JD, Moliterno DJ, Willard JE, et al. Influence of labetalol on cocaine-induced coronary vasoconstriction in humans. *Am J Med* 1992;94:608–610.
17. Briggs, RS, Birtwell AJ, et al. Hypertensive response to labetalol in phaeochromocytoma. *Lancet* 1978;1:1045–1046.
18. Hollander JE, Burstein JL, Shih ED, et al. Cocaine-associated myocardial infarction. Clinical safety of thrombolytic therapy. Cocaine Associated Myocardial Infarction (CAMI) Study Group. *Chest* 1995;107(5):2137–2141.
19. Simpson DD, Joe GW, Fletcher BW, et al. A national evaluation of treatment outcomes for cocaine dependence. *Arch Gen Psych* 1999;56: 507–514.

34

"Chest Pain" in Patients with Congenital Heart Disease

Joseph K. Perloff, MD

General Considerations

In patients with congenital cardiovascular disease, chest pain can originate in the myocardium, the great arteries, the pericardium, or the pleura (see Table 34–1).

Clinical Setting

The patients may be young or old, depending on the type of malformation causing the pain and the survival time associated with it.

Characteristics of the "Chest Pain"

The characteristics of the "chest pain" due to myocardial ischemia in patients with congenital heart disease is similar to the description offered in Chapters 29 and 30 and is illustrated in Figures 34–1 and 34–2.

The location of "chest pain" due to dissection of the aorta in patients with a congenital bicuspid aortic valve is shown in Figure 34–3. Other features of the chest pain are similar to the description offered in Chapter 43.

The characteristics of the "chest pain" due to pericarditis in patients with congenital heart disease is similar to the description offered in Chapter 27.

The characteristics of the "chest pain" due to pleural disease is similar to the description offered in Chapter 14.

From: Hurst JW, Morris DC (eds): *"Chest Pain"* →. © Futura Publishing Co., Inc., Armonk, NY, 2001.

Table 34–1.

Congenital Heart Disease That May Cause "Chest Pain."

1. Myocardial Ischemia
   a) Intrinsically abnormal coronary arteries
   b) Intrinsically normal coronary arteries
2. Great Arteries
   a) Dissecting aneurysm above a bicuspid aortic valve
   b) Rupture of a sinus of Valsalva aneurysm
3. Pericardial Disease
   a) Absence of pericardium—partial, complete
   b) Ebstein's anomaly
4. Pleural Disease
   a) Pulmonary arteriovenous fistulae

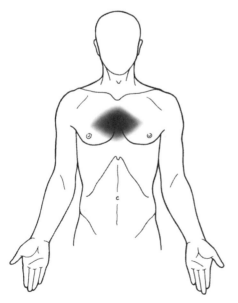

Figure 34–1. Usual location of angina pectoris.

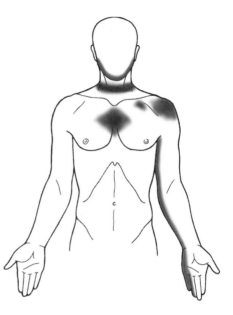

Figure 34–2. Common location of the radiation of angina pectoris.

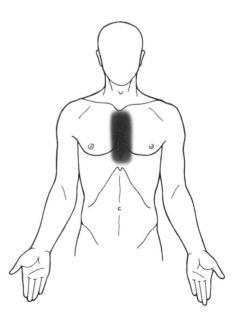

Figure 34–3. Location of the "chest pain" due to dissection of the aorta just distal to congenital bicuspid aortic valve stenosis.

Etiology and Basic Mechanisms Responsible for the "Chest Pain"

The etiologies of "chest pain" caused by congenital cardiovascular disease are diverse (Table 34–1). The symptoms of the pain itself are, for the most part, similar to those caused by acquired disease. However, it is not generally appreciated that certain types of congenital heart disease can cause chest pain. With this in mind it seems appropriate to discuss "chest pain" within the context of congenital heart disease itself.

Myocardial Ischemia

Pain due to myocardial ischemia occurs with intrinsically abnormal (see Table 34–2) or intrinsically normal coronary arteries (see Table 34–3).

Intrinsically abnormal coronary arteries

Anomalous origin of left coronary artery from pulmonary trunk: This is the most common clinically important congenital malformation of the coronary circulation.[1] Myocardial ischemia is initially caused by decreased *antegrade* perfusion of the anomalous left coronary artery but is subsequently caused by *retrograde* flow via intercoronary anastomoses acting as low-resistance channels that function as a coronary steal.[1]

Affected infants appear normal at birth and generally remain so for about 2 months, after which they experience ischemic pain and cardiac failure manifested by irritability, dyspnea, wheezing, cough, ashen gray color, and diaphoresis precipitated or aggravated by feeding, crying or a bowel movement. Conversely, angina pectoris may be deferred until the teens or young adulthood when clinical suspicion of the congenital coronary malformation is heightened by angina pectoris (see Figures 34–1 and

---

Table 34–2.

Myocardial Ischemia.
Intrinsically Abnormal Coronary Arteries.

1. Anomalous origin of left coronary artery from pulmonary trunk
2. Coronary arteriovenous fistula
3. Congenitally hypoplastic coronary arteries
4. Coarctation of the aorta, supra-valvular aortic stenosis
5. Coronary ectasia

Table 34–3.
Myocardial Ischemia.
Intrinsically Normal Coronary Arteries.

1. Proximal left coronary artery courses between aorta and pulmonary trunk
2. Increased ventricular mass—aortic or pulmonary stenosis, pulmonary hypertension

---

34–2) in a relatively young individual with no risk factors for premature atherosclerotic coronary artery disease.[1]

The diagnosis is supported by the murmur of mitral regurgitation caused by ischemic papillary muscle dysfunction and by a continuous murmur via intercoronary anastomoses.

The electrocardiogram exhibits Q waves that are typically *deep* rather than broad, and characteristically appear in leads 1, aVL and V_{5-6}. Voltage and repolarization criteria for left ventricular hypertrophy reflect a regional increase in left ventricular mass due to myocyte replication in response to hypoxemia in the immature heart.[2]

Two-dimensional echocardiography identifies the aortic origin of the right coronary artery, while Doppler interrogation and color flow imaging identify diastolic, systolic, or continuous flow entering the pulmonary trunk via the anomalous left coronary artery just distal to the pulmonary valve.[1]

Selective injection of contrast material into the *right* coronary artery shows dilatation, intercoronary anastomosis communicating with the left coronary artery, and retrograde flow into the pulmonary trunk.[1]

Two tasks confront the surgeon[2]: 1) repair of the basic coronary anomaly, and 2) the potential need for repair of mitral regurgitation. The anomalous coronary artery is ligated. Revascularization is achieved using either a reversed saphenous vein graft or the internal mammary artery.[2]

Coronary arteriovenous fistulae: Both coronary arteries arise from the aorta, but a fistulous branch of one or more of these arteries communicates directly with a cardiac chamber or with the pulmonary trunk, coronary sinus, vena cava or pulmonary vein.[1] The *drainage* site is of greater clinical and physiologic importance than the artery of origin. The coronary artery that forms the fistula is dilated, elongated and tortuous, and commonly contains saccular aneurysms that may be aneurysmal.[1] The physiologic consequences reflect the volume of blood flowing through the fistulous communication, the chamber or vessel into which the fistula drains, and myocardial ischemia that results from a coronary steal which sets the stage for angina pectoris[1] (see Figures 34–1 and 34–2).

A continuous murmur is the auscultatory hallmark of coronary arterial fistulae. The location of the murmur depends upon the chamber or vessel that receives the fistulous communication, not upon the coronary artery of origin.[1]

The electrocardiogram may be normal.

Radiologic features are determined by the volume and duration of blood flow and the site of drainage.

Two-dimensional electrocardiography with Doppler interrogation and color flow imaging establish the origin, course and site of drainage of the fistula, and assess its hemodynamic consequences.[1]

Selective coronary angiography identifies the coronary artery or arteries of origin, the morphology of the fistulous coronary bed, and the drainage site, setting the stage for surgical intervention or device occlusion.[2]

Congenitally hypoplastic coronary arteries: This condition is caused by underdevelopment of one or more coronary arteries or their major branches.[3] Patients tend to be young adults who are more apt to experience sudden cardiac death instead of chest pain. Should chest pain occur, it is likely to reflect myocardial infarction rather than angina pectoris (see Chapter 30).[3]

The echocardiogram identifies regional or global wall motion abnormalities but not their cause.

Selective coronary arteriography is definitive, disclosing hypoplasia of specific coronary arteries, with no significant response to intracoronary infusion of nitroglycerin. Treatment is medical (supportive).

Coarctation of the aorta: Premature coronary atherosclerosis occurs with coarctation of the aorta because the accompanying hypertension is a risk factor.[1,2] Symptomatic myocardial ischemia takes the form of angina pectoris (see Figures 34–1 and 34–2).

Stress electrocardiography discloses ST-T wave changes of myocardial ischemia, and exercise radionuclide perfusion localizes the sites of hypoperfusion.

Selective coronary angiography provides the definitive anatomic diagnosis.

Treatment is interventional catheterization with balloon dilatation and stent placement, or coronary artery bypass grafting.

Supravalvular aortic stenosis: In this malformation, the coronary ostia are proximal to the zone of obstruction. Hypertension in that segment causes premature atherosclerosis and angina pectoris[1,2] (see Figures 34–1 and 34–2). Coronary artery obstruction also occurs when a distorted aortic leaflet or a thickened ridge of aortic medial proliferation encroaches upon a coronary ostium.[1]

Radionuclide stress images identify regional abnormalities of myocardial perfusion.

Coronary angiography discloses coronary atherosclerosis as well as ostial obstruction.

Bypass grafting is used during surgical repair of the supravalvular stenosis.[2]

Coronary artery ectasia: In adults with cyanotic congenital heart disease, the extramural coronary arteries are typically dilated, often tortuous, and occasionally ectatic.[2,4] Dilatation results in an increase in resting myocardial blood flow which, however, does not compromise perfusion reserve.[5] Accordingly, myocardial ischemia is not a consequence, and ischemic chest pain is not a feature.

Intrinsically normal coronary arteries

Anomalous course of a major proximal coronary artery: Ectopic origin of a coronary artery is relatively common, but the *proximal course* of an anomalous coronary artery is more important than its ectopic origin.[5] Angina pectoris and myocardial infarction (see Figures 34–1 and 34–2) or sudden death are, with few exceptions, reserved for an aberrant coronary artery that courses between the aorta and pulmonary trunk.[1,5] Risk is greatest when the *left main coronary artery* arises from the right aortic sinus and passes between the aorta and the right ventricular outflow tract.[1,5] Acute angulation of the aortic origin of the anomalous coronary artery results in a slit-like ostium, and expansion of the aortic root and pulmonary trunk during exercise increases the angulation and reduces the slit.[1,5]

Myocardial ischemia is confirmed by an exercise stress electrocardiogram or radionuclide perfusion imaging.

The anomaly is identified by selective coronary angiography. Treatment is bypass grafting.

Increased ventricular mass: Afterload imposed upon the immature heart—as in congenital aortic stenosis—results in myocyte replication with appropriate angiogenesis, so capillary density remains normal.[1,6]

Accordingly, chest pain (myocardial ischemia) is uncommon in contrast to adults with acquired calcific aortic stenosis which is discussed elsewhere.

Coronary arterial embolus: This is a rare form of occlusive coronary artery disease.[7] The embolus generally arises from within the left heart, but in patients with cyanotic congenital heart disease (reversed shunt), the embolus may be paradoxical, announced by chest pain of acute myocardial infarction[7] (see Figures 34–1 and 34–2). Coronary embolization results in death in over 90% of cases because the embolus usually finds its way into the left main or anterior descending coronary artery.[7]

Selective angiography confirms the diagnosis,[7] setting the stage for intracoronary thrombolysis.

Great Arteries

Dissecting aneurysm above a bicuspid aortic valve

The ascending aorta above a bicuspid aortic valve is dilated whether the valve is stenotic, incompetent or functionally normal.[8] The dilatation is not "poststenotic," but instead is due to abnormalities of ascending aortic medial smooth muscle, elastin, collagen and ground substance.[8] Because the medial abnormality is confined to the ascending aorta, the dissection is confined to that site, so the chest pain is anterior not posterior (see Figure 34–3). Rupture is accompanied by the sudden onset of excruciating pain that may be preceded by lesser pain caused by predissection dilatation or tear.

The premorbid chest x-ray shows a convex (dilated) ascending aorta.

Two-dimensional echocardiography and magnetic resonance imaging determine aortic root dimensions and identify the dissection.

The risk of dissection increases significantly when the adult ascending aortic diameter reaches or exceeds 5 centimeters.

Rupture of a sinus valsalva aneurysm

A large acute rupture initiates a dramatic clinical picture.[1] A previously healthy, young adult, usually male, develops sudden pain that is retrosternal in addition to epigastric and in the base of the neck (see Figure 34–4).

The pain is accompanied by dyspnea, a loud continuous murmur and relentless cardiac failure.[1] The arterial pulse resembles that of aortic regurgitation, the jugular venous pressure is elevated, and biventricular impulses are prominent. The continuous murmur is louder in either systole

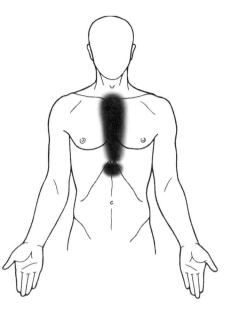

Figure 34–4. Distribution of "chest pain" caused by the rupture of a sinus of Valsalva.

or diastole, and is typically maximal below the third intercostal space along the right or left sternal border.

The chest x-ray initially exhibits pulmonary venous congestion, but subsequently exhibits increased pulmonary arterial blood flow with dilatation of both ventricles and enlargement of the right atrium and occasionally the left.

Two-dimensional echocardiography with color flow imaging and Doppler interrogation identifies the ruptured sinus of Valsalva aneurysm[1] and the chamber that receives the perforation.

Treatment is surgical closure of the perforation.[2] Rarely, an unruptured aortic sinus aneurysm compresses a coronary artery and causes angina pectoris or myocardial infarction.[1]

Pericardial Disease

Partial absence of pericardium

Agenesis of the pericardium is usually partial and left-sided.[9] Partial left-sided pericardial defects set the stage for herniation (incarceration) of the left atrial appendage. Stabbing, sharp precordial chest pain of brief duration and variable severity tends to be positional (postural).

The x-ray shows the herniated left atrial appendage confirmed by magnetic resonance imaging.[9]

Surgical repair is curative.[9]

Total absence (agenesis) of pericardium[9]

This condition results in striking mobility of the heart. Infrequent to recurrent sharp stabbing, precordial chest pain triggered by the supine or left lateral recumbent position varies from mild to severe.[9]

Magnetic resonance imaging confirms complete absence of the pericardium together with unusual positions of each of the four cardiac chambers.[9]

The etiology of the chest pain is unclear but has been assigned to torsion of the great arteries.[9] Attempts at surgical stabilization of the heart have met with tentatively encouraging results.[9]

Ebstein's anomaly of the tricuspid valve

This malformation is occasionally accompanied by chest pain located behind the sternum, in the right or left anterior chest, or in the epigastrium[10] (see Figure 34–3). Certain features suggest serous surface origin; a fibrinous pericardium has occasionally been found over the atrialized right ventricle.[1,10]

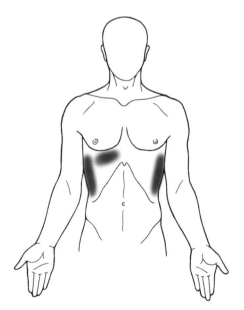

Figure 34–5. Location of "chest pain" due to congenital pulmonary arteriovenous fistulae. The "pain" is usually felt in only one of the areas of the chest indicated in the illustration.

Pleural Disease

Pulmonary arteriovenous fistulae

The substantial majority of these fistulae involve the lower lobes or right middle lobe.[1] The fistula replaces the pulmonary capillary bed and consists of a thin aneurysmal sac or a tangle of distended, tortuous vascular channels. Hemothorax occasionally results from rupture of a fistulous site on the pleural surface. Pleuritic pain overlies the lower lobes or right middle lobe that harbor the fistulae (see Figure 34–5).

Pulmonary arteriovenous fistulae usually come to light because of an abnormal shadow on chest x-ray, because of cyanosis, or because of bleeding caused by mucocutaneous telangiectasia (Rendu, Osler, Weber syndrome, tiny ruby lesions on the mucous membranes, lips and skin).[1]

Murmurs are systolic or continuous, and are often overlooked because they are faint and confined to atypical chest wall sites, i.e., over the lower lobes or right middle lobe.

Diagnosis is based upon selective pulmonary angiography during which the fistula or fistulae can be coil embolized.[2] Recurrence is common.[1,2]

References

1. Perloff JK. *The Clinical Recognition of Congenital Heart Disease, 4th ed*. Philadelphia. WB Saunders Co. 1994, pp. 91, 132, 546, 562, 581, 714.
2. Perloff JK, Child JS. *Congenital Heart Disease in Adults 2nd ed*. Philadelphia, WB Saunders Co., 1998.
3. Roberts WC, Glick BN. Congenital hypoplasia of both right and left circumflex coronary arteries. *Am J Cardiol* 1992;70:121–123.
4. Brunken RC, Perloff JK, Czernin J, et al. Adult patients with cyanotic congenital heart disease have a normal hyperemic coronary blood flow response. *J Am Coll Cardiol* (in press).
5. Roberts WC, Shirani J. Four subtypes of anomalous origin of the left main coronary artery from the right aortic sinus (or from the right coronary artery). *Am J Cardiol* 1992;70:119–121.
6. Rakusan K, Flanagan MF, Geva T, et al. Morphometry of human coronary capillaries during normal growth and the effect of age in left ventricular pressure-overload hypertrophy. *Circulation* 1992;86:38–46.
7. Gerber RS, Sherman CT, Sack JB, et al. Isolated paradoxical embolus to the right coronary artery. *Am J Cardiol* 1992;70:1633–1635.
8. Niwa K, Perloff JK, Bhuta SM, et al. Structural abnormalities of great arterial walls in congenital heart disease—prospective light and electron microscopic analyses. *Circulation* 2001;103:393–400.
9. Gatzoulis MA, Munk M, Merchant N, et al. Isolated congenital absence of the pericardium. *Ann Thorac Surg* 2000;69:1209–1215.
10. Bialostozky D, Horitz S, Espino-vela J. Ebstein's malformation of the tricuspid valve. A review of 65 cases. *Am J Cardiol* 1972;29:826–836.

35

"Chest Pain" in Patients with Aortic Valve Stenosis

Douglas C. Morris, MD

General Considerations

The chest pain customarily associated with aortic valve stenosis is secondary to myocardial ischemia. Since the cause of myocardial ischemia does not influence the features of cardiac ischemic pain, the characteristics of the pain accompanying aortic valve stenosis conforms; in general, to Heberden's description of angina pectoris (see Chapter 29).

Clinical Setting

Patients with angina pectoris and aortic valve stenosis are commonly older than 50 years of age. The condition occurs more commonly in males than females.

Characteristics of the "Pain"

The patient's characterization of the "chest pain," the common location of the "chest pain" (see Figures 35–1 and 35–2), the uncommon location of the "chest pain" (see Figure 35–3), the size of the "painful" area (see Figures 35–1 to 35–3), the duration of the "painful" sensation, the absence of tenderness of the chest wall, and the relief of the "chest pain" are similar to that of angina pectoris caused by obstructive coronary atherosclerosis. The precipitating cause of angina pectoris related to aortic stenosis is, however, almost always physical effort. Baker and Somerville emphasized

From: Hurst JW, Morris DC (eds): *"Chest Pain"* →. © Futura Publishing Co., Inc., Armonk, NY, 2001.

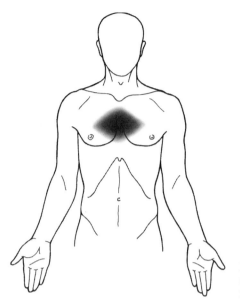

Figure 35–1. The usual location and size of the "chest pain" that is designated angina pectoris.

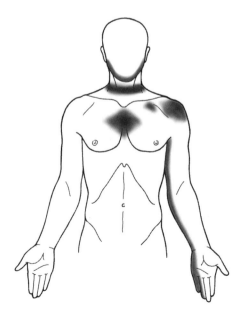

Figure 35–2. Common locations of the radiation of the "chest pain" that is designated angina pectoris. Note the radiation to the neck, jaw, left upper chest, left shoulder, inner surface of the left arm, left little finger, and left ring finger.

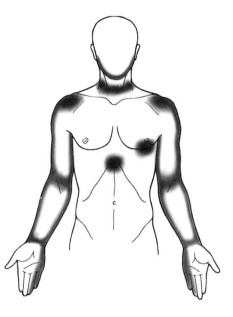

Figure 35–3. Unusual locations of the "pain" that is designated angina pectoris. The discomfort may be limited to the neck, jaw, right or left shoulder, left pectoral region, epigastrium, inner or outer surface of the right or left arms, elbows, wrists, or ring and little finger.

that, unlike angina pectoris caused by obstructive coronary atherosclerosis, that angina due to severe aortic valve stenosis was always provoked by effort, and not by emotional turmoil, exposure to cold, or following meals.[1] Also, the "pain" may not resolve as quickly as with the usual attacks of angina pectoris due to obstructive coronary atherosclerosis. This feature of the chest pain is of limited diagnostic value. Sublingual nitroglycerin must be used cautiously in the patient with aortic stenosis as it may produce syncope.

Associated Symptoms

Unlike the situation with coronary atherosclerosis, angina pectoris secondary to aortic stenosis is often associated with dyspnea and/or syncope or near syncope. These three symptoms are the cardinal features of severe aortic valve stenosis. This constellation of symptoms transiently experienced by the patient may explain why the patient on occasions may not perceive classic angina. The perception of one sensation may be overwhelmed, distorted, or obscured by a more intense unpleasantness. Angina and syncope are the consequences of left ventricular outflow obstruction and develop when the outflow obstruction is severe, but when left ventricular function is still adequate. These symptoms are characteristic of this condition and are rarely present in diseases of other heart valves.

The development of dyspnea often heralds the onset of left ventricular dysfunction.

Associated Signs

Physical examination

The physical signs associated with severe aortic valve stenosis reflect the pathophysiologic consequences of outflow obstruction of the left ventricle.[2] The amplitude of the pulse pressure is generally reduced secondary to a depression of the systolic pressure. In the elderly patient, however, the pulse pressure may be 60 mmHg or more, reflecting their less distensible arterial tree. Palpation of the carotid arteries may reveal pulsus parvus et tardus (small amplitude, gradual upslope, and gradual downslope pulse contour). Again the poorly distensible vessels of the elderly will obscure these alterations in the arterial pulse. Palpation of the chest will characteristically reveal a sustained, or "heaving," apical impulse. In addition to this heaving left ventricular impulse, there is often, but not invariably, a palpable presystolic pulsation. A systolic thrill may be felt in the second right intercostal space near the sternum.

The four characteristic auscultatory signs of aortic valve stenosis are the aortic ejection sound, the spindle-shaped systolic murmur, a delayed aortic valve closure sound with decreased intensity, and an early diastolic murmur of slight aortic regurgitation. The aortic ejection sound is a high-frequency sound occurring 0.04 to 0.08 seconds after the onset of the first sound, and is usually louder at the apex. As the aortic leaflets become calcified, the ejection sound will disappear. It is heard in less than one-third of adults with aortic valve stenosis.[3] The most consistent physical finding of aortic valve stenosis is a basal systolic murmur. The only invariable feature of this murmur is its diamond, spindle, or crescendo-decrescendo shape. The murmur is typically harsh, but may be higher pitched in the elderly. The murmur is generally loudest in the second right intercostal space near the sternum, but may be equally loud at the apex in the elderly. The murmur of aortic valve stenosis heard at the cardiac apex may be higher pitched than at the base of the heart and is not transmitted laterally like the murmur of mitral regurgitation. Although intensity, duration, and configuration of the murmur do not necessarily relate to the severity of the stenosis, some general conclusions can be drawn. The longer and louder the murmur and the later its systolic peak, the more likely that the stenosis is severe. The second heart sound is generally single (reflecting delayed aortic closure), occasionally paradoxically split, and infrequently physiologically split. One-third to one-half of patients with essentially "pure" aortic stenosis will have an early diastolic murmur audible at the base. Generally, this high-pitched decrescendo murmur reflects mild, inconsequential aortic valve regurgitation.[4]

Routine laboratory tests

Sinus rhythm is the rule in isolated aortic valve stenosis regardless of severity. Atrial fibrillation suggests coexisting mitral valve disease unless it occurs in the elderly in whom atrial fibrillation is common. The P waves in the electrocardiogram may demonstrate a left atrial abnormality as a consequence of severe left ventricular hypertrophy. The sequential changes in the QRS and T wave generally reflect the course and severity of aortic stenosis. With mild to moderate aortic valve stenosis, the electrocardiogram may be normal, but with severe stenosis the electrocardiogram reveals signs of left ventricular hypertrophy due to systolic pressure overload of the left ventricle. The mean spatial ST and T wave vectors are often directed 60° to 180° away from the spatial direction of the mean QRS vector. The QRS complexes reveal an increase in size with the 12-lead amplitude being greater than 180 millimeters. The mean QRS vector is usually directed normally: the so-called abnormal left axis deviation of the QRS vector is not a useful sign of left ventricular hypertrophy.

The cardiac silhouette on chest x-ray film is only mildly to moderately enlarged. There may be an abnormal contour of the cardiac silhouette caused by a convex bulging of the lower one-third of the left cardiac border secondary to concentric hypertrophy of the left ventricle. The other alteration in structural configuration commonly noted with aortic stenosis is dilatation of the ascending aorta. While this poststenotic dilatation is a common feature of aortic stenosis (75% to 85%), the degree of dilatation does not reflect the severity of the stenosis.[1,3,4] Calcification of the aortic valve is occasionally apparent on the lateral chest x-ray film, but is consistently present on fluoroscopy in the patient over age 40.

Exceptions to the Usual Manifestations

The exceptions to the usual manifestations of aortic valve stenosis occur generally in the elderly patient. The changes characteristic of the carotid pulse may be obscured and "normalized" by the rigid, noncompliant vessels of the elderly. Moreover, the rigid shelves of tissue, without commissural fusion, which are found in the elderly will likely produce a more high-pitched, musical type murmur. This murmur may be as loud or louder at the apex as at the second intercostal space.

Differential Diagnosis

The differential diagnosis of "chest pain" occurring in patients with aortic valve stenosis is similar to the differential diagnosis of "chest pain" in patients without aortic valve stenosis (see Chapter 29).

The determination of etiology of the systolic murmur in the second right intercostal space requires additional discussion. The differential diagnosis in the child and the young adult is between valvular aortic stenosis, subvalvular stenosis, and, much less likely, supravalvular aortic stenosis. Subvalvular stenosis could be either hypertrophic cardiomyopathy or membraneous subaortic stenosis. Neither of these forms of obstruction will present with an ejection sound. Hypertrophic subaortic stenosis rarely has an associated aortic regurgitation murmur, whereas such a murmur is common in patients with membraneous subaortic stenosis. The carotid pulse contour should also serve as a distinguishing feature between valvular and hypertrophic subaortic stenosis. Unlike valvular aortic stenosis, the upstroke of the carotid pulse in the latter rises abruptly and, frequently, there is pulsus bisferiens.

In the elderly patient, the differential diagnosis is between symptomatic severe valvular aortic valve stenosis and aortic valvular sclerosis with associated coronary atherosclerosis causing angina, or another comorbid condition causing syncope. The systolic murmur of aortic valve sclerosis peaks early in systole and the aortic valve closure sound is normal. The systolic murmur of severe aortic valve stenosis peaks in late systole and the aortic valve closure sound is faint. Paradoxical splitting of the second sound may be present in patients with severe aortic valve stenosis. Left ventricular hypertrophy is frequently present in patients with aortic valve stenosis. This finding, however, is not totally reliable in the elderly as it may be absent even in the presence of aortic stenosis, and may be present in the elderly patient with valvular sclerosis and longstanding systemic hypertension. The height of the systolic blood pressure may clarify the situation as it is rarely above 180mmHg in severe aortic stenosis. Patients with aortic valve sclerosis must be followed carefully because they commonly develop aortic valve stenosis as well as coronary atherosclerotic heart disease.

Other Diagnostic Testing

Cardiac catheterization with simultaneous recording of pressures in the left ventricular chamber and the proximal aorta remains the most accurate means of determining the severity of aortic valve stenosis. Contrast ventriculography coupled with measurement of diastolic left ventricular pressures will provide an accurate assessment of the state of ventricular function.

All patients with angina pectoris and aortic valve stenosis should have cardiac catheterization including coronary arteriography. The objective of the latter is to ascertain if the angina pectoris is due to aortic valve stenosis without obstructive coronary artery disease, or if the angina is due to obstructive coronary artery disease in addition to aortic valve stenosis. This information is needed to guide the cardiac surgeon.

Echocardiography is extremely helpful in both differentiating valvular aortic stenosis from the other conditions described above and in assessing the severity of the stenosis. The eccentric opening of a bicuspid aortic valve can be visualized with echocardiography as well as thickening, fibrosis, and calcification of the leaflets. In addition, the consequences of the stenosis such as concentric hypertrophy of the left ventricle or decreased systolic function will be apparent. Doppler echocardiography when applied by capable personnel is reliable in defining the valve gradient and the aortic valve area. The aortic valve area can be calculated using the continuity equation by measuring the velocity of the jet across the aortic valve with continuous-waveform Doppler; the velocity of the left ventricular outflow tract just proximal to the valve with pulse-form Doppler; and by measuring the area of the opening of the valve on cross-section echocardiographic view.[5–7]

Etiology and Basic Mechanisms Responsible for the "Pain"

The etiology of aortic valve stenosis is: congenital bicuspid valve stenosis which may become calcified in later life, rheumatic heart disease which has almost disappeared in the United States, aortic valve stenosis of the elderly that evolves from aortic valve sclerosis, which may be related to hyperlipidemia and the atherosclerotic process, and drug induced aortic valve stenosis from anti-appetite drugs.

Angina pectoris may occur in patients with aortic valve stenosis for two reasons. The patient may have sufficient coronary atherosclerosis in addition to aortic valve stenosis to produce angina pectoris, or the patient may have severe aortic valve stenosis and left ventricular hypertrophy with little or no evidence of obstructive coronary atherosclerosis or coronary arteriography.

The mechanism of anginal pain in patients with aortic valve stenosis who have no obstructive coronary disease is as follows. The increased left ventricular muscle mass, elevation of left ventricular pressures (the elevated left ventricular end-diastolic pressure lowers the diastolic aortic-left ventricular pressure gradient), and prolongation of the systolic ejection time all contribute to an increase in myocardial oxygen requirements with severe aortic valve stenosis. Futhermore, while total coronary blood flow is increased due to the left ventricular hypertrophy; coronary blood flow per given quantity of ventricular mass is reduced. Consequently, subendocardial blood flow is inadequate at rest; and because the cardiac output is relatively fixed by the left ventricular outflow obstruction, myocardial blood flow relative to need is reduced further during exertion. An impairment in coronary artery reserve has been established in patients with aortic stenosis and is probably an important contributor to the pathogenesis of angina in these patients. One explanation proposed is that the growth of coronary-resistance vessels does not keep pace with the increase in left ventricular mass.[8] Other factors which are specific to aortic stenosis, which have been proposed as contributing to diminished coronary reserve, include: prolongation of systole at the expense of diastole (80% of coronary flow to the left ventricle occurs in diastole); the possibility that the Venturi phenomenon may impair inflow into the coronary orifice; and the possibility that the hypertrophied myocardium compresses the intramyocardial arteries.[3]

The afferent pathway for the transmission of nociception associated with ischemia are the small sympathetic nerve fibers running parallel to the coronary arteries. These nerve fibers enter the spinal cord in the C8-T4 segment. Experimental validation of this pathway lies in the fact that thoracic sympathectomy or section of the higher thoracic dorsal roots was capable of relieving anginal pain.[4] The impulses are then transmitted through the spinal cord to the thalamus and cerebral cortex. Angina pectoris, like other pain of visceral origin, is often poorly localized and is commonly referred to the corresponding segmental dermatones.

Treatment

Exercise restrictions are recommended for all patients with aortic valve stenosis except those with mild disease. Careful follow-up is mandatory because the development of symptoms, including angina pectoris, in patients with severe aortic valvular stenosis demand valve replacement. There is no suitable nonsurgical solution for the patient with symptomatic severe aortic stenosis including those with angina pectoris. Sublingual nitroglycerin fails to consistently relieve angina as it does in patients who only have coronary atherosclerotic heart disease. In addition, sublingual nitroglycerin may precipitate syncope in patients with aortic valve stenosis. All other drugs used for the relief of angina are less valuable than they are in angina that is not associated with aortic valve stenosis and their undesirable side effects are greater. Balloon valvuloplasty is a risky, palliative procedure at its best. Whether valve replacement is warranted in the asymptomatic patient with severe aortic stenosis is debatable, but a reasonable case can be made for those patients with a valve area of less than

0.5 cm^2 and left ventricular hypertrophy with secondary ST-T wave changes in the electrocardiogram.

References

1. Baker C, Somerville J. Clinical features and surgical treatment of fifty patients with severe aortic stenosis. *Guys Hosp Rep* 1959;108:101.
2. Selzer A. Changing aspects of the natural history of valvular aortic stenosis. *N Engl J Med* 1987;317:91–98.
3. Wood P. Aortic stenosis. *Am J Cardiol* 1958;1:553–571.
4. Crawley IS, Morris DC, Silverman BD. Valvular heart disease. In Hurst JW, Logue RB, Schlant RC, et al. (eds): *The Heart Arteries and Veins*. McGraw-Hill Book Company, New York, 1978, pp. 992–1081.
5. Feigenbaum H. *Echocardiography*. Baltimore, Williams and Wilkins, 1993, pp. 239–349.
6. Marcus ML, Doty DB, Hiratzka LF, et al. Decreased coronary reserve: A mechanism for angina pectoris in patients with aortic stenosis and normal coronary arteries. *N Engl J Med* 1982;307:1362–1367.
7. Hakki A-H, Kimbiris D, Iskandrian AS, et al. Angina pectoris and coronary artery disease in patients with severe aortic valvular disease. *Am Heart J* 1980;100:441–448.
8. Malliani A. The elusive link between transient myocardial ischemia and pain. *Circulation* 1986;73:201–204.

36

"Chest Pain" in Patients with Aortic Valve Regurgitation

Douglas C. Morris, MD

General Considerations

There are many causes of acute and chronic aortic valve regurgitation (see Table 36–1). The most common causes of severe aortic regurgitation in the United States are the floppy valve syndrome with associated aortic root/annular dilatation and congenital bicuspid aortic valve. The floppy valve is characterized by myxomatous transformation of the leaflets and cystic medial necrosis of the aortic root.[1] Other relatively common causes include infective endocarditis and rheumatic valvulitis.

Clinical Setting

Both the bicuspid valve and severe myxomatous changes are more common in men. Accordingly, aortic valve regurgitation is predominantly a disease of men. The reported prevalence of angina pectoris in patients with aortic regurgitation is 3% to 30% as compared to a prevalence of 40% to 80% in patients with predominant aortic stenosis.[2] The prevalence of angina associated with aortic valve regurgitation, as well as any symptom, has been markedly reduced by the general endorsement of the concept that patients with chronic severe aortic regurgitation should have valve replacement prior to the development of symptoms.

Characteristics of the "Pain"

The patient's characterization of the "chest pain," the common location of the "chest pain" (see Figures 36–1 and 36–2), the uncommon loca-

From: Hurst JW, Morris DC (eds): *"Chest Pain"* →. © Futura Publishing Co., Inc., Armonk, NY, 2001.

Table 36–1.
Causes of Aortic Valve Regurgitation.

Chronic causes of aortic valve regurgitation.

Systemic hypertension
Rheumatic heart disease
Syphilitic aortitis
Annuloaorto ectasia
Bicuspid aortic valve (congenital)
Aortic valve stenosis of the elderly
Osteogenesis imperfecti
Kyphoscoliosis
Marfan syndrome

Acute causes of aortic valve regurgitation.

Infective endocarditis of the aortic valve
Dissection of the proximal aorta
Marfan syndrome
Trauma

Note that some of the causes of aortic valve regurgitation are listed under chronic and acute causes. Angina pectoris only occurs in patients with rather severe aortic regurgitation.

tion of the "chest pain" (see Figure 36–3), the size of the "painful" area, the lack of tenderness of the chest wall, and the relief of the "chest pain" are similar to angina pectoris due to coronary atherosclerosis. The duration of angina pectoris, the propensity to nocturnal angina, and the lack of prompt relief of angina pectoris with sublingual nitroglycerin are more common in patients with aortic valve regurgitation than it is with angina pectoris due to coronary atherosclerosis.[3]

Associated Symptoms

Chronic aortic regurgitation is generally characterized by a prolonged course with little disability for a number of years. The very observant patient may first become aware of the *increased force of cardiac contraction* as manifest by visible or palpable precordial or cervical pulsations. If there is associated ventricular ectopy, the hyperdynamic pulsations are even more disturbing.[4] If the disease is allowed to progress long enough, the patient will develop exertional dyspnea, orthopnea, paroxysmal nocturnal dispense, and easy fatigability as a result of elevated pulmonary venous pressure. Severe *dyspnea* occurs abruptly in acute severe aortic valve regurgitation as a consequence of the imposition of a severe diastolic overload on a relatively unprepared left ventricle.

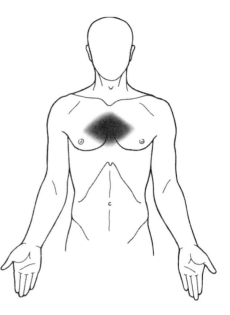

Figure 36–1. The common location of the "chest pain" due to angina pectoris in patients with aortic valve regurgitation.

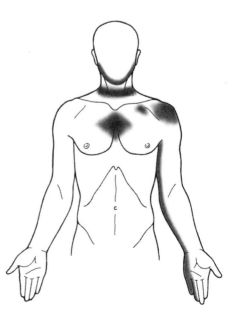

Figure 36–2. The common location of the radiation of "chest pain" due to angina pectoris in patients with aortic valve regurgitation.

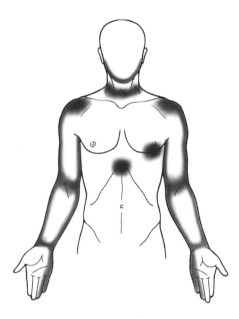

Figure 36–3. The uncommon locations of the chest pain due to angina pectoris in patients with aortic regurgitation. The "pain" may be limited to any one of the areas illustrated above.

Associated Signs

Physical examination

The physical findings in the patients with aortic regurgitation reflect the wide pulse pressure, the volume overload of the left ventricle, and the diastolic return of blood into the left ventricle. The pulse pressure is typically greater than one half of the systolic blood pressure and produces a number of peripheral manifestations such as Corrigan's pulse, Quincke's sign, Muller's sign, de Musset's sign, and Duroziez's murmur. The volume overloaded left ventricle is manifested as an overactive and inferiorly and laterally displaced apical impulse. The regurgitant blood flow produces a high-frequency decrescendo diastolic murmur along the left sternal border. This murmur is often accompanied by a systolic murmur reflecting the increased volume of blood being ejected from the left ventricle. Severe aortic regurgitation may cause a diastolic rumble (Austin Flint murmur) at the apex.

"Routine" laboratory tests

The *electrocardiogram* in patients with chronic aortic valve regurgitation may reveal evidence of left ventricular hypertrophy. A left atrial abnormality may be present. The QRS amplitude may be increased, although the mean QRS vector is commonly directed normally. Diastolic overload of the left ventricle produces a different affect on the repolarization process than systolic pressure overload. The large left ventricular cavity with its increase in surface area of the endocardium may produce a large initial QRS force, and large mean ST and T wave vectors that are generally relatively parallel to the large QRS vector. Later in the course of the aortic valve regurgitation the mean ST and T vectors will drift 90° to 180° away from the mean QRS vector and simulate the electrocardiographic changes of systolic pressure overload of the left ventricle as discussed in Chapter 32.

The electrocardiogram of acute aortic valve regurgitation may initially reveal no abnormalities.

The only noteworthy change on the *chest x-ray film* in patients with aortic valve regurgitation is enlargement of the left ventricle with inferior and lateral elongation of the cardiac apex. The ascending aorta is not typically dilated in patients with aortic valve regurgitation unless the etiology of the regurgitation is disease of the aortic root, such as aorto-annular ectasia or proximal aortic dissection.

Differential Diagnosis

Probably the most difficult differential to make with regard to aortic regurgitation is differentiating pure aortic regurgitation and combined aortic valvular disease. The wide pulse pressure is the hallmark of chronic severe aortic regurgitation and is absent when both conditions are present. A palpable fourth heart sound and calcified aortic valve leaflets are features of the other two conditions and not aortic regurgitation.

The regurgitant murmur of severe aortic valve regurgitation is distinguished from the pulmonic valve regurgitant murmur by the widened pulse pressure. Occasionally, the point of maximal intensity of the diastolic murmur will distinguish aortic root disease from aortic valvular disease. In patients with valvular lesions, the murmur is usually maximal intensity at the lower left sternal border or midsternal border. If the regurgitation is related to dilatation of the ascending aorta, the murmur is commonly loudest along the right sternal border.

Other Diagnostic Testing

Echocardiography/Doppler is beneficial in establishing the presence and severity of aortic regurgitation, defining its etiology, and determining the appropriate timing of surgery based upon left ventricular volume and function.[5] A marker of regurgitant severity is the rapidity with which the aortoventricular pressure gradient falls during diastole. The accepted index is the time required for half of the initial gradient to equilibrate. An index (pressure half-time) of less than 250 milliseconds is associated with moderate to severe aortic regurgitation. An end-systolic dimension of the left ventricle that is greater than 55mm, or an ejection fraction of less than 50% in the patient with chronic aortic regurgitation warrant vale replacement.

Cardiac catheterization allows for left ventriculography to define left ventricular size and function, aortography to define the dimensions of the aortic root and provide a semiquantitative assessment of the severity of the regurgitation, and coronary angiography to define the coronary anatomy.

Etiology and Basic Mechanisms Responsible for the "Pain"

There are numerous causes of aortic valve regurgitation (see Table 36–1). Angina pectoris is uncommon in patients with mild aortic valve regurgitation unless there is associated coronary atherosclerosis.

The obvious reason for angina pectoris in the majority of patients with aortic regurgitation is the associated presence of coronary atherosclerosis.[3] Angina pectoris in patients without coronary atherosclerosis is usually ascribed to reduced effective coronary blood flow secondary to a low diastolic aortic pressure coupled with an increase in wall tension secondary to increased left ventricular volume load.[4] Furthermore, much like the situation with aortic stenosis, a reduced capacity for augmenting coronary blood flow to meet the demands of exercise seems to exist in some patients.

The inclination for patients with moderately severe aortic valve regurgitation to have angina pectoris at rest and nocturnally has been explained as follows. Such patients have an increase in afterload when they are at rest or sleeping. In addition, patients with severe aortic valve regurgitation may experience an exaggeration of the physiologic derangement of heart failure during sleep.[3]

Treatment

The usual pharmacological treatment of angina pectoris in patients with severe aortic valve regurgitation is not satisfactory. Such patients need aortic valve surgery.

All patients with chronic aortic regurgitation require endocarditis prophylaxis. Patients with mild aortic regurgitation require no other treatment. The asymptomatic patient with severe aortic regurgitation benefits in terms of reducing the likelihood of symptoms and need for valve replacement from long-term administration of long-acting nifedipine or an ACE inhibitor.

A logical extension of this assertion is to apply the same therapy to the patient with moderate aortic regurgitation.

Decisions about valve replacement in aortic regurgitation should be based on the New York Heart Association's clinical functional class, electrocardiographic changes, and left ventricular dimensions and ejection fraction.

For details on management of aortic regurgitation see Bonow RO, Carabello B, de Leon AC Jr., et al: ACC/AHA guidelines for the management of valvular heart disease. J Am Coll Cardiol 1998.

References

1. Read RC, Thal AP, Wendt VE. Symptomatic valvular myxomatous transformation (the floppy valve syndrome): A possible forme fruste of the Marfan syndrome. *Circulation* 1965;32:897.
2. Hakki A-H, Kimbiris D, Iskandrian AS, et al. Angina pectoris and coronary artery disease in patients with severe aortic valvular disease. *Am Heart J* 1980;100:441–448.
3. Basta LL, Raines D, Najjar S, et al. Clinical, haemodynamic and coronary angiographic correlates of angina pectoris in patients with severe aortic valve disease. Br Heart J 1975;37:150–157.
4. Crawley IS, Morris DC, Silverman BD. Valvular heart disease. In: Hurst JW, Logue RB, Schlant RC, et al. (eds): *The Heart.* New York: McGraw-Hill Book Company, 1978, pp. 992–1081.
5. Donovan CL, Starling MR. Role of echocardiography in the timing of surgical intervention for chronic mitral and aortic regurgitation. In: Otto CM (ed): *The Practice of Clinical Echocardiography.* Philadelphia: WB Saunders Company, 1997, pp. 327–354.

"Chest Pain" in Patients with Rheumatic Mitral Valve Stenosis

Douglas C. Morris MD

General Considerations

Unlike the situation with aortic valve disease, particularly aortic valve stenosis, angina pectoris is uncommon in patients with mitral valve disease. Less than 10% of patients with rheumatic mitral stenosis experience chest pain indistinguishable from angina pectoris due to coronary atherosclerosis.

Clinical Setting

Clinically manifested rheumatic mitral stenosis usually takes about 10 years from the occurrence of rheumatic fever to develop, and 20 years to become symptomatic. Therefore, symptomatic mitral valve stenosis usually appears in the third or fourth decade of life.[1] Two important variations on this natural history have become apparent in recent years. The first is the development of severe mitral valve stenosis in the very young. This variation is isolated to the underdeveloped countries. The reasons for the early appearance of the disease are unclear, but the possibilities include occurrence of rheumatic fever at a very early age, multiple bouts of rheumatic fever, or lack of treatment. The clinical manifestations are comparable to mitral valve stenosis in the adult, except that growth retardation is a prominent feature.[2] The other variation is that mitral valve stenosis may be initially recognized in the elderly patient. Elderly patients seldom provide a reliable history of previous rheumatic fever and physicians may forget to ask about the symptoms of chorea.

From: Hurst JW, Morris DC (eds): *"Chest Pain"* →. © Futura Publishing Co., Inc., Armonk, NY, 2001.

Characteristics of the "Pain"

Patients with rheumatic mitral valve stenosis may have "chest pain" secondary to the recumbent cough reflecting pulmonary venous hypertension, the development of pneumonia to which patients with mitral valve stenosis are predisposed, and pulmonary emboli secondary to atrial fibrillation. In each of these circumstances, the patient is pleuritic and isolated to a particular area of the chest. The chest "pain" associated with pulmonary embolism is discussed in Chapter 16. The presence of typical angina pectoris in a patient with mitral valve stenosis warrants an evaluation to exclude the existence of coronary atherosclerosis. The purpose of this chapter is to discuss the occurrence of angina pectoris in patients with mitral valve stenosis who may experience the "pain" secondary to pulmonary hypertension.

The patient's characterization of the "chest pain"

The common location of the "chest pain" (see Figure 37–1), the uncommon location of the "chest pain," the size of the painful area, the duration of the "chest pain," the lack of tenderness of the chest wall, the precipitating causes of the "chest pain," and the relief of the "chest pain" are similar to angina pectoris due to coronary atherosclerosis (see Chapter 29) with a few exceptions. The "chest pain" due to pulmonary hypertension may be pre-

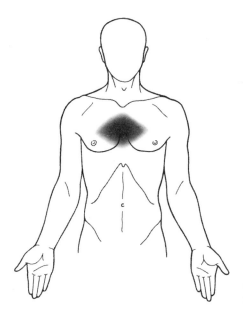

Figure 37–1. The usual location and size of the "chest pain" that is designated angina pectoris.

cipitated by effort, but it is almost always associated with severe dyspnea and seems to last longer than the "pain" of angina due to coronary athero-sclerosis. Atrial fibrillation with a rapid rate may precipitate "chest pain" that lasts longer than angina due to coronary artery disease. Finally, sublin-gual nitroglycerin does not seem to relieve the discomfort as promptly as it does with angina due to coronary atherosclerosis.

A cardinal feature of mitral valve stenosis is dyspnea. The patient may describe this subjective awareness of an increased work of breathing as chest discomfort. This discomfort is usually perceived as a diffuse precor-dial sensation related to exertion but also to recumbent position. It usually appears and abates more insidiously than angina pectoris. Sublingual ni-troglycerin may afford some relief by reducing the left atrial hypertension and reducing pulmonary congestion. The discomfort of dyspnea does not radiate outside the confines of the precordium.

Associated Symptoms

Angina pectoris occurs in a small percentage of patients with mitral stenosis. Patients with angina pectoris due to pulmonary hypertension al-most always have other symptoms of mitral valve obstruction in addition to angina pectoris. The most frequent symptomatic manifestations of mi-tral valve stenosis are dyspnea and fatigue. The dyspnea usually develops gradually. Initially, it occurs only with exertion, but later is expressed as orthopnea and paroxysmal nocturnal dyspnea. The dyspnea may, how-ever, develop abruptly in concert with the appearance of atrial fibrillation. It is also striking that many patients with mitral valve stenosis gradually curtail their physical activity in response to the increased respiratory work without ever actually perceiving the sensation of dyspnea.

Fatigue, the clinical correlate of a low cardiac output, often appears as the dyspnea dissipates. The reduced cardiac output is usually precipitated by the development of atrial fibrillation or right ventricular decompensation.[2]

Associated Signs

In the patient with mitral stenosis, the *jugular venous waves* reflect the presence and degree of pulmonary hypertension (large A wave), right ven-tricular failure (large A and V waves), and tricuspid regurgitation (large V wave). The apical impulse would only be remarkable if it is displaced or diffuse, as the left ventricle should not be affected by mitral valve stenosis. Noteworthy findings on palpation of the chest in mitral valve stenosis are a palpable first sound, a palpable pulmonary valve closure sound, and a palpable right ventricular lift along the left sternal border.

The *auscultatory hallmarks* of mitral valve stenosis are a loud first sound, an opening snap (heard over the anterior chest), a diastolic rumble (heard only at the apex), and accentuation of the pulmonary valve closure sound. The most sensitive auscultatory index of the severity of mitral valve stenosis is the aortic valve closure to opening snap interval, except when there is high left ventricular diastolic pressure from aortic valve disease which alters the left atrial/left ventricular diastolic pressure gradient. Also, in older patients a long interval may occur despite severe mitral valve stenosis. The existence of pulmonary hypertension is evidenced by the accentuation of the pulmonary valve closure sound. An accentuated pulmonic valve closure sound is heard at the apex where it is not normally heard.

In sinus rhythm, the *electrocardiogram* shows left atrial abnormality and a vertical mean QRS vector that remains posteriorly directed. In atrial fibrillation, the fibrillatory waves are usually coarse. As time passes the mean QRS vector shifts to the right and anteriorly, signifying the presence of right ventricular hypertrophy.

The *chest x-ray film* in the patient with mitral valve stenosis usually demonstates evidence of left atrial enlargement and pulmonary venous congestion. The left atrial appendage may be seen along the left cardiac border just below the enlarged main pulmonary artery. Calcification of the mitral valve and Kerley B lines may be seen.

Differential Diagnosis

The recognition of angina pectoris in patients with mitral valve stenosis leads to the following problem: Is the angina pectoris caused by the pulmonary hypertension secondary to severe mitral valve stenosis only, or does the patient with mitral valve stenosis have additional coronary atherosclerosis? Regardless of whether there are clues to the presence of pulmonary hypertension, one should assume that additional coronary atherosclerosis might be present and plan diagnostic testing, including a coronary arteriogram.

If the patient is a female under the age of 40 years and there is evidence of pulmonary hypertension, the angina pectoris is probably caused by pulmonary hypertension. When the patient is a male this assumption is not as reliable as it is in females.

Since angina pectoris is relatively infrequent in patients with mitral stenosis, its presence may call into question the correctness of the diagnosis of mitral valve stenosis. The three cardiac conditions, which to some degree may mimic mitral stenosis, are severe chronic aortic valve regurgitation, secundum atrial septal defect, and left atrial myxoma.

Severe aortic regurgitation may present with a late diastolic rumble at the cardiac apex (Austin Flint murmur) reflecting partial closure of the anterior mistral leaflet due to regurgitation flow. In such patients, however, there should be clear evidence of an enlarged, volume overloaded left ventricle and no opening snap.

In the patient with a *large secundum atrial septal defect*, there might be a diastolic rumble reflecting increased flow across the tricuspid valve. Again, there will be no opening snap, but there will be fixed splitting of the second sound (not the case with mitral valve stenosis). The rumble across the tricuspid valve is usually more medium pitched in comparison to the mitral low-pitched rumble. The chest x-ray film does not demonstrate left atrial enlargement or pulmonary venous hypertension in patients with a secundum atrial septal defect. The main pulmonary arteries and its branches are large while the aortic knob is small. While most secundum atrial septal defects are not large enough to produce a tricuspid rumble, the echocardiogram (see below) is especially useful in making the distinction between a secundum atrial septal defect and mitral valve stenosis when the need arises.

An *atrial myxoma* mimics mitral stenosis only in that it produces evidence of left atrial outflow obstruction. The tumor plop is a generally low-pitched thud rather than the high-pitched opening sound associated with mitral valve stenosis. Furthermore, the symptoms and auscultatory sounds associated with an atrial myxoma are more paroxysmal or episodic than is the case with mitral valve stenosis.

Other Diagnostic Testing

Patients with rheumatic mitral stenosis may have additional coronary atherosclerosis. Accordingly, it is essential to separate the patients with angina pectoris due to pulmonary hypertension from the patients with mitral valve stenosis who may also have coronary atherosclerosis. Patients who are older than 40 years should have coronary arteriograms performed prior to mitral valve surgery. Patients under age 40 should have coronary arteriography only if they have chest pain compatible with angina pectoris.

As alluded to in the preceding section, echocardiography is the most effective means of confirming or establishing the diagnosis of mitral valve stenosis. The pathologic changes associated with rheumatic valvulitis are all visible on transthoracic echocardiography. These changes include fusion of the commissures, thickening and calcification of the valve leaflets, and fusion and shortening of the chordae tendineae. An echocardiographic scoring based upon leaflet motion, leaflet thickening, subvalvular disease, and commissural calcium serves as a guide for the selection of patients for percutaneous valvuloplasty. Echocardiography can also exclude the existence of an atrial mass (myxoma), volume overload of the right ventricle (typical of secundum atrial septal defect), and diastolic fluttering of the anterior mitral leaflet (seen in aortic regurgitation). Doppler flow velocity tracings accurately measure the left atrial-left ventricular diastolic pressure gradient. The Doppler pressure half-time gradient defined as the rate at which the mitral valve gradient declines to one-half the initial value can be used to calculate the mitral valve area. The mitral valve area can also be calculated using the Doppler continuity equation.

Etiology and Basic Mechanisms Responsible for the "Pain"

Angina pectoris occurs in patients with mitral stenosis only if they have pulmonary hypertension, right ventricular systolic hypertension, and right ventricular hypertrophy or have associated coronary atherosclerosis. The systolic right ventricular intracavitary pressure is an important determinant of right ventricular coronary blood flow. Unlike left ventricular coronary blood flow, which is confined almost exclusively to diastole, right ventricular systolic and diastolic pressures being normally less than the systolic and diastolic pressure in the aorta allows for continuous coronary blood flow. When the systolic pressure within the right ventricle becomes elevated the pressure gradient between aorta and right ventricle decreases and coronary blood flow decreases to the right ventricular myocardium. In addition, with severe pulmonary hypertension, the diastolic pressure in the right ventricle may increase to the point that it lowers the aortic to right ventricular diastolic pressure gradient and reduces the coronary flow to the right ventricular myocardium.[3] Rarely, the myocardial ischemia is caused by coronary embolization.

Patients with mitral valve stenosis who have angina pectoris *and* coronary atherosclerosis are usually recognized by coronary arteriography. The mechanism of "chest pain" is similar to that discussed in Chapter 27. In addition to the usual mechanism responsible for angina pectoris, the patient with significant mitral valve stenosis may be unable to increase their cardiac outputs with effort. (Refer to Chapter 27 for a discussion of the afferent nerve pathways for the perception of pain of myocardial ischemia).

Treatment

The immediate management approach to those patients experiencing angina as a consequence of pulmonary hypertension is to have them curtail those activities eliciting angina pectoris followed by urgent percutaneous or surgical intervention.

Any patient with symptomatic mitral stenosis, *including those patients with angina pectoris due to right ventricular hypertension,* warrants valvuloplasty or valve replacement. The expectation is that successful intervention will result in resolution of the pulmonary hypertension over the ensuing few months. The one possible exception to this management approach is the patient with new onset atrial fibrillation. In these patients, cardioversion or rate control might afford resolution of their symptoms. Regardless of the patient's response to cardioversion, the appearance of atrial fibrillation usually implies the development of atrial enlargement and atrial myopathy. Such a development is a reason to consider intervention on the valve.

References

1. Rowe JC, Bland EF, Sprague HB, et al. The course of mitral stenosis without surgery: Ten- and twenty-year perspectives. *Ann Intern Med* 1960;52:741–749.
2. Reichek N, Shelburne JC, Perloff JK. Clinical aspects of rheumatic valvular disease. *Prog Cardiovasc Dis* 1973;15:491–502.
3. Ross RS. Right ventricular hypertension as a cause of precordial pain. *Am Heart J* 1961;61:134–135.

38

"Chest Pain" in Patients with Hypertrophic Cardiomyopathy

Douglas C. Morris, MD

General Consideration

The clinical diagnosis of hypertrophic cardiomyopathy is based upon the presence of a thicker than normal left ventricular wall associated with a nondilated left ventricular cavity in the absence of any cardiac or systemic process capable of producing the hypertrophy. Most commonly, the pattern of hypertrophy is diffuse and concentric involving both the septum and the lateral free wall. Less frequently, the hypertrophy is asymmetrical. Ventricular septal hypertrophy is by far the most common type of asymmetrical hypertrophy, with midventricular and apical hypertrophy being less common.

Hypertrophic cardiomyopathy is a heterogeneous disease of the sarcomeres that basically follows a mendelian dominant inheritance. While the inheritance of hypertrophic cardiomyopathy is heterogeneous, so are the phenotypic manifestations.[1] There are frequent, sporadically appearing cases that are subsequently transmitted with the same pattern of inheritance. "Chest pain" is one of the most common symptoms in patients with hypertrophic cardiomyopathy and is the presenting symptom in approximately 10 percent of the patients.[2]

Clinical Setting

The disease has a bimodal distribution of appearance, either between the early teenage years and age 35 or after age 60. The condition occurs more commonly in males than females.

From: Hurst JW, Morris DC (eds): *"Chest Pain"* →. © Futura Publishing Co., Inc., Armonk, NY, 2001.

Characteristics of the "Pain"

Regional myocardial ischemia occurs in hypertrophic cardiomyopathy and is responsible for the chest pain. As emphasized in other sections of this book, "chest pain" due to myocardial ischemia will always be perceived the same regardless of its etiology. The "pain" is located in the area illustrated in Figure 38–1. Therefore, the patient's characterization of the "chest pain," the common location of the "chest pain" (see Figures 38–1 and 38–2), the uncommon locations of the "chest pain," the size of the painful area, and the lack of tenderness of the chest wall, are similar to the description of angina pectoris discussed in Chapter 29. There are three important exceptions. They are: the "chest pain" may last longer than the chest pain due to obstructive coronary atheroslcerosis; the "chest pain" often occurs at rest rather than with effort; and the "chest pain"may not be relieved with nitroglycerin.[3]

Each of these exceptions is accounted for by the pathophysiological features of the disease, which give rise to the angina. (Refer to section on Etiology and Basic Mechanisms Responsible for the "Pain.") While patients with outflow obstruction and those without obstruction may have angina, the patients with nonobstructive hypertrophic cardiomyopathy present with angina less frequently.[1]

Pasternac and associates make an important distinction between the "chest pain" generally associated with hypertrophic cardiomyopathy and that generally associated with a dilated cardiomyopathy by declaring that,

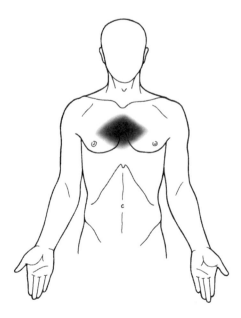

Figure 38–1. The usual location and size of the "chest pain" that is due to angina pectoris in patients with hypertrophic cardiomyopathy. The location of the "pain" is similar to that produced by obstructive coronary disease.

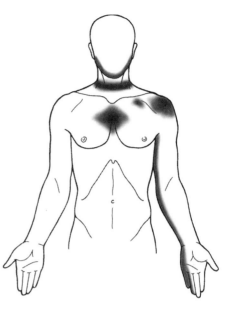

Figure 38–2. The usual distribution of the radiation of the "chest pain" that is characteristic of angina pectoris is shown in this illustration. The radiation of angina pectoris due to hypertrophic cardiomyopathy is similar to that produced by obstructive coronary disease.

"39% to 72% of patients with idiopathic hypertrophic cardiomyopathy experience anginal pain and as many as 52% of patients with congestive cardiomyopathy report vague chest pain."[4]

Associated Symptoms

The clinical symptomatology of hypertrophic cardiomyopathy and valvular aortic stenosis has been considered to be indistinguishable. *Dyspnea*, *angina pectoris*, and *syncope* are the predominant symptoms in both. The major symptomatic difference in the two diseases is in the presenting symptom. Exertional angina is the initial symptom in the majority of patients with valvular aortic stenosis, while exertional dyspnea is the first complaint in approximately two-thirds of the patients with hypertrophic cardiomyopathy.[2]

The *syncope* associated with hypertrophic cardiomyopathy also tends to present under different circumstances than is the case with valvular aortic stenosis. The syncope with valvular aortic stenosis predictably occurs with exertion and carries a rather ominous prognosis. In hypertrophic cardiomyopathy, syncope is not necessarily associated with hemodynamic evidence of severe obstruction. Patients with hypertrophic cardiomyopathy may experience post-tussive syncope and sudden assumption of the erect position often results in dizziness, if not outright loss of consciousness. Some patients with hypertrophic cardiomyopathy experience syncope immediately after the cessation of exertion rather than during the actual physical effort.[2]

Palpitations, either secondary to ventricular ectopy or to atrial fibrillation, while an infrequent complaint in the patients with hypertrophic cardiomyopathy, are rarely mentioned by the patient with valvular aortic stenosis.

Associated Signs

Physical examination

The left ventricular hypertrophy is reflected by a variably displaced and forceful apical impulse and a fourth heart sound that is often palpable. Patients with nonobstructive hypertrophy have either no murmur or a faint grade 1/6 apical systolic murmur. Patients with outflow obstruction have a grade 3/6 to 4/6 systolic murmur generally of rather uniform intensity throughout the precordium. With appropriate provocation, such as the inhalation of amyl nitrite, assuming the upright posture, or the Valsalva maneuver, the murmur intensifies.[1] The response to Valsalva maneuver will distinguish hypertrophic cardiomyopathy from the murmur of valvular aortic stenosis. Another distinguishing feature is rapidly rising carotid pulse and pulsus bisferens in patients with hypertrophic cardiomyopathy which is unlike the slow rising, low amplitude carotid pulse that is typical of valvular aortic stenosis.

"Routine" laboratory tests

The electrocardiographic abnormalities produced by hypertrophic cardiomypathy are: a left atrial abnormality, increase in the amplitude of the QRS complexes, an abnormally directed initial QRS force producing abnormal Q waves, and a mean T vector directed 90° to 180° away from the mean QRS vector. A persistent ST segment vector may be directed toward the ventricular epicardium suggesting epicardial injury, and a huge T wave vector may be directed to the right upper quadrant in patients with apical hypertrophic cardiomyopathy. These abnormalities can simulate myocardial infarction leading to a serious diagnostic error.

The cardiac silhouette on the *chest x-ray film* is mildly or moderately enlarged with perhaps increased convexity to the left heart border. The elderly patient with obstructive cardiomyopathy may demonstrate a calcified mitral valve annulus on the chest x-ray film.

Differential Diagnosis

Hypertrophic cardiomyopathy has been referred to as the "great masquerader." The murmur associated with this condition can be misinterpreted as the murmur of aortic valvular disease, the murmur of pure mitral regurgitation, or the murmur of a ventricular septal defect. The angina pectoris is commonly thought to be a manifestation of coronary artery disease, particularly, if Q waves on the electrocardiogram are diagnosed as a previous myocardial infarction.

Other Diagnostic Testing

Echocardiography is the most useful diagnostic technique for establishing the presence of hypertrophic cardiomyopathy and for defining the anatomical changes associated with the condition and the physiologic consequences of the changes. *Exercise electrocardiography or ambulatory monitoring* may be of value in establishing the presence of and defining the extent of ventricular ectopy. *Cardiac catheterization* is only necessary to define coronary anatomy in certain select patients, to define the outflow tract gradient before contemplated septal ablation or myomectomy, and to exclude associated coronary atheroslcerosis.

Etiology and Basic Mechanisms Responsible for the "Pain"

Exertional myocardial ischemia can be precipitated by myocardial oxygen requirements in excess of the capacity of normal coronary blood flow to deliver oxygen. The possible contribution of this mechanism to myocardial ischemia in patients with hypertrophic cardiomyopathy is suggested by the augmented myocardial oxygen requirements documented under basal conditions in this disease.[5] This increased basal oxygen requirement probably results from the increased muscle mass and partly from the elevated left ventricular pressures in patients with outflow obstruction. The latter component perhaps accounts for the clinical observation that patients with obstructive hypertrophic cardiomyopathy are more likely to experience angina than those patients with the nonobstructive variety. The demonstration that patients with hypertrophic cardiomyopathy may have an inadequate increase in coronary blood flow with exercise[5] suggests that additional explanations such as inadequacy of capillary density with respect to the increased muscle mass, the presence of abnormally narrowed small intramural coronary arteries, or systolic compression of large intramyocardial coronary arteries.[3] An increase in the intimal and medial components of small intramural coronary arteries and frequent narrowing of the lumens has been found in a majority of patients with hypertrophic cardiomyopathy studied at autopsy.[3] Systolic compression of the large intramyocardial coronary arteries is a frequent angiographic observation in patients with obstructive hypertrophic cardiomyopathy. The myocardial ischemia may be accentuated or more sustained if the already abnormally elevated left ventricular diastolic pressure is increased further and results in a decrease in coronary blood flow. In conclusion, myocardial ischemia associated with hypertrophic cardiomyopathy seems to be multifactorial. Factors such as exaggerated basal oxygen demands, impaired coronary flow reserve, and reduced diastolic aortic-left ventricular gradient are all important, but there exact interplay is not completely defined.

Treatment

Treatment for hypertrophic cardiomyopathy should be directed toward relief of symptoms, as there is no evidence that treatment prolongs life. Initially, relief of dyspnea and angina is usually achieved with administration of a beta-blocker or verapamil. Disopyramide is an acceptable alternative in the female patient whose symptoms are refractory to these drugs. The patient judged to be at high risk of sudden death from ventricular arrhythmias should be considered for amiodarone or an implantable defibrillator. Pacemaker implantation, while still controversial, is championed by some investigators as beneficial in those patients refractory to medical therapy. Ventricular septal myomectomy or the still investigative technique of septal ablation should be reserved for those patients refractory to all the above approaches. The production of infarction by injecting alcohol into the first septal perforator artery to produce necrosis and decrease contractility of the hypertrophied septum is currently being studied.

References

1. Wigle ED, Rakowski H, Kimball BP, et al. Hypertrophic cardiomyopathy: Clinical spectrum and treatment. *Circulation* 1995;92:1680–1690.
2. Braunwald E, Lambrew CT, Rockoff SD, et al. Idiopathic hypertrophic subaortic stenosis: I. A description of the disease based upon an analysis of 64 patients. *Circulation* 1964;29(Suppl IV):IV3–IV119.
3. Maron BJ, Bonow RO, Cannon RO III, et al. Hypertrophic cardiomyopathy: Interrelations of clinical manifestations, pathophysiology, and therapy. *N Engl J Med* 1987;316:780–789.
4. Pasternac A, Noble J, Streulens Y, et al. Pathophysiology of chest pain in patients with cardiomyopathies and normal coronary arteries. *Circulation* 1982;65:778–789.
5. Cannon RO III, Rosing DR, Maron BJ, et al. Myocardial ischemia in patients with hypertrophic cardiomyopathy: Contribution of inadequate vasodilator reserve and elevated left ventricular filling pressures. *Circulation* 1985;71:234–243.

39

"Chest Pain" in Patients with Dilated Cardiomyopathy

Douglas C. Morris, MD

General Considerations

Dilated cardiomyopathy is a condition characterized by left ventricular dilatation and eventually by symptoms of left ventricular dysfunction. Most of the patients ultimately develop enlargement of all four *cardiac chambers* and intractable heart failure. Although the etiology is commonly not definable, the myocardial dysfunction probably represents a final common pathway that is the end result of damage from any one of a number of agents, including toxins, metabolic derangement, or infectious agents.

Clinical Setting

Although the condition might develop in patients of any age, it most commonly occurs in the middle ages of life and is more frequent in men.[1]

Characteristics of the "Pain"

Occasionally, a patient with a dilated cardiomyopathy will experience pleuritic "chest pain" due to a pulmonary embolus (see Chapter 16). In addition, right upper quadrant abdominal or epigastric discomfort due to congestive hepatomegaly may also occur. The "chest pain" experienced by patients with dilated cardiomyopathy is, according to Massumi, "vague and nonspecific in character, often of an aching quality and widely distributed over the anterior chest. No relationship to effort could be established. . . ."[2] Characteristically, chest pain appeared with onset of failure

From: Hurst JW, Morris DC (eds): *"Chest Pain"* →. © Futura Publishing Co., Inc., Armonk, NY, 2001.

and subsided with it."[2] The location of this type of "chest pain" is shown in Figure 39–1.

About 10% of patients have angina pectoris.[1,3,4] The patient's characterization of the chest pain, the common location of the "chest pain" (see Figures 39–2 and 39–3), the uncommon location of the "chest pain," the size of the "painful" area, the duration of the "chest pain," the lack of tenderness of the chest wall, the precipitating cause of the "chest pain," and the relief of the "chest pain" are, for the most part, similar to those discussed in Chapter 29. It has been noted that most patients with dilated cardiomyopathy and angina experienced a marked variability in the amount of exercise necessary to precipitate angina.[5] Patients with exertional angina pectoris associated with a dilated cardiomyopathy usually have associated dyspnea because heart failure (as noted above) is commonly present. Also, the angina pectoris may last longer than angina pectoris caused by coronary atherosclerosis because all of the normal recovery mechanisms are not intact. Relief of the angina pectoris related to dilated cardiomyopathy with standard therapy is not as predictable as it often is when coronary atherosclerotic heart disease is responsible for the myocardial ischemia.

Associated Symtpoms

The most striking symptoms associated with dilated cardiomyopathy are those of left ventricular failure. *Dyspnea*, initially with exertion and

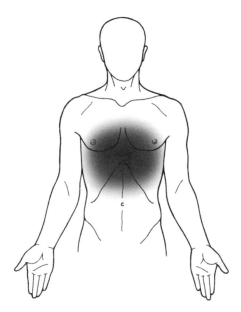

Figure 39–1. The "chest pain" associated with dilated cardiomyopathy is commonly widely distributed over the anterior portion of the chest. The "pain" may occur with heart failure and subside as the failure subsides.

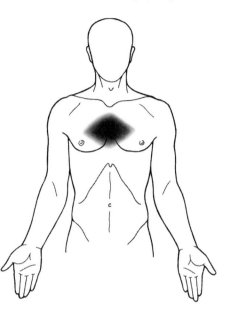

Figure 39–2. "Chest pain" characteristic of angina pectoris may occur in a small percentage of patients with dilated cardiomyopathy. The common location of the "pain" is shown in this illustration.

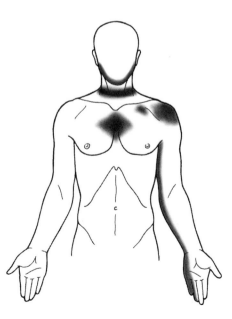

Figure 39–3. The common location of the radiation of "chest pain" due to angina pectoris is shown in this illustration. The radiation of the "pain" is similar to that produced by obstructive coronary artery disease.

eventually with recumbency, is the usual initial symptom and ultimately is present in almost all patients. *Generalized weakness* and exertional related fatigue or exhaustion due to diminished cardiac output is common. Right heart failure is a late consequence of this condition and carries a very grave prognosis. The appearance of right heart failure is frequently associated with a lessening of the dyspnea at the expense of the development of ascites and lower extremity edema, and worsening fatigue. *Syncope,* or near syncope, may be experienced by those patients who develop episodes of ventricular tachycardia. Other arrhythmias such as *atrial fibrillation* or *ventricular ectopy* are common and may be perceived as palpitations. *Lightheadedness or dizziness* due to postural hypotension is a common complaint, particularly in those patients being aggressively treated with diuretics and/or vasodilators.

Associated Signs

Physical examination

The findings on physical examination will typically reflect the left ventricular dilatation and decompensation of the ventricles. The dilated left ventricle is manifest by a larger than normal, laterally displaced, apical impulse, and possibly a palpable presystolic impulse.

The clinical manifestations of a decompensated left ventricle include a left ventricular gallop, reduced blood pressure with a narrowed pulse pressure, and pulsus alternans. The decompensated right ventricle usually results in elevated jugular venous waves, an engorged liver, peripheral edema, and ascites.

Systolic murmurs are common in these patients usually due to mitral regurgitation and less frequently tricuspid regurgitation. Tricuspid regurgitation can also lead to a pulsatile liver.

"Routine" laboratory tests

Early in the course of this disease, the *chest x-ray film* may only show mild left ventricular enlargement. As the disease progresses, the chest x-ray film will portray generalized cardiomegaly and pulmonary venous hypertension, interstitial pulmonary edema and, at times, alveolar pulmonary edema.

Usually by the time the disease is apparent on physical examination, *the electrocardiogram* will demonstrate some of the following: atrial fibrillation, intraventricular conduction defects, complicated bundle branch block, and diffuse low voltage. The abnormal direction of the initial QRS forces produce abnormal Q waves that may simulate myocardial infarcts. The combination of abnormal Q waves and "chest pain" may lead the physician to suspect the presence of coronary atherosclerotic heart disease.

Differential Diagnosis

The important differential to make in patients with an apparent dilated cardiomyopathy is between those patients who have a potentially reversible situation and those patients whose condition is irreversible. Women who develop a dilated cardiomyopathy during the peripartum period will fully recover about 50% of the time. Patients who develop a dilated cardiomyopathy in the setting of an acute myopericarditis will, on occasions, recover. If recognized early enough, cardiomyopathy due to hemochromatosis will respond to removal of excess body iron and sarcoid cardiomyopathy may improve with corticosteroids. Most importantly, it is imperative to recognize the patient with a globally dysfunctioning left ventricle due to "hibernation" due to diffuse, severe coronary atherosclerosis. The reestablishment of adequate coronary blood flow by bypass coronary surgery to the hibernating regions of myocardium may improve left ventricular function.

Other Diagnostic Testing

Echocardiography is the standard means of establishing the presence of a dilated, poorly contractile left ventricle. The other high-tech procedures available to exclude a reversible etiology are *thallium scanning,* which is useful in excluding sarcoid, myocardial biopsy which may identify sarcoidosis, hemochromatosis, or acute myocarditis, and *coronary arteriography* which is necessary to absolutely exclude coronary atherosclerosis.

Etiology and Basic Mechanisms Responsible for the "Pain"

As stated in the beginning, dilated cardiomyopathy may be caused by toxins, metabolic derangement, or infectious agents. Many times the cause is never established.

The pathogenesis of angina pectoris in patients with dilated cardiomyopathies remains unresolved. Pasternac and associates found reduced coronary blood flow at rest and during pacing in patients with a cardiomyopathy.[6] Opherk and associates, however, reported normal basal coronary perfusion but limited pharmacologic flow reserve compared with control subjects. The dipyridamole-induced increase in coronary resistance correlated directly with the basal left ventricular end-diastolic pressure.[7] Nitenberg and associates found a limited flow response to dipyridamole in patients with dilated cardiomyopathy but no correlation with left ventricular filling pressures.[8] Perhaps, the most complete study of the problem is by Cannon and associates at the National Heart, Lung and Blood Institute.[5] These investigators found no differences in the basal and pacing-stimulated coronary flows between patients with dilated cardiomyopathy and angina pectoris and those without angina pectoris. The patients with chest pain did have a lower peak coronary flow and higher absolute coronary resistance after dipyridamole infusion. These same patients demonstrated a significantly greater restriction in coronary flow response to pacing following the administration of ergonovine.[5] While this limited flow reserve could be due to an elevated left ventricular filling pressure causing extravascular compression of the coronary microvasculature, it is more likely due to an abnormality of the microvasculature itself. In the study by Cannon and associates, there was no morphologic evidence of disease of small coronary vessels on myocardial biopsy suggesting that the increases in coronary vascular resistance occur in the intermediate-sized vessels.[5] The response to dipyridamole also suggests that this is the site of the increased coronary resistance.

Treatment

While standard therapy for angina pectoris may be tried, the response to such treatment is poor. This is probably true because of the complex mechanisms responsible for angina in patients with dilated cardiomyopathy.

Therapy in the patient with a dilated cardiomyopathy should be focused upon reduction of symptoms of heart failure, halting the progression of ventricular dysfunction and prolongation of survival.

The vague "chest pain" that does not have the diagnostic features of angina pectoris may be relieved by the intensive treatment of heart failure.

In the asymptomatic patient the angiotensin-converting enzymes inhibitors are the only drugs to have established benefit. In patients with heart failure due to a poorly contractile, dilated left ventricle, filling pressures should be reduced by vasodilators and diuretics and cardiac output improved by afterload reduction with vasodilators (first choice—angiotensin-converting enzymes inhibitors). Digitalis in the symptomatic patient improves functional status, decreases clinical deterioration, and reduces the need for hospitalization for heart failure.

In selected patients with heart failure, beta-adrenergic blocking agents improve ventricular function, retard disease progression, and improve survival. Spironolactone when added to therapy with angiotensin-converting enzymes inhibitors, digoxin, and loop diuretics also improves survival. The value of dual chamber pacemakers is now being studied in a selected group of patients.

Cardiac transplantation is indicated for heart failure that is intractable in patients who are in the proper age group and have no comorbid disqualifying disease.

References

1. Oakley C. Diagnosis and natural history of congested (dilated) cardiomyopathies. *Post Grad Med J* 1978;54:440–447.
2. Massumi RA, Rios JC, Gooch AS, et al. Primary myocardial disease: Report of fifty cases and review of the subject. *Circulation* 1965;31:19–40.
3. Hatle L, Orjavik O, Storstein O. Chronic myocardial disease. *Acta Med Scand* 1976;199:399–405.
4. Komajda M, Jais JP, Reeves F, et al. Factors predicting mortality in idiopathic dilated cardiomyopathy. *Euro Heart J* 1990;11:824–831.
5. Cannon RO, Cunnion RE, Parrillo JE, et al. Dynamic limitation of coronary vasodilator reserve in patients with dilated cardiomyopathy and chest pain. *J Am Coll Cardiol* 1987;10:1190–1200.
6. Pasternac A, Noble J, Streulens Y, et al. Pathophysiology of chest pain patients with cardiomyopathies and normal coronary arteries. *Circulation* 1982;65:778–789.
7. Opherk D, Schwarz F, Mall G, et al. Coronary dilator capacity in idiopathic dilated cardiomyopathy: Analysis of 16 patients. *Am J Cardiol* 1983; 51:1657–1662.
8. Nitenberg A, Foult J-M, Blanchet F, et al. Multifactorial determinants of reduced coronary flow reserve after dipyridamole in dilated cardiomyopathy. *Am J Cardiol* 1985;55:748–754.

40

"Chest Pain" in Patients with Restrictive Cardiomyopathy

Douglas C. Morris, MD

General Considerations

Restrictive cardiomyopathy is the least common of the cardiomyopathies. The primary disorder is impaired diastolic function that may result from a process involving the endocardium, the myocardium, or both. The most commonly encountered myocardial disorders are amyloidosis and idiopathic myocardial fibrosis. The condition can, however, result from a number of other diseases including scleroderma, sarcoidosis, hemochromatosis, Fabry's disease, endomyocardial fibrosis, hypereosiniphilic syndrome, and carcinoid.

Clinical Setting

Restrictive cardiomyopathy should be considered in any patient who exhibits unexplained congestive heart failure.

Characteristics of the "Pain"

Patient's characterization of the "chest pain"

When "chest pain" is present the patient describes it as discussed in Chapter 29.

Common location of the "chest pain"

See Figures 40–1 and 40–2.

From: Hurst JW, Morris DC (eds): *"Chest Pain"* →. © Futura Publishing Co., Inc., Armonk, NY, 2001.

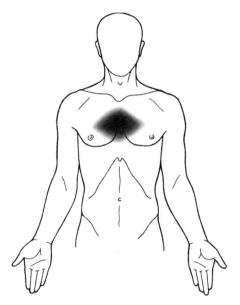

Figure 40–1. The usual location and size of the "chest pain" that is characteristic of angina pectoris.

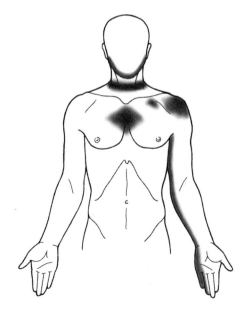

Figure 40–2. Common locations of the radiation of the "chest pain" that is characteristic of angina pectoris. Note the radiation to the neck, jaw, left upper chest, left shoulder, inner surface of the left arm, left little finger, and left ring finger.

Uncommon locations of the "chest pain"

The "chest pain" may be located rarely in the right arm or limited to the left or right shoulder, elbow, or wrist, as discussed in Chapter 29.

Size of the "painful" area

See Figures 40–1 and 40–2.

Duration of the "chest pain"

Angina pectoris produced by effort lasts 2 to 3 minutes, 10 minutes at the most, when precipitated by effort. The "chest pain" associated with restrictive cardiomyopathy tends to last longer than the "pain" of angina due to coronary atherosclerotic heart disease.

Tenderness of the chest wall

The chest wall is not tender.

Precipitating causes of the "chest pain"

The "chest pain" is precipitated by exercise and its onset often occurs immediately after the exercise rather than during it as it commonly does in patients with coronary atherosclerotic heart disease.

Associated Symptoms

The most pronounced symptoms are those of left heart failure including *exertional dyspnea, orthopnea,* and *nocturnal dyspnea.* Exercise intolerance due to easy fatigability is also frequently present secondary to a further compromise in diastolic filling of the ventricle by the tachycardia produced by exertion. Often, however, right heart failure predominates as manifested by *ankle swelling* and *abdominal discomfort.*

Associated Signs

Physical examination

The jugular venous pressure is elevated and the jugular venous pulse waves show a rapid x and y descent. The most prominent venous movement, however, is the y descent. The jugular venous pulse may actually rise during inspiration (Kussmaul's sign). The apical impulse is usually normal. Auscultation of the heart usually reveals murmurs of mitral and tricuspid regurgitation. There is usually a left ventricular gallop sound, and less often a fourth sound.[2] In advanced cases, the femoral pulse will demonstrate pulsus alternans. Peripheral edema and ascites are also present in advanced cases, and the liver is enlarged and pulsatile. Up to one-third of patients with restrictive cardiomyopathy will present with signs of thromboembolic events.[2]

Additional physical findings may be tied to the other organ systems involved by the systemic process causing the restrictive cardiomyopathy, such as polyneuropathy with amyloidosis, cutaneous flushing and diarrhea with the carcinoid syndrome, and increased skin pigmentation in hemochromatosis.

"Routine" laboratory tests

The *electrocardiogram* is almost always abnormal. Most often the electrocardiogram shows nonspecific ST and T wave abnormalities. With infiltrative processes such as amyloidosis, there will likely be diffuse low voltage, depolarization abnormalities ("pseudoinfarction pattern"), and conduction abnormalities including atrioventricular block. Atrial fibrillation is common. The *chest x-ray film* usually demonstrates a normal size heart with possible atrial enlargement. Later the heart may become larger than normal. Pulmonary congestion is often present, as well as interstitial edema and Kerley B lines in the more severe cases. Pleural effusions may be present.

Differential Diagnosis

The presence of angina pectoris warrants an investigation to exclude the co-existence of coronary atherosclerosis. Angina pectoris, in the absence of coronary atherosclerosis, renders hereditary amyloidosis as the likely etiology of the restrictive cardiomyopathy.

The establishment of a diagnosis of restrictive cardiomyopathy demands the exclusion of constrictive pericarditis. The findings in restrictive cardiomyopathy (prominent y descent in the jugular venous waves, Kussmaul's sign, ascites, and peripheral edema) are the same as those in constrictive pericarditis. No single finding or diagnostic technique is totally reliable in establishing the diagnosis. The distinction between these two conditions is usually based upon a series of findings as outlined in Table 40–1.

Table 40–1.

The Differential Diagnosis of Restrictive Cardiomyopathy and Constrictive Pericarditis.*

Type of Evaluation	Restrictive Cardiomyopathy	Constrictive Pericarditis
Physical examination	Kussmaul's sign may be present Apical impulse may be prominent S3 may be present, rarely S4 Regurgitant murmurs common	Kussmaul's sign usually present Apical impulse usually not palpable Pericardial knock may be present Regurgitant murmurs uncommon
Electrocardiography	Low voltage (especially in amyloidosis),pseudo-infarction, left axis deviation, atrial fibrillation, conduction disturbances common	Low voltage ($<$ 50 percent)
Echocardiography	Increased wall thickness (especially thickened interatrial septum in amyloidosis) Thickened cardiac valves (amyloidosis) Granular sparkling texture (amyloid)	Normal wall thickness Pericardial thickening may be seen Prominent early diastolic filling with abrupt displacement of interventricular septum
Doppler studies	Decreased RV and LV velocities with inspiration Inspiratory augmentation of hepatic-vein diastolic flow reversal Mitral and tricuspid regurgitation common	Increased RV systolic velocity and decreased LV systolic velocity with inspiration Expiratory augmentation of hepatic-vein diastolic flow reversal
Cardiac catheterization	LVEDP often $>$ 5 mmHg greater than RVEDP, but may be identical	RVEDP and LVEDP usually equal RV systolic pressure $<$ 50 mmHg RVEDP $>$ one third of RV systolic pressure
Endomyocardial biopsy	May reveal specific cause of restrictive cardio-myopathy	May be normal or show nonspecific myocyte hypertrophy or myocardial fibrosis
CT/MRI	Pericardium usually normal	Pericardium may be thickened

*LV denotes left ventricular, RV right ventricular, LVEDP left ventricular end-diastolic pressure, RVEDP right ventricular end-diastolic pressure, CT computed tomography, and MRI magnetic resonance imaging.

Source: Kushwaha SS, Fallon JT, Fuster V. Restrictive cardiomyopathy. N Engl J Med 1997;336(No. 4): 267–276. Copyright © 1997 Massachusetts Medical Society. All rights reserved. Used with permission.

Other Diagnostic Testing

The other modes of establishing the diagnosis of restrictive cardiomyopathy are located in Table 40–1.

On *Doppler echocardiography,* the pattern of mitral-inflow velocity in restrictive cardiomyopathy is a combination of increased early diastolic filling velocity, decreased atrial filling velocity, an increased ratio of early diastolic filling to atrial filling, a decreased deceleration time, and a decreased isovolumic relaxation time. Flow testing in the pulmonary-vein or hepatic-vein demonstrates that systolic forward flow is less than diastolic forward flow. Also, during inspiration there is increased reversal of diastolic flow after atrial contraction in the hepatic and pulmonary veins.

During *cardiac catheterization,* the hemodynamic hallmark of a restrictive cardiomyopathy is the so-called "dip and plateau." The "dip and plateau" is characterized by a deep and rapid early decline in ventricular pressure at the onset of diastole, with a rapid rise to a plateau in early diastole. Although exceptions occur, there is generally not equalization of the diastolic pressures (unlike constrictive pericarditis). The left ventricular end diastolic pressures are characteristically 5mmHg or more higher than the right ventricular end-diastolic pressures. In those situations in which the distinction between restrictive cardiomyopathy and constrictive pericarditis remains uncertain, magnetic resonance imaging to evaluate for pericardial thickness or endomyocardial biopsy should be considered.

Etiology and Basic Mechanisms Responsible for the "Pain"

A rapid deceleration of diastolic flow, reduction of peak hyperemic flow velocity, and restriction of coronary flow reserve characterize coronary blood flow in restrictive cardiomyopathy.[3] The rapid deceleration of diastolic flow is partially due to an elevation of zero-flow pressure, in turn, due to a markedly elevated end-diastolic ventricular pressure. Amyloidosis imposes two other burdens on the coronary circulation that probably account for association of angina pectoris with restrictive cardiomyopathy of this particular etiology and not with other etiologies. In amyloidosis, there is increased ventricular wall tension during diastole due to infiltration of the interstitial space between myocardial cells and reduced blood flow through small distal coronary arterioles, the lumens of which may be partially obliterated by amyloid.[1] The infiltration of intramural coronary arteries and luminal narrowing of the microvessels resulting in increased microvascular resistance also contributes to the rapid deceleration of diastolic flow.

Treatment

The cornerstone of therapy in the patient with a restrictive cardiomyopathy is diuretics. Diuretics are used to control the venous congestion in both the pulmonary and systemic circulation. These patients, however, generally require a slightly elevated left ventricular filling pressure in order to maintain maximal cardiac output. Overdiuresis will result in reduced cardiac output and symptoms of fatigue and lightheadedness. Digoxin should be used cautiously as it is potentially arrhythmogenic in patients with amyloidosis. The loss of the atrial contribution to ventricular filling during atrial fibrillation will further compromise the cardiac output. Consequently, it is important to maintain sinus rhythm even if amiodarone is required. Since the stroke volume is relatively fixed in restrictive cardiomyopathy, the onset of bradyarrhythmias may require atrial and ventricular pacing. Anticoagulation with warfarin is recommended because of the propensity for thrombus formation in the atrial appendages and subsequent emboli.[2] Some patients with restrictive cardiomyopathy due to conditions other than amyloid or some other systemic disease, may be candidates for cardiac transplantation.

References

1. Booth DR, Tan SY, Hawkins PN, et al. Cellular and molecular cardiology: A novel variant of transthyretin, $59^{Thr \rightarrow Lys}$, associated with autosomal dominant cardiac amyloidosis in an Italian family. *Circulation* 1995;91:962–967.
2. Kushwaha SS, Fallon JT, Fuster. Medical progress: Restrictive cardiomyopathy. *New Engl J Med* 1997;336:267–276.
3. Akasaka T, Yoshida K, Yamamuro A, et al. Phasic coronary flow characteristics in patients with constrictive pericarditis: Comparison with restrictive cardiomyopathy. *Circulation* 1997;96:1874–1881.

41

"Chest Pain" in Patients with Pulmonary Hypertension

Robert C. Schlant, MD and J. Willis Hurst, MD

General Considerations

There are many causes of pulmonary artery hypertension (see Table 41–1). "Chest pain" (simulating the pain of myocardial ischemia) that is directly due to the persistent increase in pulmonary artery pressure is the subject of this chapter. Chest pain due to acute pulmonary embolism is discussed in Chapter 16 and the pleuritic chest pain of pulmonary infarction is discussed in Chapter 14.

It seems likely, as discussed later, that the "chest pain" with a persistent elevation in pulmonary artery pressure is due to right ventricular ischemia. All patients with pulmonary artery hypertension do not have "chest pain," suggesting that the chest pain occurs most often in patients with considerable pulmonary artery pressure *and* rather marked right ventricular hypertrophy.

Clinical Setting

Today "chest pain" due to pulmonary artery hypertension and right ventricular hypertrophy is often seen in patients with primary (unexplained) pulmonary artery hypertension. This condition occurs more commonly in young women than young men. Repeated pulmonary emboli may produce a similar condition and must always be ruled out in patients thought to have unexplained pulmonary artery hypertension.

Pulmonary artery hypertension also occurs in patients with collagen disease such as lupus erythematosis or progressive systemic sclerosis.

From: Hurst JW, Morris DC (eds): *"Chest Pain"* →. © Futura Publishing Co., Inc., Armonk, NY, 2001.

Table 41–1.

Causes of Persistent Pulmonary Artery Hypertension.

☐ Primary (unexplained) Pulmonary Artery Hypertension
☐ Lung Disease
  • Obstructive lung disease (bronchitis and emphysema)
  • Interstitial lung disease
  • Repeated pulmonary emboli
  • Pulmonary vascular disease (lupus, progressive systemic sclerosis) and antiappetite drugs.
  • Alveolar hypoventilation (sleep apnea, abnormal chest bellows, and abnormal respiratory control)
☐ Heart Disease
  • Mitral valve disease (especially mitral stenosis)
  • Heart failure due to left ventricular disease
  • Congenital heart disease (Eisenmenger physiology)
☐ Disease of the Pulmonary Veins (rare)

The condition under discussion also occurs in children and young adults with congenital heart disease who have Eisenmenger physiology.

In years past, the "chest pain" associated with pulmonary artery hypertension occurred in occasional patients with rheumatic mitral stenosis. While this condition still occurs in patients with mitral stenosis, it occurs much less often because patients with mitral stenosis are subjected to mitral valve surgery or balloon valvuloplasty much earlier than they were formerly.

Patients with severe forms of pulmonary disease may develop chest pain related to pulmonary artery hypertension, but such patients are greatly limited by dyspnea and the type of pain discussed here may not occur.[1,2]

Pulmonary artery hypertension secondary to heart failure, with the exception of heart failure due to mitral stenosis, rarely causes "chest pain."

The "chest pain" associated with the sudden development of pulmonary artery hypertension that occurs with large pulmonary emboli is discussed in Chapter 16.

Characteristics of the "Chest Pain"

Patient's characterization of the "chest pain"

Chest pain may simulate angina pectoris (see Chapter 29).

Common location of the "chest pain"

The usual location of the "chest pain" is shown in Figure 41–1.

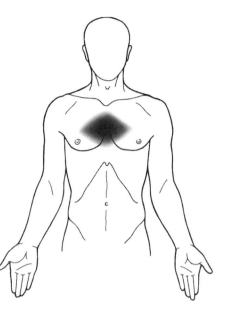

Figure 41–1. The location of the "chest pain" is believed to be due to right ventricular ischemia in patients with severe pulmonary hypertension.

Uncommon locations of the "chest pain"

It is uncommon for the chest pain to radiate beyond the anterior portion of the chest.

Size of the painful "area"

The approximate size of the painful area is shown in Figure 41–1.

Duration of the "chest pain"

"Chest pain" provoked by effort subsides in several minutes after the patient ceases the effort. The "chest pain" related to pulmonary artery hypertension that is produced by effort may last longer than the usual episode of angina pectoris due to atherosclerotic coronary heart disease.

Tenderness of the chest wall

There is no tenderness of the chest wall.

Precipitating causes of the "chest pain"

The chest pain is commonly produced by effort. This is to be expected because the pulmonary pressure in these patients is increased by physical effort. In this regard the "chest pain" does not differ from that of effort angina due to atherosclerotic coronary heart disease. The "chest pain" may occur at rest in severe situations, especially if there is systemic hypotension or hypoxia.

Relief of the "chest pain"

The pain is not as predictably relieved by nitroglycerin as is angina pectoris due to coronary atherosclerotic heart disease.
Any drugs known to cause pulmonary hypertension must be stopped.

Associated Symptoms

Dyspnea invariably accompanies the "chest pain" associated with persistent pulmonary artery hypertension. In fact, the patient may develop dyspnea with effort and stop before "chest pain" develops.
Syncope commonly occurs in patients with chronic pulmonary hypertension.

Associated Signs

Physical examination

Generalized cyanosis may be detected. This occurs late in the course of patients with primary pulmonary hypertension when the right atrial pressure exceeds the left atrial pressure and produces a right-to-left shunt through a patent foramen ovale. A similar physiologic condition may prevail when the right atrial pressure becomes elevated in patients with pulmonary hypertension from any cause.

Cyanosis and clubbing of the fingers and toes are always observed in patients with Eisenmenger physiology. When a patent ductus is responsible for the Eisenmenger physiology, the marked elevation of pulmonary pressure produces a severe right-to-left shunt into the aorta, which produces more cyanosis and clubbing of the toes than of the fingers.

A large A wave is seen in the deep jugular venous pulse. A large V wave is usually seen when there is tricuspid regurgitation.

An anterior movement of the anterior chest wall may be detected; it is due to right ventricular hypertrophy. The prominent pulsation of the pulmonary artery itself can be felt in the second left intercostal space near the sternum.

On auscultation the pulmonary valve closure sound may be as loud as, or louder than, the aortic valve closure sound in patients with pulmonary artery hypertension. A loud pulmonary valve closure sound may be heard at the cardiac apex where it is rarely heard normally; this signifies the presence of pulmonary artery hypertension.

There may be a right atrial gallop sound in patients with right ventricular hypertrophy due to pulmonary artery hypertension. In addition, the murmur of tricuspid regurgitation may be heard. The murmur of pulmonary valve regurgitation may be noted along the left sternal border.

The usual murmur of a patent ductus or ventricular septal defect will not be present in patients with Eisenmenger physiology because the pulmonary artery hypertension and right ventricular hypertension decreases the pressure gradients responsible for the usual murmurs in such cases.

Late in the course of the disease the patient develops edema, a large liver, and ascites.

"Routine" laboratory tests

Erythrocytosis may be present in patients with a right-to-left shunt, either late in the course of primary pulmonary artery hypertension or throughout the course of patients with Eisenmenger physiology. The arterial oxygen saturation may be lower than normal.

Chest x-ray films commonly reveal right atrial enlargement in the frontal view and right ventricular enlargement in the lateral view. The main pulmonary artery is always larger than normal. The right and left branches of the pulmonary artery are larger than normal. It is useful to measure the diameter of the tracheal air column in the frontal x-ray film; the diameter of the right pulmonary artery measured near the cardiac border should not normally be wider than the trachea. The right and left branches of the pulmonary artery taper rather quickly, indicating pulmonary artery hypertension.

The abnormalities noted on the chest x-ray film of patients with mitral stenosis are discussed in Chapter 34.

The *electrocardiogram* of patients with moderate pulmonary hypertension may reveal a right atrial abnormality and signs of systolic pressure overload of the right ventricle.

The mean QRS vector may initially be directed vertically and slightly posteriorly when patients develop right ventricular hypertrophy *after* normal left ventricular dominance has developed. This is commonly the case with severe primary pulmonary artery hypertension. As time passes, and the right ventricular hypertrophy increases, the mean QRS vector will be directed more to the right *and* anteriorly where the right ventricle is located. The mean T vector is directed 90° to 180° away from the mean QRS vector.

The electrocardiogram rarely shows signs suggesting coronary disease.

Exceptions to the Usual Manifestations

The clinical picture described here has few exceptions.

Differential Diagnosis

The presence of pulmonary artery hypertension is easily identified using the history, physical examination, chest x-ray film, and electrocardiogram.

The "chest pain" associated with pulmonary hypertension must be separated from angina pectoris due to atherosclerotic coronary heart disease. Atherosclerotic coronary heart disease is rare in young people and the separation of the two conditions is not a problem in that group of patients. Severe pulmonary artery hypertension in older patients can produce pain simulating that of angina pectoris due to atherosclerotic coronary heart disease, but coronary arteriography is rarely justified.

Other Diagnostic Testing

In general, stress electrocardiograms, nuclear studies aimed at detecting myocardial ischemia, and coronary arteriograms are not performed on patients with obvious severe pulmonary artery hypertension. *An echocardiogram and right and left cardiac catheterization* may be indicated to identify Eisenmenger's physiology or left ventricular disease, and to measure the degree of pulmonary hypertension. Coronary arteriography is rarely indicated in such patients.

Etiology and Basic Mechanisms Responsible for the "Pain"

The normal pulmonary artery pressure in subjects at sea level is 25 mmHg systolic and 15 mmHg diastolic. The normal pulmonary artery pressure may be 10 mmHg higher than that in subjects who live at high altitude. The pulmonary artery pressure rises very little as the result of exercise in normal subjects.

Patients with mild to moderate pulmonary arterial hypertension as occurs in patients with heart failure due to left ventricular disease rarely develops "chest pain" with effort unless the left ventricular disease is due to coronary artery disease of some type, or cardiomyopathy. Of these causes, coronary disease is the most common cause of the "chest pain" produced by effort.

Years ago we believed that the "chest pain" due to pulmonary arterial hypertension was due to abrupt distention of the pulmonary artery itself, which was believed to be due to the rise in pulmonary artery pressure with exercise.

Currently we believe the "chest pain" that simulates angina pectoris due to coronary atherosclerosis that occurs in patients with moderate to severe pulmonary hypertension is likely due to myocardial ischemia of the right ventricle.[3]

The perfusion of blood to the left ventricle occurs mainly during mechanical diastole and little during systole. This is because the systolic pressure in the coronary artery is the same as the systolic pressure in the left ventricle; there is no pressure gradient to ensure coronary blood flow. During mechanical diastole the diastolic pressure in the coronary artery may be normally about 60 to 80 mmHg whereas the diastolic pressure within the normal left ventricle is 10 mmHg or less. Accordingly, with such a large diastolic pressure gradient the coronary flow to the left ventricle is adequate for rest and exercise.

The myocardial perfusion of blood to the right ventricle by the coronary arteries is quite different to the perfusion of the left ventricle by the coronary arteries. This is because the systolic pressure in the coronary arteries may be 130 mmHg during mechanical systole and 80 mmHg during mechanical diastole, while the systolic pressure in the right ventricle is normally 25 mmHg during systole and the diastolic pressure in the right ventricle is normally about 5 mmHg or less during diastole. Accordingly, there is a large pressure gradient during both systole and diastole, permitting right ventricular perfusion to occur during both mechanical systole and mechanical diastole.

When severe pulmonary artery hypertension develops, the systolic pressure within the right ventricle becomes markedly elevated, decreasing the normal pressure gradient between the systolic pressure in the coronary artery and the systolic pressure within the right ventricle. The same is true when the diastolic pressure in the right ventricle becomes elevated; in this situation the pressure gradient between the coronary artery and the right ventricle decreases in diastole. So, the coronary blood flow is markedly decreased in systole and to some degree in diastole.

In addition, the thick right ventricle needs more coronary blood flow than a normal ventricle—just as a hypertrophic left ventricle needs more coronary blood flow than a normal left ventricle.

Couple this anatomic-physiologic rearrangement with the fact that the pulmonary artery pressure increases with exercise in patients with pulmonary arteriolar disease who have an increase in pulmonary arteriolar resistance. This causes a rapid elevation of pulmonary artery pressure with exercise in patients with pulmonary hypertension thereby preventing adequate myocardial perfusion of the right ventricle during exercise.

In addition to the factors mentioned above, the patient may be hypoxic and an erythrocytosis may develop.

All of the factors listed above conspire to produce angina of the right ventricle.

Finally, an argument exists as to whether or not primary (unexplained) pulmonary hypertension is due to pulmonary emboli. The question is difficult to answer because, at autopsy, patients who are believed to have primary pulmonary hypertension may have evidence of pulmonary emboli, but that does not answer the question—are the emboli in such patients the cause of the pulmonary arteriolar disease or are they secondary to the problem.

Treatment

The treatment of the "chest pain" that seems to be angina pectoris of the right ventricle is poor. Nitroglycerin, beta-blockers, and calcium channel-blockers all fail consistently to reduce the "pain." In fact, these drugs may cause some harm, including the precipitation of syncope in patients with primary pulmonary hypertension.

Other drugs have been reported to lower the pulmonary artery pressure of such patients. This should decrease the physiologic derangement that causes the "chest pain," but thus far the perfect drug has not been found. Any drug that lowers peripheral resistance along with lowering the pulmonary arteriolar resistance can produce syncope.

Pulmonary transplantation and cardiopulmonary transplantation are successful in the treatment of carefully selected patients with severe pulmonary hypertension. The problems here are the availability of donors, the likelihood of rejection, and cost.

References

1. Szidon JP, Fishman AP. Approach to the pulmonary patient with respiratory Signs and symptoms. In: Fishman AP (ed): *Pulmonary Diseases and Disorders, 2nd edition.* New York, McGraw-Hill, 1988, pp. 313–366.
2. Fishman AP. Pulmonary hypertension and cor pulmonale. In Fishman AP (ed): *Pulmonary Diseases and Disorders, 2nd edition.* New York, McGraw-Hill, 1988, pp. 999–1048.
3. Ross RS, Baker BM. Right ventricular hypertension as a cause of angina pectoris (abstract). *Circulation* 1960;22:801–802.

42

"Chest Pain" in Patients with Systemic Hypertension

J. Willis Hurst, MD

General Considerations

Patients with systemic hypertension and left ventricular hypertrophy may have "chest pain" due to: dissection of the aorta (see Chapter 43), angina pectoris, and infarction due to associated atherosclerosis of the coronary arteries (see Chapter 29), and angina pectoris with normal or near normal coronary arteriograms. The latter condition is discussed in this chapter.

Clinical Setting

A small percentage of patients with systemic hypertension due to any cause who develop left ventricular hypertrophy may have angina pectoris with normal coronary arteriograms.

Characteristics of the "Pain"

The patient's characterization of the "chest pain," the common location of the "chest pain" (see Figures 42–1 and 42–2), the uncommon location of the chest pain (see Figure 42–3), the size of the painful "area," the duration of the "chest pain," the lack of tenderness of the chest wall, the precipitating causes of the "chest pain," and relief of the "chest pain" are similar to that of angina pectoris due to coronary atherosclerotic heart disease (see Chapter 29).

From: Hurst JW, Morris DC (eds): *"Chest Pain"* →. © Futura Publishing Co., Inc., Armonk, NY, 2001.

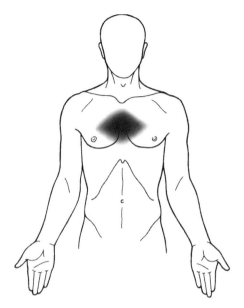

Figure 42–1. The usual location and size of the "chest pain" that is designated angina pectoris.

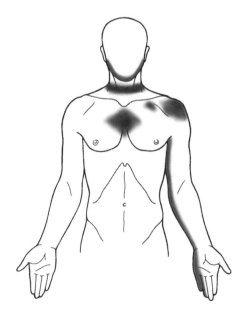

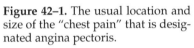

Figure 42–2. Common locations of the radiation of the "chest pain" that is designated angina pectoris. Note the radiation to the neck, jaw, left upper chest, left shoulder, inner surface of the left arm, left little finger, and left ring finger.

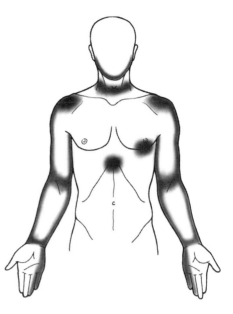

Figure 42–3. Unusual locations of the "pain" that is designated angina pectoris. The discomfort may be limited to the neck, jaw, right or left shoulder, left pectoral region, epigastrium, inner or outer surface of the right or left arms, elbows, wrists, ring and little finger.

Associated Symptoms

Some patients may complain of poor mentation, slight perspiration, slight dyspnea, and near syncope during an episode of angina. Patients commonly dislike the discomfort even though it may be mild. Patients with hypertensive heart disease may complain of dyspnea that seems out of proportion to findings on physical examination of the lungs and chest roentgenogram because of high left ventricular filling pressures (diastolic dysfunction).

Associated Signs

Physical examination

The classification of systemic hypertension has changed considerably in the last few years.[1] Currently, the following classification is recommended. The optimal blood pressure is < 120 mmHg systolic and < 80 mmHg diastolic. Normal blood pressure is defined as < 130 mmHg systolic and < 85 mmHg diastolic. High-normal is defined as being 130–139 mmHg or 85–89 mmHg diastolic. Hypertension is divided into stages. Stage 1 is defined as being 140–159 mmHg systolic or 90–99 mmHg diastolic. Stage 2 is defined as being 160–179 mmHg systolic or 100 to 109 mmHg diastolic. Stage 3 is defined as being ≥ 180 mmHg systolic or ≥ 110 mmHg diastolic.

The blood pressure should be recorded in both arms. The blood pressure is usually higher in the legs than in the arms unless there is coarctation of the aorta or severe peripheral vascular disease due to atherosclerosis.

The cardiac apex impulse may be displaced leftward beyond the left mid clavicular line. The size of the apex impulse may be larger than a quarter, and the apex impulse may be sustained longer in systole than normal.

A left ventricular atrial gallop is commonly heard at the cardiac apex due to a poorly compliant left ventricle. Later, a left ventricular gallop sound may be heard signifying the presence of left ventricular dysfunction.

"Routine" laboratory tests

The electrocardiogram: The electrocardiogram may show signs of left ventricular hypertrophy including a left atrial abnormality, increase in QRS amplitude with a normally directed mean spatial QRS vector, and S-T and T wave changes that, when represented as mean spatial vectors, gradually become directed away from the mean spatial QRS vector. These electrocardiographic abnormalities are typical of those seen in patients with systolic pressure overload of the left ventricle.

The chest x-ray film: The chest x-ray film may be normal, showing no cardiac enlargement, because there is concentric hypertrophy of the left ventricle and little dilatation. As time passes the left ventricle may not only be thicker than normal, but may become dilated as well. At this point in time it is possible to detect left ventricular enlargement on the chest x-ray film. As more times passes the left atrium, the right atrium, and right ventricle also may become enlarged. Radiographic signs of heart failure may eventually develop.

The routine laboratory tests: There may be no abnormalities of the blood or urine detected early in the course of hypertension unless the condition is caused by primary renal disease. Later in the course of hypertension from any cause there may be evidence of renal failure and electrolyte abnormalities.

Exceptions to the Usual Manifestations

There are few, if any, exceptions to the usual manifestation describe above.

Differential Diagnosis

The purpose of this chapter is not to discuss the various causes of systemic hypertension or to elaborate on all of the causes of chest pain in hypertensive patients. Rather, it is to discuss angina pectoris in patients with systemic hypertension who have left ventricular hypertrophy and normal or near normal coronary arteriograms.

Other Diagnostic Testing

When the physician interprets the patient's complaint of "chest pain" to be characteristic of angina pectoris with a predictive value of 90%, it is proper to recommend a coronary arteriogram rather than a stress electrocardiogram or nuclear study.

The S-T and T wave abnormalities of left ventricular hypertrophy, when present, may interfere with the interpretation of an exercise electrocardiogram. Therefore, an exercise electrocardiogram is not the best test to use when the predictive value of the history is in the 50% range (see Chapter 29). Also, a nuclear test may not solve the problem because such tests may reveal a false-negative response. This occurs because the myocardial ischemia in these patients tends to be generalized and a nuclear scan identifies the difference in the uptake of the nuclear material in various parts of the myocardium. If there is poor uptake of the nuclear material throughout the myocardium the nuclear scan may not detect the areas of ischemia. Accordingly, a coronary arteriogram is usually needed to exclude the presence of atherosclerotic plaques in the coronary arteries.

Etiology and Basic Mechanisms Responsible for the "Pain"

Three different mechanisms combine to produce angina pectoris in hypertensive patients with left ventricular hypertrophy who have normal, or near normal, coronary arteriograms.[2]

- The hypertrophied left ventricular myocardium requires more coronary blood flow than normal myocardium.
- Most patients with hypertension will, during some stage of their disease, have an increase in peripheral resistance. The resistant coronary arterioles located in the deeper portion of the left ventricular myocardium participates in this generalized physiologic reaction. This leads to the inability of the penetrating coronary arterioles to dilate

with exercise as they do normally. This abnormal inability to dilate when they should can be identified in other vascular beds as well as in the heart.

- The requirements of the myocardium for an increase in coronary blood flow when physical effort increases the work of the heart triggers the development of myocardial ischemia. This added to the two factors mentioned above produces angina pectoris in patients with hypertension and left ventricular hypertrophy who have normal or near normal coronary arteriograms.

Treatment

The angina pectoris occurring in patients with left ventricular hypertrophy and normal or near normal, coronary arteriograms can be relieved by the following approach.

The patient's hypertension must be controlled and the usual drugs, including nitroglycerin, beta-blockers, calcium antagonists, etc. will commonly relieve patients with angina pectoris in patients with left ventricular hypertrophy and normal, or near normal, coronary arteriograms. The angina may be gradually relieved as the left ventricular hypertrophy diminishes.

References

1. Canzanello VJ, Sheps SG. The sixth report of the Joint National Committee on Prevention, Detection, Evaluation, and Treatment of High Blood Pressure. *Cardiol Rev* 1998;6(No. 5):272–277.
2. Schlant RC, Alexander RW. Diagnosis and management of patients with chronic ischemia heart disease. In: Alexander RW, Schlant RC, Fuster V (eds). *Hurst's The Heart*. New York: McGraw-Hill, 1998, p. 1293.

Part XI

"Chest Pain" Caused by Diseases of the Aorta

Although the definition of "chest pain"→ is discussed in Chapter 1, the definition is repeated here so that communication is clear.

The quotation marks around "chest" imply that different patients have different definitions of the word "chest." Here we use the word to indicate pain located above the waist. Then, too, *angina pectoris* is not always located in the pectoral region—it may be felt only in the jaw, neck, shoulder, elbow, or wrist. Therefore, the word "chest" implies that other parts of the upper body may also be involved with painful syndromes.

The quotation marks around "pain" imply that patients may assign other terms to their discomfort, such as indigestion, burning, ache, etc.

The arrow after "chest pain" implies that the physician initially may not know the cause of the symptom, so a differential diagnosis must be established that fits the available information.

43

"Chest Pain" in Patients with Aortic Dissection

Joseph Lindsay, Jr., MD

General Considerations

Aortic dissection, splitting of the aortic wall in its long axis by a column of blood, is a process akin to that by which fire wood splits when attacked with wedge and maul. It must not be confused with aortic aneurysm. The latter differs from dissection both in pathogenetic mechanism and in clinical presentation.

Clinical Setting

The condition creates a dramatic clinical syndrome that almost invariably includes chest pain. Most common in individuals with systemic hypertension, especially men in mid and late life, it may also be expected in patients with congenital and/or heritable weakness of the aortic media. For example, patients with Marfan's Syndrome and those with aortic coarctation or bicuspid aortic valve have an increased risk of aortic dissection.

Characteristics of the "Pain"

Patient's characterization of the "chest pain"

All but a small minority of patients with acute aortic dissection present because of pain in the trunk.[1,2] Two characteristics of the "pain" set it apart: first, the pain produced by aortic dissection is almost always very intense and often agonizing. Patients may indicate that it is the worst they have ever ex-

From: Hurst JW, Morris DC (eds): *"Chest Pain"* →. © Futura Publishing Co., Inc., Armonk, NY, 2001.

perienced. Second, suddenness of onset is typical. Moreover, the characteristic gradual crescendo to maximum intensity, typical of other pain syndromes, is absent. Thus, from a position of relative comfort the patient is abruptly in agony. Many reviews of the subject suggest that patients use descriptors such as "tearing" or "ripping." While these adjectives are occasionally spontaneously reported, this writer has often wondered whether these characteristics were inferred by the clinician based on a knowledge of the pathogenesis of the disorder. Thus, the intensity of the pain and its sudden onset combined with location of the pain in more than one site on the torso (see below) should alert the examiner to the likelihood of aortic dissection.

A neurosurgeon with a career-long interest in the mechanisms of pain provided this first-hand description,[3] " . . . I was taking a nap in a New York hotel room prior to going out for that evening. . . . I turned over in bed and had the sudden onset of a severe pain just medial to and above the scapula. . . . the intensity of the pain rapidly reached a level I had rarely experienced before." He went on to describe the pulsatile nature of his discomfort, a seldom emphasized feature of the pain of this disorder. "I noticed at once that the pain was pulsating slowly, varying from great intensity to negligible, in a cyclical manner. I soon realized that this was my pulse rate, surprisingly slow at about 40 beats per minute. . . . I was beginning to believe that these symptoms could only be the result of a dissecting aneurysm of the aorta." He was correct in his self-diagnosis.

Common location of the "chest pain"

The pain of aortic dissection occurs predictably in the midline of the torso in one or more of the following areas: the anterior chest, the interscapular region, the epigastrium, and the lumbar area (see Figures 43–1 and 43–2). Most characteristically, it involves more than one of these locations, either simultaneously or sequentially. So characteristic is the involvement of multiple sites that it constitutes an important signal to the examiner. In a review of our experience we found that only about a third of patients had pain isolated to one of the four sites mentioned, about a third had pain in two sites, and the final third had discomfort in three or four sites. Three-quarters of all patients with dissection had discomfort in the anterior chest, hence the first diagnostic thought upon presentation is often myocardial infarction, a condition far more common than aortic dissection. This mimicry may be enhanced in some patients with aortic dissection who report pain in the neck and throat. The examiner must, therefore, recognize that accompanying pain in the interscapular, epigastric, or lumbar areas may be signaling the less common condition.

Some authors have reported interscapular pain to be a hallmark of

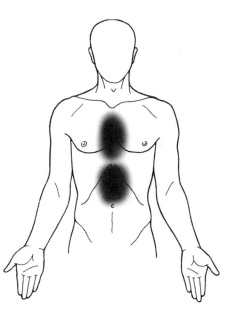

Figure 43–1. The "chest pain" caused by dissection of the ascending aorta may be located in the thorax (see upper dark area). The "chest pain" caused by dissection of the abdominal aorta may be located in the epigastrum as illustrated in the lower dark area shown.

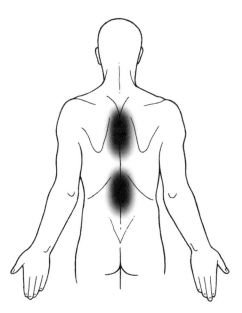

Figure 43–2. The "chest pain" caused by dissection of the ascending aorta may be located in the upper portion of the back (see upper dark area). In fact, the pain due to dissection of the aorta may be felt more severely in the back. The "chest pain" caused by dissection of the abdominal aorta may be located in the lower portion of the back (see lower dark area).

distal aortic dissection. (i.e., the process begins beyond the arch vessels.) Slater and DeSanctis[2] found that 94% of their patients with distal dissection had interscapular pain as compared to 50% of patients in whom the dissection involved the ascending aorta. Pain in that location without pain in the anterior chest was rare in proximal dissection while pain in the anterior chest without interscapular pain provided a clue to involvement of the ascending aorta. Practically, these hints as to the location of the process are of little use since an adequate diagnostic approach nearly always requires imaging to identify the site of the dissection.

Uncommon locations of the "chest pain"

Pain limited to sites other than the four mentioned above is rare. Discomfort in the jaw, throat, neck, or shoulder in association with anterior chest pain has already been commented upon. While not frequent, the potential for confusion with the radiation of myocardial infarction (MI) pain makes it important to recognize. The retropubic region is another rare location of the pain of aortic dissection.

Size of the painful "area"

In keeping with its visceral origin, the pain of aortic dissection is sensed over relatively large areas of the torso.

Duration of the "chest pain"

From a diagnostic standpoint, the duration of the pain is not helpful. As described above, aortic dissection is a sudden, catastrophic event and not a recurring symptom of a chronic illness. In patients for whom intensive antihypertensive therapy is chosen over operative treatment, continued pain despite adequate blood pressure control may constitute an indication for operative intervention. External rupture or a major stroke may result in cessation of pain but both are preterminal events.

Tenderness of the chest wall

Tenderness of the chest wall is not a characteristic feature of the pain of aortic dissection.

Precipitating causes of the "chest pain"

Unlike effort angina, the pain of aortic dissection is not predictably triggered by any specific activity or event. An exception may be the occasional report of its onset during intense isometric exercise, for example, straining to lift a heavy object. It could be suggested that the systemic hypertension resulting from such a maneuver triggers the dissection, but the symptoms of the vast majority of aortic dissections begin with the victim at rest or engaged in ordinary activity. The use of cocaine can precipitate aortic dissection undoubtedlyu as the result of an abrupt elevation of blood pressure.

Relief of the "chest pain"

The pain of acute aortic dissection is not relieved by a change in body position or any other action on the part of the patient.

Associated Symptoms

Other than pain, syncope is the only symptom of aortic dissection occurring with any frequency. It may follow an episode of pain, but its occurrence may prevent the patient from perceiving the pain or may cloud his or her memory for it. Although relatively unusual as the sole manifestation of this disorder, recognition of its importance is crucial. Syncope and its frequent companion, hypotension, almost invariably are associated with rupture of the ascending aorta into the pericardial space. Thus, the occurrence of syncope identifies a patient in need of emergency surgical intervention.

A few patients complain of weakness of the legs at the same time as the "chest pain." Spinal cord ischemia, reflecting involvement by the dissection of the origin of one or more of the spinal arteries, may be the source. Similarly bilateral or unilateral leg weakness can result from obstruction of one or both of the iliac branches by the dissection.

Associated Signs

Physical examination

Two principal physical findings that can support the suspicion of aortic dissection should be specifically sought. First, a murmur of aortic regurgitation, attributable to distortion of the aortic root and undermining of the support for the aortic valve, will be found in about half of all patients with dissection beginning in the ascending aorta. Second, absence or diminution of a femoral, radial, or carotid pulse can also be identified in about half of patients with ascending dissection so that all but a small minority of individuals with dissection involving the ascending aorta will not have one or both of these findings.[1] In contrast, a majority of patients whose dissection spares the ascending aorta have neither of these signs. The murmur of aortic regurgitation is quite infrequent and pulse loss less frequent than in proximal dissection.[1]

Many patients with acute aortic dissection are hypertensive on admission in keeping with the risk of this process in hypertensive patients. A small number are alarmingly hypertensive. Diastolic blood pressures of 150–160 mmHg are sometimes encountered. It has been postulated that renal ischemia accounts for this. Twenty percent of patients with ascending dissection are hypotensive. Most or all of these have rupture into the pericardial space.

"Routine" laboratory tests

Among the customary "routine" laboratory examinations only the *chest x-ray film* is of practical importance for the diagnosis of aortic dissection. The aortic silhouette is abnormal in up to 90% of patients with acute dissection.[2] Dissection of the proximal aorta results in protrusion of the aortic shadow from the right side of the mediastinum, and distortion of the aortic knob is typical of distal dissection. Unfortunately, these findings are nonspecific and the quality of the film is often less than ideal in these acutely ill patients. Despite these limitations, in an appropriate clinical setting the x-ray finding of an abnormal mediastinal contour increases the likelihood of the diagnosis.

The electrocardiogram often demonstrates left ventricular hypertrophy. Hypertrophy-associated ST-T changes may entice the unwary to diagnose MI and administer thrombolytic therapy, a potentially calamitous decision. In rare instances compromise of an aortocoronary ostium by the dissection may, in fact, produce an acute infarction with diagnostic electrocardiographic findings. Fortunately, this is a rare event.

Exceptions to the Usual Manifestations

A small minority of patients do not report pain. Some will have experienced syncope and will either not remember or not have appreciated the discomfort. Others will have had a major neurologic event as an early complication of their disease and be unable to provide a history. Truly painless dissections are most often small and limited, but even extensive ones occasionally turn up as surprise findings on autopsy or radiographic examination.

Evidence of occlusion of an aortic branch may dominate the clinical picture. Sudden hemiparesis or paraparesis, a consequence of cerebral or spinal cord ischemia may make the presentation appear to be a stroke.

Rarely, symptoms related to an ischemic limb or evidence of severe aortic regurgitation may dominate the picture.

Also infrequent are patients who appear with chest pain typical of pericarditis. Their presentation may include a friction rub and electrocardiographic changes typical of that disorder. "Weeping" from the external surface of the affected ascending aorta into the pericardial space probably accounts for this presentation.

Differential Diagnosis

The diagnosis of acute aortic dissection can be strongly suspected on clinical grounds in most instances *if it is considered.* If the possibility is not considered, important physical findings may be missed. Nearly all patients present with acute pain. Failure to suspect dissection occurs because more common illnesses (e.g., acute MI, pulmonary embolism, cholecystitis, perforated abdominal viscus, or lumbosacral strain) may be simulated. The characteristics of the pain that should alert the examiner to the possibility of dissection are listed in Table 43–1.

Once the identifying characteristics of the pain are recognized, the physical examination can be focused on a search for the murmur of aortic regurgitation or alterations in the radial, femoral, or carotid pulses. Such an examination and study of the chest radiograph for evidence of distortion of the aortic silhouette will nearly always point the way to the diagnosis.

Other Diagnostic Testing

For confirmation of the diagnosis, either computed tomography *after bolus administration of contrast material* or *transesophageal echocardiography* may be used with confidence. Both have high sensitivity and high specificity. Some believe magnetic resonance imaging to be even more accurate; however, its value is limited in acutely ill patients because of the longer imaging time and the inaccessibility of patients during image acquisition.

Aortography, once the standard definitive test, is seldom required.

Table 43–1.

Characteristics of Pain Suggesting Aortic Dissection.

Abruptness of onset
Maximal intensity from inception
Excruciating in nature
Occurring simultaneously or sequentially in more than one location

Only when detailed knowledge of the status of the branch vessels is important to the surgeon will it be mandatory before operative treatment. Since aortography allows visualization primarily of the lumen of the aorta, it may in fact not identify a recently appreciated variant of aortic dissection, *medial hematoma*. As is true of classic dissection, in this condition there is a collection of blood separating the layers of the aortic media. Unlike the typical situation no visible connection to the aortic lumen is present. Consequently, no opacification of the medial cleavage may occur and the presence of this "false" lumen may be missed. Computed tomography, transesophageal echocardiography, or magnetic resonance imaging will identify this lesion.

Etiolology and Basic Mechanisms Responsible for the "Pain"

A predilection for aortic dissection appears to result from a weakened aortic media in individuals with certain heritable disorders and in others with congenital abnormalities of the aorta and/or the aortic valve. The great risk of aortic dissection in Marfan's syndrome has long been known and the increased incidence of dissection in patients with aortic coarctation or bicuspid aortic valve have recently been well established. The underlying basis for an abnormal aortic media in Marfan's syndrome has been identified. A genetic mutation(s) results in abnormal fibrillin, an interstitial protein closely related to elastin. As of this writing, no underlying abnormality of the aortic media has been identified in the majority of patients with dissection who have none of these conditions. Since most are hypertensive it is an open question as to whether the process develops solely because of the abnormally high aortic wall stress or whether the increased stress uncovers a latent weakness. A light microscopic abnormality of the aortic media, "cystic medial necrosis," described 75 years ago by Erdheim, was long considered emblematic of a diseased aortic wall. Recent systematic studies suggest that it is a nonspecific finding reflecting an aorta that has been subjected to prolonged wear and tear.

It seems likely, though there have not been systematic studies, that the splitting of the elastic lamina of the aortic media by the dissecting column of blood is the direct cause of the pain. Two observations lead this writer to that conclusion. First, the pain is difficult to relieve with analgesics, even with narcotics. However, it often subsides with appropriate antihypertensive treatment (see below), making it reasonable to presume the relief to be attributable to the effect of the treatment in halting the progression of the medial hematoma and reducing the pressure for expansion of the false channel. Second, in many patients pain occurs sequentially over the thorax from chest to back or abdomen as if tracking the progress of the process.

Treatment

Symptomatic relief of the "chest pain" may be very difficult even with narcotics. Pharmacological reduction in the arterial pressure, for example with nitroprusside or beta-adrenergic blocking drugs, is more consistently effective. There are, however, even more urgent reasons for instituting aggressive antihypertensive treatment, either as a prelude to surgery or as the fundamental treatment strategy. This is true since sudden life-threatening complications, particularly external rupture with cardiac tamponade or exsanguination, threaten. Untreated, the mortality of those with involvement of the ascending aorta is about one per cent per hour for the first 48 hours. For this reason aggressive antihypertensive therapy with beta-adrenergic blocking drugs and/or a potent vasodilator such as nitroprusside are begun at once for all individuals in whom the blood pressure is elevated. The goals of such treatment are to halt the progression of the medial split and to prevent external rupture of the false channel. Urgent operative management of nearly all dissections involving the ascending aorta is indicated. The surgeon will resect the aortic segment containing the entry tear and replace it with a graft. For dissections not involving the ascending aorta the risk of rupture is much less, and continued aggressive blood pressure control is the strategy of choice. Complications such as occlusion of an artery to a major branch vessel or continued pain may dictate an operative approach. If so, the surgeon will adopt the same strategy as in ascending dissection, that is, removal of the aortic segment containing the entry tear. Surgery for dissection in the descending thoracic aorta is more morbid than that in the proximal segment. Paraplegia is a complication in about 10%.

References

1. Lindsay J Jr, Hurst JW. Clinical features and prognosis in dissecting aneurysm of the aorta. *Circulation* 1967;35:880–888.
2. Slater EE, DeSanctis RW. The clinical recognition of dissecting aortic aneurysm. *Am J Med* 1976;60:625–633.
3. Hunt WE, Wooley CF. The pulsatile pain of acute aortic dissection: A neurosurgeon's personal experience. *Am Heart J* 1996;132:1267–1268.
4. Armstrong WF, Bach DS, Carey LM, et al. Clinical and echocardiographic findings in patients with suspected acute aortic dissection. *Am Heart J* 1998;136:1051–1060.
5. Lindsay J Jr. Diagnosis and treatment of diseases of the aorta. *Current Prob Cardiol* 1997;22:506–518.

44

"Chest Pain" in Patients with Aortic Aneurysms

Joseph Lindsay, Jr, MD

General Considerations

Aneurysms, areas of focal or diffuse dilatation of the aorta, develop at sites of congenital or acquired medial weakness.[1] The dilatation may be circumferential (fusiform) or balloon-like (saccular). Aneurysms may be located at any position along the aorta's long axis, but they are most frequent below the renal arteries and at the aortic root. Expansion and rupture are nearly inevitable unless the patient succumbs to an intercurrent illness before this can occur.

Clinical Setting

Aneurysms are uncommon before middle and late life except in patients with identifiable congenital syndromes associated with connective tissue weakness.

Characteristics of the "Pain"

Patient's characterization of the "chest pain"

Unlike the situation with angina pectoris and aortic dissection, no typical chest pain of aortic aneurysm can be described. Furthermore, the absence of pain prior to impending rupture is the rule rather than the exception. Thus, the onset of pain signals an important turning point in the natural history of such lesions. *When chest or back pain (abdominal or back*

From: Hurst JW, Morris DC (eds): *"Chest Pain"* →. © Futura Publishing Co., Inc., Armonk, NY, 2001.

pain in the case of abdominal aneurysm) can be clearly associated with an aneurysm, it should be assumed that expansion is occurring and that rupture has either taken place or is impending. Similarly, the threat of rupture must be considered when any pain in a patient with aortic aneurysm cannot be clearly demonstrated to originate in another process. Available descriptions of the discomfort almost universally use the adjectives "deep" and "aching," but these nonspecific descriptors of visceral pain are not particularly useful and variations on the theme are frequent. For instance, pleuritic pain may reflect leak into the pleural space or mediastinum and pain originating from bony structures may result from erosion of bone.

Common location of the "chest pain"

The location of the pain depends upon the site of the aneurysm and the periaortic structures upon which it is impinging. As with aortic dissection it is typically reported along the course of the aorta in the midline of the trunk. The location of the "chest pain" due to rupture of an aneurysm of the ascending aorta might mimic the "pain" of myocardial infarction, pericarditis, or dissection of the aorta (see Figures 44–1, 44–2, and 44–3). Pain from an expanding aneurysm of the descending segment of the aorta may produce back or left chest pain (see Figure 44–4). Expansion or rupture of an infrarenal aneurysm may mimic an acute abdominal process (see Figure 44–5).

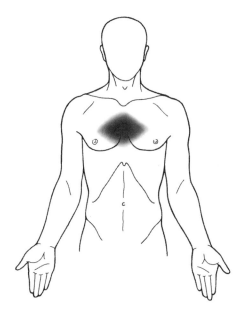

Figure 44–1. The pain associated with an expanding or a ruptured thoracic aneurysm may be located in the area of the chest shown in the above illustration. The location of the pain is similar to that of myocardial infarction.

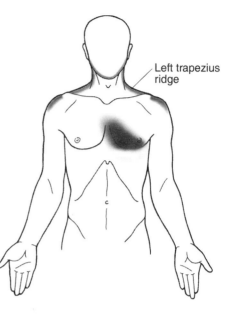

Figure 44–2. The *location* of the pain of an expanding or a ruptured thoracic aortic aneurysm may be similar to that of pericarditis. The pain of a ruptured thoracic aortic aneurysm is usually constant, but it may be aggravated by inspiration.

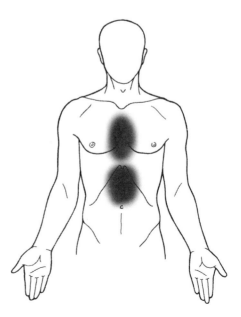

Figure 44–3. The location of the pain of an expanding or a ruptured aortic aneurysm may be similar to the location of the pain produced by dissection of the aorta. The upper dark area illustrates the location of the pain due to an expanding or a ruptured aneurysm of the thoracic aorta. The lower dark area illustrates the location of the pain due to an expanding or a ruptured aneurysm of the abdominal aorta.

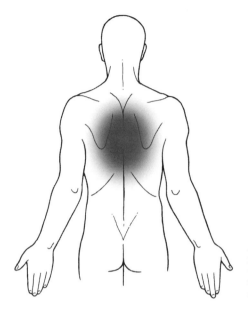

Figure 44–4. The dark area shown illustrates the location of pain produced by an expanding or a ruptured descending thoracic aortic aneurysm.

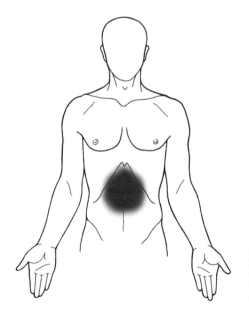

Figure 44–5. The dark area shown illustrates the location of the pain due to an expanding or a ruptured abdominal aortic aneurysm.

Uncommon locations or features of the "chest pain"

Aneurysms of the aortic arch and those of the descending thoracic aorta are of particular interest. Fixed by the arch vessels, they lie in a position to compress mediastinal structures or to erode the thoracic spine. Pain in the back or in a variety of locations in the rib cage may result.

Size of the "painful" area

Unlike the pain originating in the chest wall, "pain" originating in an expanding aortic aneurysm is typically deep and visceral in nature and is experienced over a substantial area of the surface of the torso.

Duration of the "chest pain"

In as much as pain associated with aortic aneurysm indicates expansion or impending rupture of the aorta, it often precedes more overt evidence of rupture by a few hours. The pain is usually persistent with slight waxing and waning until rupture develops. Occasionally, it may persist for several days and rarely for a few weeks. Only when the pain results from erosion of the vertebrae or rib cage is it likely to be chronic.

Tenderness of the chest wall

Tenderness of the chest wall is characteristic of a process originating in those structures and not of an expanding aneurysm. In the unusual case of an aneurysm eroding a rib or vertebra, some tenderness may be detected in the area of erosion.

Precipitating causes of the "chest pain"

No consistent precipitating cause has been connected with aortic aneurysm rupture and therefore there are no obvious precipitating causes of the "pain."

Relief of the "chest pain"

There is no typical and therefore no diagnostically helpful maneuver or drug for the relief of pain associated with aortic aneurysm.

Associated Symptoms

Aneurysms involving the aortic arch, positioned as they are adjacent to a variety of mediastinal structures, may produce symptoms by compression of these structures. Tracheobronchial compression may produce a chronic cough, dyspnea, or wheezing. Compression of the recurrent laryngeal nerve as it loops around the arch may produce hoarseness. Esophageal compression may produce dysphagia. Compression of the great veins in the thorax may produce signs of obstruction of the superior vena cava. In fact, aortic aneurysm is among the most common causes of this dramatic clinical syndrome. Descending thoracic aortic aneurysms may become adherent to adjacent lung. Massive hemoptysis is the usual consequence of rupture, but recurrent smaller amounts of hemoptysis can precede the final event by days or weeks. Finally, it is important to remember that rupture of an aneurysm may be heralded by syncope.

Associated Signs

Physical examination

Detection of a pulsating mass in the epigastrium in the course of a routine physical examination is frequently the way in which abdominal aortic aneurysms are detected. In fact, unless the patient is particularly obese, this finding can be detected in nearly all patients with abdominal aneurysms of appreciable size.

Physical findings are not frequent with thoracic aneurysms. However, pulsatile lifting of one of the sternoclavicular joints—a rarely sought physical sign—can raise the suspicion of a thoracic aortic aneurysm. Rarely, tracheal deviation or a tracheal "tug" can be detected in aneurysms involving the aortic arch. Detection of the murmur of aortic regurgitation frequently leads to the identification of an aortic root aneurysm.

Evidence of acute blood loss often dominates the clinical presentation when an aneurysm has ruptured. Pallor, hypotension, and tachycardia provide testimony to the event. Massive hematemesis or hemoptysis accompanies rupture into the esophagus or tracheobronchial tree. Abdominal pain and tenderness, usually moderate, accompanies rupture of an abdominal aneurysm.

"Routine" laboratory tests

As has been stated, most aortic aneurysms are asymptomatic and therefore come to the attention of the physician because of an examination or a laboratory study that was ordered to solve another clinical problem. Standard radiographic examinations commonly detect such unexpected lesions and are the most useful routine test for identifying aortic aneurysm if symptoms suggest the possibility of rupture. Posterior-anterior films of the chest may, in many instances, identify aneurysms involving the arch and descending thoracic aorta, but those of the aortic root (anuloaortic ectasia) may not be seen since their intrapericardial location results in their being obscured by the cardiac silhouette. Anterior-posterior or cross table lateral films of the abdomen may identify the "egg-shell" calcification that is common in the wall of abdominal aortic aneurysms.

Ultrasound examinations are often useful when plain radiographs do not provide the needed information. Aortic root aneurysm is often first identified during a two-dimensional echocardiogram conducted because of the murmur of aortic regurgitation or an unrelated cardiac condition. Abdominal ultrasound can confirm the presence of an abdominal aneurysm that is suspected from physical examination. Ultrasound examinations also provide a useful estimate of the size of an aneurysm.

Exceptions to the Usual Manifestations

Complications of an aortic aneurysm may produce clinical presentations that do not initially draw attention to the presence of the aortic dilatation. Embolization of plaque material and thrombus from the "raw" surface of the atherosclerotic aorta is frequent and may be the initial manifestation of a previously unrecognized aneurysm. Emboli to the lower extremities or the abdominal viscera are most common, but stroke attributable to embolism to the brain can also occur. Moreover, rupture of an aneurysm into an adjacent venous structure, the pulmonary artery, or a cardiac chamber may produce circulatory decompensation and a continuous murmur. Rarely an abdominal aneurysm ruptures or leaks into the duodenum resulting in a picture of gastrointestinal hemorrhage. Although the hemorrhage is usually massive, it can be in smaller amounts and intermittent. Such aortoduodenal fistulae are somewhat more common as a late complication of graft replacement of an abdominal aortic aneurysm.

Differential Diagnosis

An expanding or ruptured thoracic aneurysm may produce "chest pain" that requires the examiner to consider a variety of diagnoses. The presence of circulatory signs of blood loss is always important but this may be initially confusing. The "chest pain" may have features suggestive of a pleuritic process and thus require that the diagnosis of pulmonary embolism/infarction, pneumonia, or pericarditis be considered. A musculoskeletal source can be suggested particularly if the aneurysm is producing bony erosion. Myocardial infarction may be suggested when rupture of an aneurysm of the aortic root occurs. Fortunately for the examiner, a chest radiograph is most often among the first diagnostic tests obtained in patients with "chest pain" and typically leads to an appreciation of the nature of the process.

The pain of aortic dissection, described in Chapter 43, is distinctive. Abrupt expansion or rupture of a pre-existing aneurysm can be similar. A formerly popular designation of aortic dissection as "dissecting aortic aneurysm" reflects this potential confusion. While the diagnostic strategy and therapy may be similar, the pathogenetic bases for the two conditions are sufficiently dissimilar as to make the distinction important.

Just as rupture of an aneurysm in the thorax raises a broad differential diagnosis, rupture of one in the abdomen can provide an equally troublesome diagnostic dilemma. If the possibility occurs to the examiner, the diagnosis can, however, be relatively easy. Abdominal distress, the source of which is not initially clear, in a man older than 55 or 60 years should be a warning flag. Evidence of blood loss, not a feature of many acute abdominal conditions, is a further cause to consider this entity.

Other Diagnostic Testing

Computed radiographic tomography, magnetic resonance imaging or angiography, and transesophageal echocardiography are all valuable, but the latter two methods of examination have limitations. Transesophageal echo is largely useful for the thoracic aorta and magnetic resonance examinations are not available in all institutions and are limited in their applicability in acutely ill patients. Thus, computed tomography is often the most readily available imaging modality and, when technically satisfactory, almost always provides the necessary diagnostic information.

Etiology and Basic Mechanisms Responsible for the "Pain"

The medial weakness underlying an aneurysm may be heritable (e.g,. Marfan's syndrome), associated with a congenital anomaly (e.g., coarctation, or bicuspid aortic valve), acquired from an infectious process (eg. luetic or bacterial aortitis), or from noninfectious aortitis (e.g., Takayasu's or giant cell). Aneurysms also commonly occur at the site of medial weakness created by previous aortic dissection. Most often, however, the etiology is not obvious. When this is the case, aneurysms have often been labeled "atherosclerotic," but this assumption is now challenged by those who believe that as yet unidentified defects in the media are required for aneurysm formation. The challengers contend that the atherosclerosis covering the luminal surface of the aneurysm results from the altered flow patterns that follow aortic dilatation.

No detailed study of the mechanisms of pain in patients with expanding or ruptured aortic aneurysm has been reported. It is intuitively attractive to believe that the discomfort results from pressure by the expanding aneurysm on afferent nerves in the aortic wall and periaortic tissue.

Treatment

The treatment of aortic aneurysms is surgical. In order to prevent rupture, asymptomatic aneurysms should be removed when they reach a size at which the risk of rupture exceeds operative risk. Currently, thoracic aneurysms that are 6 cm in diameter or abdominal aneurysms that reach 5 cm in diameter are considered to meet this threshold, but operation may be delayed in patients with multiple comorbid conditions. Moreover, many surgeons recommend operation even before aneurysms reach these sizes in younger, "good risk" subjects. In patients with Marfan's syndrome resection of an ascending aortic aneurysm of 5 cm (rather than 6 as recommended for the patient without this condition) has been advocated. In most instances the aneurysm is resected and replaced with a graft of synthetic material. The operative approach and its complexity varies with the location of the structure.

References

1. Lindsay J Jr. Diagnosis and treatment of diseases of the aorta. *Current Prob Cardiol* 1997;22:506–518.

Part XII

"Chest Pain" Related to Emotional or Psychiatric Conditions

Although the definition of "chest pain"→ is discussed in Chapter 1, the definition is repeated here so that communication is clear.

The quotation marks around "chest" imply that different patients have different definitions of the word "chest." Here we use the word to indicate pain located above the waist. Then, too, *angina pectoris* is not always located in the pectoral region—it may be felt only in the jaw, neck, shoulder, elbow, or wrist. Therefore, the word "chest" implies that other parts of the upper body may also be involved with painful syndromes.

The quotation marks around "pain" imply that patients may assign other terms to their discomfort, such as indigestion, burning, ache, etc.

The arrow after "chest pain" implies that the physician initially may not know the cause of the symptom, so a differential diagnosis must be established that fits the available information.

45

"Chest Pain" in Patients with Anxiety Disorders

Bernard L. Frankel, MD

General Considerations

In 1871, Jacob Da Costa described a cluster of symptoms (including chest pain, palpitations, rapid pulse, headaches, dizziness, fatigue, gastrointestinal symptoms, sleep difficulties, etc.) which subsequently came to be known by terms such as Da Costa's syndrome, soldiers' heart, effort syndrome, irritable heart, neurasthenia, and most commonly, neurocirculatory asthenia.[1,2] A sine qua non of this disorder has always been the absence of significant cardiac pathology, particularly coronary artery disease, as an etiologic factor. As a result of more recent studies, it is generally accepted that a primary psychiatric diagnosis accounts for most cases of this condition.[3]

Coronary arteriography has documented the absence of significant coronary atherosclerotic heart disease as the cause of chest pain in patients who, in the past, might have been diagnosed with neurocirculatory asthenia. Studies have consistently shown that in 10% to 40% of patients with chest pain who are evaluated with coronary arteriography, there is no evidence of clinically significant coronary antherosclerosis.[4] Despite the normal arteriograms and the low risk of future myocardial infarctions, as many as 70% of these patients continue to complain in follow-up studies of chest pain with associated significant social and occupational disability.[5]

Clinical Setting

Not surprisingly, there is a high prevalence of psychiatric disorders, especially *anxiety and depressive disorders,* in patients with noncardiac chest

From: Hurst JW, Morris DC (eds): *"Chest Pain"* →. © Futura Publishing Co., Inc., Armonk, NY, 2001.

pain.[6] The most common psychiatric disorder diagnosed in patients with such pain is *panic disorder,* its prevalence in these patients ranging from 25% to 60%.[7] In these patients, panic disorder tends to be associated with being female and younger than 45. There is often a family history of panic disorder or other anxiety disorders. Risk factors for coronary atherosclerosis are often absent. Patients with panic disorder often have a past history of *generalized anxiety disorder* or *major depressive disorder,* and/or have either of these disorders comorbidly with panic disorder. They also are likely to have associated past or current social or occupational difficulties, contact with mental health professionals, and/or use of psychotropic drugs compared to patients with angina pectoris and *without* panic disorder.

Characteristics of the "Pain"

Patients' characterization of the "chest pain"

Patients with anxiety disorders may describe the pain as "sticking," "stabbing," and/or a "dull ache." They may refer to chest "discomfort" or "tightness" rather than "pain." Most characteristic of *panic disorder* is the pain's onset during a panic *attack,* the diagnosis of which requires the acute onset of intense fear or discomfort with at least four of the 13 symptoms in Table 45–1 developing abruptly and reaching a peak within 10 minutes. This

---

Table 45–1.

Criteria for Panic Attack.

A discrete period of intense fear or discomfort, in which four (or more) of the following symptoms developed abruptly and reached a peak within 10 minutes:
  (1) palpitations, pounding heart, or accelerated heart rate
  (2) sweating
  (3) trembling or shaking
  (4) sensations of shortness of breath or smothering
  (5) feeling of choking
  (6) chest pain or discomfort
  (7) nausea or abdominal distress
  (8) feeling dizzy, unsteady, lightheaded, or faint
  (9) derealization (feelings of unreality) or depersonalization (being detached from oneself)
  (10) fear of losing control or going crazy
  (11) fear of dying
  (12) paresthesias (numbness or tingling sensations)
  (13) chills or hot flushes

Source: Reprinted with permission from the Diagnostic and Statistical Manual of Mental Disorders, Fourth Edition. Washington, DC, American Psychiatric Association, 1994.

attack usually lasts from 5 to 20 minutes and rarely as long as an hour. Recurrent and unexpected panic attacks are the key features of panic disorder.[8]

Common location of the "chest pain"

"Chest pain" related to a panic attack is sometimes localized to the retrosternal region, especially if the sensation of choking, dyspnea, or smothering is also prominent. Generally, however, "chest pain" due to a psychiatric disorder does not have characteristic locations or patterns of radiation which help distinguish it from angina pectoris (see Figures 45–1, 45–2, and 45–3.)

Uncommon locations of the "chest pain"

Because some very anxious patients with psychiatric disorders are prone to misinterpret the significance of trivial somatic sensations in any area of the upper torso as "chest pain," unusual sites may occasionally be cited (see Figure 45–4.)

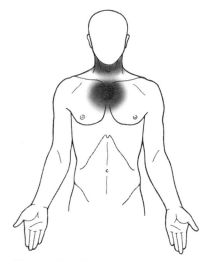

Figure 45–1. This figure shows the location of the "chest pain" sometimes associated with panic attacks. It may be felt anteriorly (rather than retrosternally) and in the neck.

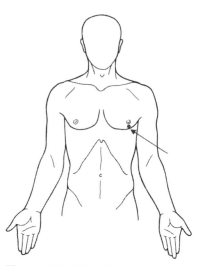

Figure 45–2. The "chest pain" associated with anxiety may be located as shown in this diagram. The size of the area may be no larger than the tip of the finger.

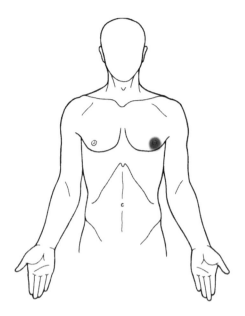

Figure 45–3. The "chest pain" associated with anxiety may be located near the cardiac apex. The area of discomfort may be about half the size of the hand.

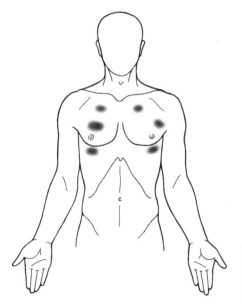

Figure 45–4. Patients with anxiety may complain of "chest pain" in any or all of the areas of the chest shown in this illustration.

Size of the painful "area"

Typically, there is no characteristic size of the area of the "chest pain" related to anxiety disorders, unless the pain is associated with chest wall tenderness, which may be very localized (e.g., "one-finger") or diffuse.

Duration of the "chest pain"

As noted above, "chest pain" due to a panic attack characteristically develops abruptly, peaks within 10 minutes, and subsides within 20 minutes. In contrast, patients with "chest pain" related to generalized anxiety disorder or hypochondriasis may describe a continuous, dull ache lasting for hours or days, or intermittent discomfort or achiness recurring over longer periods (e.g., "every day for months").

Tenderness of chest wall

Though uncommon, localized or diffuse chest wall tenderness, when present, greatly increases the likelihood of a psychiatric etiology for the "chest pain."

Precipitating causes of the "chest pain"

In patients with panic disorder, the panic attacks are recurrent and un-expected. Patients typically report no precipitants (e.g., "It came out of the blue!"). Patients with phobias (e.g., agoraphobia, claustrophobia) may have "chest pain" resulting from intense anxiety, with or without other symptoms of a panic attack, provoked by the realization that they are in-volved in the phobic situation. (Thus, this anxiety is not unexpected.) In patients with generalized anxiety disorder, who are chronically anxious, "chest pain" is often precipitated by stressful life events.[9,10] Also, general-ized anxiety disorder is often observed comorbidly with panic disorder.

Those patients with "chest pain" resulting from severe anxiety who do not have panic disorder, a generalized anxiety disorder, or a phobia, of-ten may be diagnosed with an *adjustment disorder with anxiety*. This diag-nosis indicates a significant stress has caused an abnormally high level of anxiety occurring within 3 months of the onset of the stress and lasting no longer than 6 months after the stress has terminated.[8] Stressful life events (e.g., losses, rejections, threats) are easy to ask about, yet primary care physicians, cardiologists, and other specialists do not routinely do so.

In some patients with "chest pain" due to anxiety, the condition stems from hypochrondriacal tendencies or frank hypochondriasis. Intense bodily preoccupation, strong fears or convictions of disease, and exaggerated fears of dying, for example, are typical manifestations of the abnormal attitudes, beliefs and worries which can act as precipitating and perpetuating factors for recurrent episodes of "chest pain" regardless of the initial causes.[8]

Relief of the "chest pain"

As noted above, the "chest pain" (and the other somatic symptoms) of a panic attack typically reach peak intensity within 10 minutes and last less than 20 minutes. If the chest pain is secondary to anxiety stemming from a stressful life event or phobic situation, then relief usually occurs when the stress is over or the patient leaves the phobic environment. Medications, typically benzodiazepines, are often effective. Reassurance about the absence of significant heart disease often fails to bring significant relief (see below).

Associated Symptoms

Patients with a panic attack as the cause of their "chest pain" have at least three more of the 13 symptoms listed in Table 45–1. These patients almost invariably have other cardiorespiratory symptoms: palpitations, pounding heart, increased heart rate; and shortness of breath or a smothering sensation. They often describe their fear as almost unbearably intense, terrorizing, or a sensation of doom. In addition to recurrent and unexpected panic attacks, the diagnosis of panic disorder requires that at least one of the panic attacks has been followed by at least 1 month's duration of one or more of three other symptoms: (a) persistent worry about having more attacks (i.e., anticipatory anxiety); (b) worry about the consequences or meaning of these attacks (e.g., a heart attack, loss of control, "going crazy"); and (c) a marked behavioral change caused by the attacks (e.g., about 50% develop agoraphobia within a year after onset).[8]

Because of the high prevalence of the disruption of family, social and/or occupational activities, as well as a worsening pessimism about getting an accurate diagnosis and effective treatment, significant depressive symptoms may develop. Between 50% and 65% of panic disorder patients have comorbid major depressive disorder.[8] Patients with panic disorder also have a high rate of comorbid substance abuse. Alcohol, benzodiazepines, opioid analgesies, and other drugs may be used in excess to relieve the anticipatory anxiety and/or the panic attack symptoms.

One of the most prevalent associated symptoms in patients with "chest pain" related to psychiatric disorders is disturbed respiratory function. Patients often report frequent sighing related to the feeling that they "just can't get a good breath." Feelings of suffocation, smothering, "air hunger," or shortness of breath after trivial physical exertion or a change in posture are also common. Less commonly, the *symptoms* of hyperventilation may also be associated with this "chest pain." (Hyperventilation *syndrome*, a contentious diagnosis, is probably synonymous with panic disorder.)[6, 10]

Because other functional disorders often coexist in patients with "chest pain" related to psychiatric disorders (e.g., chronic fatigue, irritable bowel, tension headaches) it is important to also inquire about noncardiac somatic symptoms. Similarly, it is of value to ask about *previous* episodes of any functional complaints (cardiac and noncardiac) and whether these or any documented physical diseases were related to stressful life events. Furthermore, patients should be asked about past physical and sexual abuse, since these are often found in patients with chronic or recurrent pain for which no physical etiology has been identified.

It is not unusual for patients with "chest pain"secondary to a psychiatric disorder to report frequent evaluations in emergency rooms and the offices of specialists (e.g., cardiologists and gastroenterologists). Many eventually come to believe that "the doctors think it's all in my head." As a result, such patients may omit or minimize any psychological symptoms and psychosocial stresses so as to decrease the likelihood that the physician will think their pain is "mental" or "psychosomatic" and, therefore, will not do a very thorough evaluation. With such patients, it is essential also to ask a close family member about anxiety and depressive symptoms and current stresses in the patient's life. Such an ancillary historian often can provide important information, previously undisclosed by the patient, which is of significant diagnostic value.

In patients whose "chest pain" is associated with generalized anxiety disorder, there are other characteristic symptoms as listed in Table 45–2. These patients, unlike those with panic disorder, may describe a dull ache lasting for hours or days that is located near the cardiac apex and is unrelated to effort (see Figure 45–3). Similar to patients with panic disorder, they are more likely to have a negative cardiac risk profile, age less than 45, and a positive past psychiatric history.

Associated Signs

Physical examination

Patients with "chest pain" related to a primary anxiety disorder may have some of the manifestations of anxiety on physical examination (e.g., hyperhidrosis or a mild tremor) since they are often anxious in medical settings (especially when they start feeling the physician doesn't think their pain is "real"). The examination of the heart is usually normal, though occasionally

---

Table 45–2.

Diagnostic Criteria for Generalized Anxiety Disorder.

A. Excessive anxiety and worry (apprehensive expectation), occurring more days than not for at least 6 months, about a number of events or activities (such as work or school performance).
B. The person finds it difficult to control the worry.
C. The anxiety and worry are associated with three (or more) of the following six symptoms (with at least some symptoms present for more days than not for the past 6 months). **Note:** Only one item is required in children.
   (1) restlessness or feeling keyed up or on edge
   (2) being easily fatigued
   (3) difficulty concentrating or mind going blank
   (4) irritability
   (5) muscle tension
   (6) sleep disturbance (difficulty falling or staying asleep, or restless unsatisfying sleep)
D. The focus of the anxiety and worry is not confined to features of an Axis I disorder, e.g., the anxiety or worry is not about having a Panic Attack (as in Panic Disorder), being embarrassed in public (as in Social Phobia), being contaminated (as in Obsessive-Compulsive Disorder), being away from home or close relatives (as in Separation Anxiety Disorder), gaining weight (as in Anorexia Nervosa), having multiple physical complaints (as in Somatization Disorder), or having a serious illness (as in Hypochondriasis), and the anxiety and worry do not occur exclusively during Posttraumatic Stress Disorder.
E. The anxiety, worry, or physical symptoms cause clinically significant distress or impairment in social, occupational, or other important areas of functioning.
F. The disturbance is not due to the direct physiological effects of a substance (e.g., a drug of abuse, a medication) or a general medical condition (e.g., hyperthyroidism) and does not occur exclusively during a Mood Disorder, a Psychotic Disorder, or a Pervasive Developmental Disorder.

Source: Reprinted with permission from the Diagnostic and Statistical Manual of Mental Disorders, Fourth Edition. Washington, DC, American Psychiatric Association, 1994.

---

there is slight tachycardia or infrequent premature contractions. The following signs, however, when present, point strongly to a psychiatric etiology of their pain: (a) localized (one-finger) or diffuse areas of chest wall tenderness; (b) obvious sighs, gasping breaths often involving the accessory neck muscles, and/or respiratory "tics" (e.g., throat-clearing); (c) an inability for patients to hold their breath at peak inspiration for more than 20 seconds. (This effort may provoke their typical pain and/or extreme breathlessness.); (d) sensations of gasping and chest tightness when lying flat (in patients without obvious pulmonary edema).[11]

Some of these patients may chronically hyperventilate but do not appear to be overbreathing to an observer.[12] When hyperventilation is suspected, it may be helpful to have the patient hyperventilate during the examination, even though about 50% of patients who attempt this will not reproduce their usual pain.[10,11] Patients who *do* experience their pain and/or other symptoms of a panic attack during this voluntary hyperventilation almost certainly have a significant anxiety disorder as the etiologic factor for their pain. This simple test is, unfortunately, commonly omitted.

"Routine" laboratory tests

Laboratory tests are usually normal.

Exceptions to the Usual Manifestations

It is likely that 20% to 30% of patients with chest pain *and* documented coronary atherosclerotic heart disease with angina pectoris have a comorbid, significant psychiatric disorder (e.g., panic disorder, generalized anxiety disorder, major depression, hypochondriasis)[13] which causes amplification of both their cardiac pathology-based symptoms and their other functional, physical symptoms stemming from their psychiatric disorder. Patients with panic disorder who also have documented coronary atherosclerotic heart disease with angina pectoris may be analogous to patients with "pseudoseizures" who also have documented epilepsy; i.e., it may be very difficult to ascertain the etiology of an episode of chest pain or a seizure unless the patient happens to be having an electrocardiogram or encephalogram, respectively, during that event.

There is no evidence that panic attacks cause significant ischemic changes in patients free of cardiovascular disease. This, however, has not been studied in patients with panic disorder and coronary atherosclerotic heart disease. It is likely, though, that the intense anxiety of a panic attack in patients with panic disorder and coronary atherosclerotic heart disease will indeed cause ischemic changes since it has been shown that laboratory-induced mental stress causes such changes in patients with this type of heart disease but without panic disorder.[14,15]

Differential Diagnosis

While most patients with recurrent and unexpected panic *attacks* have panic *disorder*, some do not. It is essential to rule out other causes of these attacks: (a) medical conditions (e.g., hyperthyroidism, temporal lobe epilepsy, pheochromocytoma); (b) substances such as prescribed medications and illicit drugs (e.g., levothyroxine, theophylline, amphetamines, alcohol, caffeine, cocaine); (c) other psychiatric disorders (e.g., posttraumatic stress disorder, major depressive disorder).

A small number of patients who appear to have severe hypochondriasis or preoccupation with disease may in fact have somatic delusions, which are manifestations of a psychotic disorder, usually a *delusional disorder* (previously known as "paranoia").[8] This illness is typically less disruptive of other aspects of their lives (and is, therefore, less recognizable) than schizophrenia, a psychotic disorder which is more likely to be detected.

Other Diagnostic Testing

Clinical rating scales (which patients may easily complete in less than 5 minutes) are often helpful in diagnosing an anxiety disorder or detecting clinically significant anxiety-related symptoms.[16, 17] More extensive psychological tests, while often more informative, especially regarding hypochondriasis and somatization, typically require a referral to a mental health professional experienced in administering such tests.

Etiology and Basic Mechanisms Responsible for the "Pain"

The intense anxiety of a panic attack causes an increase in the force of the heart's contraction and in heart rate via sympathetic arousal. It also causes bodily hypervigilance, which is a heightened awareness of physical sensations and symptoms together with selective attention to them. Moreover, somatic and visceral stimuli are perceived as more serious and menacing because patients who have panic attacks have a bias toward threatening information or dangerous situations. The panic attack has been characterized as "an acutely hypochondriacal state during which the individual misattributes benign bodily sensations to serious medical disease, 'catastrophizing' them and mistaking them as evidence of a grave medical emergency."[18]

There is also convincing evidence of other etiologic factors in panic disorder (and perhaps generalized anxiety disorder as well): (a) brain abnormalities involving a dysregulation of the noradrenaline, serotonin and gamma-aminobutyric acid (GABA) neurotransmitter systems; (b) childhood learning, conditioning, and reinforcement as a result of experiences with recurrent episodes of physical symptoms and/or close involvement with anxious, somatizing parents;[19] (c) patients' psychological need to diminish their own awareness of how emotionally upset or distressed they're actually feeling about some life situation (because, for example, such emotions are perceived as evidence of "weakness" or as otherwise stigmatizing). Panic attacks can distract patients from underlying worrisome psychological issues and re-direct their anxiety and attention to identifying and treating the assumed physical disease causing their "chest pain" before it "kills" them.

There is less evidence for significant biochemical and neuroanatomic abnormalities in generalized anxiety disorder than in panic disorder. It is more likely that patients with generalized anxiety disorder have learned early in life (usually by adolescence), typically from parents, the chronic, free-floating anxiety "about everything" that characterizes this disorder. A similar learning model probably applies to patients with hypochondriasis.

How exactly does marked anxiety, depression or other intense emotions cause this chest pain? Physicians may find it useful to remind patients about familiar physical symptoms (e.g., blushing, "butterflies in the stomach," hives, sweaty palms, increased pulse, tension headaches) that generally are known to be caused by intense emotions, especially fear or anxiety. Patients know these symptoms are transient and do not connote the presence of a serious underlying physical disease. Why one person will typically have gastrointestinal symptoms and another, dermatologic or cardiorespiratory ones, appears to depend on specific organ system vulnerabilities genetically determined or acquired by learning or conditioning early in life. Thus, normally ignored minor symptoms, which might originate from the chest wall (muscles, ligaments, etc.), the esophagus, and respiratory system are greatly magnified by the strong, anxiety-tinted "lenses" of the psychiatric disorders discussed above to the point where they are experienced as "chest pain" or discomfort and interpreted as a manifestation of a potentially lethal, underlying type of heart disease. It is this mistaken, malignant interpretation which increases the anxiety which then aggravates the chest pain, thus initiating a vicious downward spiral often leading to repeated visits to emergency rooms or physicians' offices.[20] (See Chapter 46 for further discussion of issues relevant to pain etiology and mechanisms.)

Treatment

It is critical that any patients with functional physical symptoms, but especially those who mistakenly believe their symptom, "chest pain," indicates a potentially lethal heart condition, be treated by physicians with the same respect, concern, and attention to detail they would show for angina patients whose chest pain *is* caused by coronary atherosclerotic heart disease. The pain related to a psychiatric disorder is just as "real" and legitimate as that caused by coronary atherosclerotic heart disease. That it happens to have a psychiatric etiology in no way diminishes the severity of the anguish, suffering, and interference it can cause in the lives of patients. In fact, the "chest pain" in these patients may be more severe and disabling than it is in patients with angina pectoris.

Reassurance alone is not especially helpful to patients with "chest pain" due to a psychiatric disorder. Saying, for example, that "all the tests indicate that you do not have heart disease, so there's nothing to worry about" together with *not* saying what *is* causing the pain often does little to relieve the pain. Follow-up studies have consistently shown that a large number of these patients continue for several years or longer to have chest pain sufficiently severe to significantly interfere with their work, and family and/or social relationships.[21] Continuing to believe they have or *might have* serious heart disease, they remain high utilizers of health care services and sources of frustration for their well-intentioned physicians.

In addition to reassurance about the absence of heart disease as the cause of the pain, physicians need to be able to tell patients what *is* the likely cause. They should therefore, screen patients for the presence of a significant psychiatric disorder, most often panic disorder, generalized anxiety disorder and/or major depressive disorder. They should ask patients about recent psychosocial stressors (family, love-life, occupational, financial, etc.) and, if denied, also ask a close family member. Once the physician establishes that a psychiatric disorder is the likely cause, he/she needs to empathically explain that as a result of anxiety caused by stresses in their lives, which are troubling them more than they realize, patients develop the equivalent of, for example, a "tension headache in the chest wall" or a "charley-horse in a chest muscle," and this, not heart disease, is almost certainly the cause of their pain. The physician should assure patients there is effective treatment, and refer them to a psychiatrist for psychotropic medications to help with their brain's "chemical imbalance," and for psychotherapy (or counseling) to learn to deal with their stressors. They should also be given a non-renewable, short-term prescription for a benzodiazepine if anxiety and sleep difficulties are prominent symptoms.

The benzodiazepines which appear to be most useful for panic disorder until the patient is seen by the psychiatrist are clonazepam and alprazolam. Clonazepam is preferred because it is less likely to cause a significant dependence problem. For generalized anxiety disorder and anxiety associated with major depressive disorder, any of the benzodiazepines appear to be equally efficacious in the short term. (Of note, the Food and Drug Administration has approved two selective serotonin reuptake inhibitors (SSRIs), sertraline and paroxetine, for panic disorder, and another antidepressant, venlafaxine, for generalized anxiety disorder. For long-term use, these are probably preferable to the benzodiazepines.) In general, the combination of psychotropic drugs and psychotherapy (especially cognitive therapy) appears to be more effective than drugs alone in these disorders.[22] For those patients who adamantly refuse a referral to mental health professionals because they will not accept the primacy of a psychiatric disorder (typically, patients with chronic somatization related to generalized anxiety disorder and/or hypochondriasis), regularly scheduled appointments with primary care physicians who follow the specific treatment regimen for somatizing patients as detailed elsewhere have been shown to be highly effective.[23]

References

1. Da Costa JM. On irritable heart: A clinical study of a form of functional cardiac disorder and its consequences. *Am J Sci* 1871;61:17–52.
2. Paul O. Da Costa's syndrome or neurocirculatory asthenia. *Br Heart J* 1987;58:306–315.
3. Fava GA, Magelli C, Savron G, et al. Neurocirculatory asthenia: A reassessment using modern psychosomatic criteria. *Acta Psychiat Scand* 1994;89:314–319.
4. Alexander PJ, Prabhu SGS, Krisnamoorthy ES, et al. Mental disorders in patients with noncardiac chest pain. *Acta Psychiat Scand* 1994;89:291–293.
5. Fleet RP, Beitman BD. Unexplained chest pain: When is it panic disorder? *Clin Cardiol* 1997;20:187–194.
6. Katon W, Hall ML, Russo J, et al. Chest pain: Relationship of psychiatric illness to coronary arteriographic results. *Am J Med* 1988;84:1–9.
7. Carter SC, Servan-Schreiber D, Perlstein WM. Anxiety disorders and the syndrome of chest pain with normal coronary arteries: Prevalence and pathophysiology. *J Clin Psychiat* 1997;58 suppl 3):70–73.
8. American Psychiatric Association. Diagnostic and Statistical Manual of Mental Disorders, 4th ed. Washington, DC, American Psychiatric Association, 1994.
9. Carter SC, Maddock RJ. Chest pain in generalized anxiety disorder. *Int J Psychiat Med* 1992;22:291–298.
10. Goldberg RJ, Posner DA. Anxiety in the medically ill. In: Stoudemire A, Fogel BS, Greenberg DB (eds). *Psychiatric Care of the Medical Patient. 2nd Ed.* New York, Oxford University Press, 2000, pp. 165–180.
11. Bass C. Unexplained chest pain and breathlessness. *Med Clin N Amer* 1991;75:1157–1173.
12. Okel BB, Hurst JW. Prolonged hyperventilation in man. *Arch Int Med* 1961;108:757–762.
13. Wulsin LR, Yingling K. Psychiatric aspects of chest pain in the emergency department. *Med Clin N Amer* 1991;75:1175–1188.
14. Fleet RP, Dupuis G, Marchand A, et al. Panic disorder in emergency department chest pain patients: Prevalence, comorbidity, suicidal ideation, and physician recognition. *Am J Med* 1996;101:371–380.
15. Jiang W, Babyak M, Krantz DS, et al. Mental stress-induced myocardial ischemia and cardiac events. *JAMA* 1996;21:1651–1656.
16. Spielberger CD. Manual for the State-Trait Anxiety Inventory (STAI form Y). Palo Alto, CA, Consulting Psychologists Press, 1993

17. Zung WW. A rating instrument for anxiety disorders. *Psychosomatics* 1971;12: 371–379.
18. Barsky AJ. Palpitations, cardiac awareness, and panic disorder. *Am J Med* 1992;92 (suppl 1A):31S–34S.
19. Serlie AW, Erdman RAM, Passchier J, et al. Psychological aspects of non-cardiac chest pain. *Psychother Psychosom* 1995;64:62–73.
20. Salkovskis PM. Psychological treatment of noncardiac chest pain: The cognitive approach. *Am J Med* 1992;92 (suppl 5A):114S–121S
21. Ockene IS, Shay MJ, Albert JS, et al. Unexplained chest pain in patients with normal coronary arteriograms. *N Engl J Med* 1980;303:1249–1252.
22. Frankel BL. Office of psychiatry for the internist. In: Stein SF, Kokko JP (eds). *The Emory University Comprehensive Board Review in Internal Medicine.* New York, McGraw-Hill, 2000, pp. 585–600.
23. Smith GR Jr, Rost K, Kashner M. A trial of the effect of a standardized consultation on health outcomes and costs in somatizing patients. *Arch Gen Psychiat* 1995;52:238–243.

46

"Chest Pain" in Patients with Depressive Disorders

Bernard L. Frankel, MD

General Considerations

The discussion in this chapter will emphasize the depressive disorders—especially *major depressive disorder*, but also *dysthymia* and *"minor depression"*—not only as etiologic factors in noncardiac chest pain, but also as seriously complicating factors in coronary atherosclerotic heart disease.

Among medical outpatients, there is a 2% to 16% prevalence of major depressive disorder, the most serious of the depressive disorders; and for all depressive disorders, the prevalence is 9% to 20%.[1] More than half of patients with major depressive disorder present to physicians with somatic chief complaints, some of which (e.g., insomnia, fatigue, and anorexia) are nonspecific.[2] Often, however, they are about pain (e.g., in the back, head, chest). Palpitations are also among the most common depression-related somatic symptoms.[3]

With a prevalence rate in patients with noncardiac chest pain of about 20% to 40%, major depressive disorder is close behind the anxiety disorders (especially *panic disorder*, with its prevalence rate of about 25% to 60%) as a significant etiologic factor in noncardiac chest pain.[2,4] In one study, for example, of 1000 primary care outpatients, of the 27% with unexplained chest pain, about two-thirds had a "mood disorder" (i.e., major depressive disorder, dysthymia, etc.).[5]

As noted in the previous chapter, 50% to 60% of patients with panic disorder have comorbid major depressive disorder. In about one-third of these patients with both disorders, the major depressive disorder precedes the onset of the panic disorder, while in the rest the major depressive disorder is coincident with or follows the onset of the panic disorder.[6] Thus,

From: Hurst JW, Morris DC (eds): *"Chest Pain"* →. © Futura Publishing Co., Inc., Armonk, NY, 2001.

it is not surprising that studies report more than 70% of patients with non-cardiac chest pain are likely to have either panic disorder, major depressive disorder, or both compared to less than 10% of patients with angina pectoris due to coronary atherosclerotic heart disease.[7]

Other studies of patients *with* coronary atherosclerotic heart disease have reported the prevalence of "depression" (major depressive disorder, dysthymia, minor depression) as 16% to 23%.[1] Moreover, major depressive disorder has been found to greatly increase morbidity and mortality after a myocardial infarction,[8] and also appears to be an independent risk factor in the development and progression of atherosclerotic heart disease.[1]

Clinical Setting

For major depressive disorders, the mean age of onset is the late 20s, with the highest incidence occurring in the 25- to 44-year-old range. It is 1.5 to 2 times more common in females. It is not unusual to find a history of depressive disorders or alcohol abuse in close family members since studies have established a genetic predisposition toward major depressive disorder.[6]

The diagnostic criteria for *major depressive* disorder require the presence of depressed mood for at least 2 weeks, and presence of 4 of the 8 symptoms in Table 46–1, which offers a mnemonic based on these eight symptoms: SIG: E CAPS, short for "prescribe energy capsules."[9] In patients who deny depressed mood (often the elderly, who may complain of irritability instead), anhedonia *must* be present together with four or more of the remaining seven symptoms. A final diagnostic criterion is the ruling out of three other psychiatric disorders, which may also meet the criteria listed in Table 46–1: (1) bipolar disorder, depressed; (2) substance-induced

---

Table 46–1.

Diagnostic Criteria for Major Depressive Syndrome.

Sleep	Insomnia or hypersomnia
Interests	Loss of interest or pleasure in activities
Guilt	Excessive guilt, worthlessness, hopelessness
Energy	Loss of energy or fatigue
Concentration	Diminished concentration ability; indecisiveness
Appetite	Decreased appetite, >5% weight loss or gain
Psychomotor	Psychomotor retardation or agitation
Suicidality	Suicidal thought, ideation, plan, or attempt; includes thoughts of death or preoccupation with death

Source: Wise MG, Rundell JR. Concise Guide to Consultation Psychiatry, 2nd ed. Washington, DC: American Psychiatric Press, Inc. 1994:56. Used with permission.

depressive disorder (e.g., due to prednisone); and (3) depressive disorder due to a general medical condition (e.g., hypothyroidism).[6]

Dysthymia is characterized by the presence of a depressed mood most of the day, on "more days than not," for a period of at least 2 years (in adults) during which the patient has 2 or more of the following 6 symptoms: (a) appetite disturbance; (b) sleep disturbance; (c) fatigue or low energy; (d) low self-esteem; (e) hopelessness; (f) poor concentration or indecisiveness. In addition, these symptoms must cause significant impairment in occupational, social, or other important areas of functioning. Finally, these symptoms cannot be biologically caused by the use of substances (recreational or prescribed) or by a medical disorder. Often having its onset in childhood or late adolescence, dysthymia may appear to be a pervasive feature of the patient's personality and outlook on life. Dysthymic patients are at high risk for developing major depressive disorder, with a reported lifetime prevalence of 68%.[6]

Minor depression, (formally, a "depressive disorder not otherwise specified")[6] refers to clinically significant depressive symptoms which do not meet the criteria for any other mood disorder. When a stressful life event precipitates such "minor" depressive symptoms and they last no longer than 6 months, then a diagnosis of an *adjustment disorder with depressed mood* is usually appropriate.[6]

It is more likely that an anxiety or depressive disorder, rather than coronary atherosclerotic heart disease, will turn out to be the etiologic basis for the "chest pain" if (as noted in the previous chapter) the patient is female, younger than 45, without risk factors for coronary atherosclerotic heart disease, with a past psychiatric history and a positive family psychiatric history.[10,11] While the more likely of these two psychiatric disorders is panic disorder, major depressive disorder is likely to be present comorbidly in more than half the patients with noncardiac chest pain due to panic disorder. Minor depression is probably even more prevalent than major depressive disorder as a comorbid disorder in such patients.

Characteristics of the "Pain"

Patients' characterization of the "chest pain"

While some patients with depressive disorders may describe their pain as noted in the previous chapter, they are unlikely to describe the pain's occurrence as part of a panic *attack* unless they have comorbid panic *disorder* (see Table 45–1). Patients with depressive disorders, especially major depressive disorder, are more likely than anxiety-disordered patients to describe their pain in a resigned, pessimistic, or apathetic manner, sometimes simultaneously reporting their belief that the presence of a serious heart disease is a foregone conclusion. (If they have a major depressive disorder *with psychosis,* their descriptions may be delusional and bizarre.)

In patients whose pain is known to be caused by coronary atherosclerotic heart disease, and who also have a significant depressive disorder, the characteristics of the pain may be those of angina, but the patient's manner of reporting them may communicate the presence of associated significant depression. Also, patients with angina due to coronary atherosclerotic heart disease may develop another type of chest pain that is characteristic of the comorbid depressive (or anxiety) disorder.

Common location of the "chest pain"

Chest pain related to major depressive disorder or other depressive disorders has neither characteristic locations nor patterns of radiation which would indicate any specific psychiatric disorder as its etiology. As a rule, however, the discomfort is located near the cardiac apex[12] (see Figures 46–1 and 46–2). Patients with depression may describe the "chest pain" as being retrosternal with or without the "pain" being felt in other areas of the chest. This, of course, poses a difficult diagnostic problem (see Figure 46–3). Patients with coronary atherosclerotic heart disease and a comorbid depressive disorder are, of course, more likely to describe the location of their pain as retrosternal with or without radiation to the shoulder, neck, jaw, or arms.

Uncommon locations of the "chest pain"

Patients with major depressive disorder with psychosis or with marked anxiety may indicate *any* area(s) of their chest as the site(s) of the pain (see Figure 46–4). They may also describe unusual or frankly bizarre patterns of pain radiation.

Size of the painful "area"

The painful "area" may vary in size from the circumference of a finger-tip to the entire chest. Patients with a psychotic major depressive disorder may also describe unusual *shapes* as well as sizes of the area of pain.

Duration of the "chest pain"

The duration of the pain due to a depressive disorder or discomfort is often substantially longer (e.g., hours, days, "never going away") than in patients with pain due to panic disorder or angina pectoris.

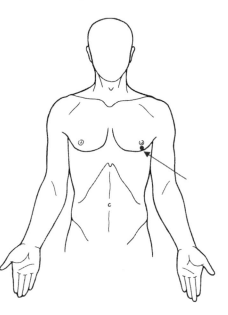

Figure 46–1. Patients with depression may describe their "chest pain' as being localized near the cardiac apex. The size of the area may be no larger than the tip of the finger. This, of course, is similar to the "chest pain" associated with anxiety.

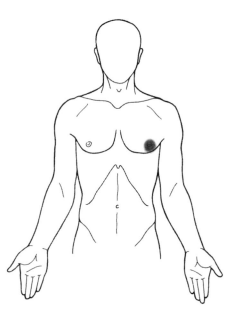

Figure 46–2. Patients with depression may describe their "chest pain" as being located near the cardiac apex and be about half the size of a hand. This, of course, is similar to the "chest pain" associated with anxiety.

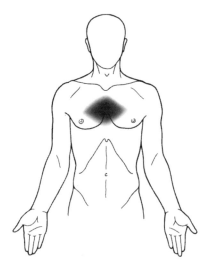

Figure 46–3. Patients with depression may describe retrosternal "chest pain." This creates a difficult diagnostic problem because the location of the discomfort may be similar to that of angina pectoris. Then, too, patients with depression and coronary atherosclerotic heart disease *and* angina may focus their attention on retrosternal discomfort which may or may not be due to myocardial ischemia.

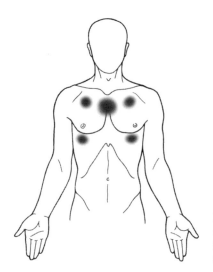

Figure 46–4. Patients with major depressive disorder with psychosis or marked anxiety may indicate *any* area(s) of their chest as the site(s) of the "pain."

Tenderness of the chest wall

As noted in the previous chapter, localized or diffuse tenderness of the chest wall, though not common, strongly points to the presence of an etilogic anxiety, depressive, or somatoform disorder.

Precipitating causes of the "chest pain"

In patients with depression-induced "chest pain," physical exertion may not be a consistent precipitant. Also, a lack of energy is a characteristic symptom of significant depression. In major depressive disorder, the "chest pain" may occur in association with an increase in the intensity of depressive symptoms, e.g., an outburst of sobbing.

While the absence of a precipitating, stressful life event does not rule out the diagnosis of major depressive disorder, many patients with this diagnosis *do* have psychosocial stressor-precipitants. In patients who have panic disorder, the "chest pain" and other symptoms of the recurrent panic attacks themselves often act as the stressful precipitant for the major depressive disorder that may develop comorbidly with or after the onset of the panic disorder. Patients with "chest pain" associated with dysthymia may also have psychosocial stressors as precipitants, especially if major depressive disorder and/or an anxiety disorder is comorbid.

Patients with angina pectoris due to coronary atherosclerotic heart disease and a comorbid depressive (or anxiety) disorder are likely to have the usual precipitants of typical angina, such as physical exertion and acute emotional distress.

Relief of the "chest pain"

There is no characteristic pattern of relief of the "chest pain" caused by depressive disorders. In those patients where the pain occurs only in relation to temporary increase in the severity of depressive symptoms (e.g., as with the onset of crying) relief may result from the return to the previous, less intense level of symptomatology. Cessation of physical exertion or reassurance is usually of little value. Only the treatment of the depressive disorder itself is likely to result in significant relief.

Associated Symptoms

Patients with major depressive disorder have at least four of the symptoms listed in Table 46–1. Because of the patient's *somatic* focus, the *psychological* symptoms (depressed mood, anhedonia, guilt, worthlessness, hopelessness, impaired concentration, indecisiveness, and suicidal ideation or recurrent thoughts of death) often remain undisclosed unless physicians specifically ask about them. They should always inquire about suicidal ideation and thoughts about death. Such thoughts are not unusual in patients who persist in believing they have a serious (and probably fatal) heart disease and feel increasingly hopeless about getting the "correct" diagnosis and treatment. Patients should also be asked routinely about substance abuse since its lifetime prevalence in major depressive disorder is about 25%.[6] In addition, patients with major depressive disorder complain of significantly more symptoms on a medical review of symptoms compared with non-depressed control patients.[13] If the major depressive disorder is of the psychotic variety, patients may have bizarre, delusional ideas about the causes of their pain or their (nonexistent) heart disease. They may complain, for example, of a heart that is literally "rotting."

Patients with depressive disorders have a greatly impaired ability to solve problems and cope with the expectations and tremendous trifles of daily life. Non-compliance with treatment regimens, therefore, is also common.

While their "chest pain" may be the most prominent symptom, patients with major depressive disorder, dysthymia, or minor depression often have other functional symptoms (e.g. headaches, gastrointestinal disturbances, musculoskeletal aches) especially where there is a history of chronic somatization. Since there is also a high prevalence of comorbid anxiety disorders in patients with depressive disorders, please see the previous chapter for the relevant associated symptoms.

Associated Signs

Physical examination

Patients who have severe major depressive disorder may convey their emotional state by their appearance and behavior. If they have psychomotor retardation, their faces may appear downcast, blank, resigned, apathetic, and expressionless. Their posture may be hunched over, almost motionless; their gait, slow. They may speak slowly, in brief phrases without emotional intonation. In contrast, psychomotor agitation is characterized by outer and inner turmoil: marked restlessness (resembling akathisia), irritability, and expressions of anguish and torment. The cardiac exam is typically normal. Since it is not unusual for patients with "chest pain" due to a significant depressive disorder to also have a comorbid anxiety disorder, especially panic disorder, please refer to the discussion of the physical examination in the previous chapter.

"Routine" laboratory tests

Laboratory tests are usually normal in otherwise healthy patients who have depressive disorders. In patients with coronary atherosclerotic heart disease and depressive disorders, the electrocardiogram and chest x-ray film may be abnormal. (See Chapters 29 and 30.)

Exceptions to the Usual Manifestations

Some patients with "chest pain" due to a major depressive disorder will deny feeling depressed and not appear depressed. If, however, physicians use the algorithm pertaining to patients who deny depression mood (as described in the legend of Table 46–1) to empathically interview such patients and a close family member, the major depressive disorder will usually be uncovered or strongly suspected.

Differential Diagnosis

In contrast to patients who bring themselves to psychiatrists because they are aware they are depressed, patients with significant depressive disorders who are being seen for "chest pain" in primary care, cardiology, or emergency settings will typically focus on the chest pain and associated physical symptoms. They will rarely mention psychosocial stressors or depressive symptoms spontaneously, and often minimize, deny, or "forget" these when directly asked about them because of underlying concerns about being perceived as "someone with a mental problem" who will be wasting the doctor's time. It is important, therefore, to question a close family member about depression and stressors in every patient who denies their presence in view of the high prevalence of depressive (and anxiety) disorders in patients with "chest pain." Physicians' interviewing styles (i.e., *how* questions are asked) are also very important in eliciting accurate information from these patients.[10]

In significantly depressed patients (even those who do not meet the criteria for a major depressive episode that are listed in Table 46–1), organic or biological causes for the depressive symptoms must be ruled out. These are medical disorders (e.g., hypothyroidism, central nervous system lesions) and substances or drugs (e.g., narcotics, alcohol, steroids). When such disorders or substances are found to be etiologic, the appropriate diagnosis is *substance-induced mood disorder* or *mood disorder due to a general medical condition*, respectively.[6]

Even if patients with "chest pain"due to depressive disorder, as well as those with angina from coronary atherosclerotic heart disease, acknowledge significant depressive *somatic* symptoms (e.g., insomnia, anorexia, fatigue, slowness), they often attribute them to the chest pain and/or heart disease. Rather than agreeing, their physicians should "count" such symptoms among the criteria required to diagnose major depressive disorder, even when such symptoms (e.g., fatigue) might reflect an organic problem (e.g., coronary atherosclerotic heart disease). The risk of *not* perceiving them as symptoms of depression (i.e., missing the diagnosis of major depressive disorder) far outweighs the risk, between about 1.5% and 8%, of erroneously counting them as depressive symptoms (i.e., mistakenly diagnosing major depressive disorder).[14] In other words, not giving a selective serotonin re-uptake inhibitor (SSRI) or another of the new-generation antidepressants to patients who have unrecognized major depressive disorder is usually much riskier than prescribing such antidepressants for patients who actually do not have major depressive disorder. Furthermore, especially with depressed patients with coronary atherosclerotic heart disease, the physician must resist the tendency to view their depression as appropriate, as though he or she were thinking, "If I had that condition, I'd be depressed, too!" In this regard, others have noted, "the most common cause for the underdiagnosis and undertreatment of depression in medical patients is the mistaken notion that if a depression is understandable, explainable, and reactive to environmental circumstances, then it is neither pathological nor requires treatment."[15]

In patients who are depressed and delusional (e.g., insisting that x-rays from the television set are damaging their heart) several diagnoses, in addition to major depressive disorder with psychosis, must be considered. They are delusional disorder, schizoaffective disorder, schizophrenia, and psychotic disorder caused by a substance or a medical condition.[6]

Depressed patients with "chest pain" who have multiple, chronic, recurrent somatic complaints in the absence of explanatory physical disease (i.e., somatizing patients) are likely to have a comorbid somatoform disorder (probably somatization disorder, undifferentiated somatoform disorder, or hypochondriasis).[6]

Other Diagnostic Testing

There are several clinical rating scales that are helpful in diagnosing a depressive disorder. The Beck Depression Inventory (BDI), Carroll Depression Rating Scale, and Zung Self-Assessment Depression Scale are among the most widely used. They can be easily completed by patients in less than 5 minutes and are easily scored.[14]

Etiology and Basic Mechanisms Responsible for the "Pain"

A model has been proposed to help understand what must be a multi-causal, biopsychosocial etiology of chest pain due to psychological factors or psychiatric disorders.[16] Its key concept is that the physical and psychological symptoms result from misinterpretating as seriously threatening, somatic sensations stemming from insignificant physical pathology or excessive awareness of normal bodily processes. Acute, *precipitating* and chronic, *predisposing* psychosocial variables increase the likelihood that patients will have such troubling misinterpretations.

The acute, precipitating variables (the "emotional arousal" group) result from the interaction between personality and stress. This group reflects the more prevalent psychological states (e.g., concern, worry, and autonomic arousal) and the less prevalent formal psychiatric diagnoses (mainly anxiety, depressive, and hypochondriacial disorders).

The chronic, predisposing psychosocial variables (the "illness knowledge and experience" group) include knowledge and family history of heart disease (and other illnesses); models of heart disease in friends, family, in the media; and general experience and level of satisfaction with physicians and medical facilities. This group also includes personality traits and attitudes towards physicians.

Once the pathogenic misinterpretation of trivial physical sensations in the chest is made, symptoms of frightening chest pain develop. This pain, now (mistakenly) assumed to reflect serious heart disease, may be maintained and reinforced not only by the two groups of variables described above, but also by other, often more powerful factors. These include secondary depression and/or anxiety and panic; the reactions and behavior of family, friends, employers, and especially physicians, whose diagnostic and therapeutic uncertainty may be particularly potent reinforcers of worsening cardiac illness behavior (e.g., the physician who reassures the patient that "nothing is wrong" with his heart and then prescribes nitrates "just to be sure").[17] With or without the addition of economic reinforcers (e.g., disability programs), these factors may quickly lead to chronic, significant physical and psychological disability in patients with "chest pain" due to depressive (or anxiety) disorders, who, as a result, have sometimes been referred to as "cardiac cripples" or "cardiophobics."[18]

As for the patients with angina pectoris due to coronary atherosclerotic heart disease, a comorbid depressive disorder may worsen their angina and coronary atherosclerotic through several mechanisms which are consequences of the depressive disorder, especially major depressive disorder: (a) non-compliance; (b) the deleterious effects of major depressive disorder-related high cortisol levels on blood vessels; (c) major depressive disorder-related increased sympathoadrenal activity's effects on cardiac function and platelets, mediated by increased catecholamines; (d) increased platelet activation and platelet secretion; and (e) decreased heart-rate variability.[1]

Treatment

Most of what is written in the first three paragraphs of the "treatment" section of the previous chapter also pertains to patients with "chest pain" due to depressive disorders. It will, therefore, not be repeated here.

With regard to medications for noncardiac chest pain patients and those with coronary atherosclerotic heart disease-related angina, it is clear that the eight new-generation antidepressants (i.e., the *non*-tricyclics and *non*-monoamine oxidase inhibitors), appear to be equally efficacious in outpatients with major depressive disorder. Thus, the choice among the current octet of drugs (four selective serotonin reuptake inhibitors: fluoxetine, sertraline, paroxetine, and citalopram; and 4 others: buproprion, venlafaxine, nefazodone, and mirtazapine) depends more on other factors such as side-effect profile, past treatment response, target symptoms, co-morbid medical disorders, and other drugs the patient is using. It is important to note that even with an optimum pharmacotherapeutic regimen, about 75% of patients with major depressive disorder treated only with antidepressants achieve a complete remission. The combination of psychotherapy (especially of the cognitive-behavioral or interpersonal kind) and antidepressants has generally been shown to be more effective than either alone.[9]

It is recommended that when physicians suspect or detect a depressive disorder in their patients with "chest pain", they empathically explain how this disorder is causing the chest pain (as described above and in the preceding chapter) *in addition to* giving the usual reassurance that no heart disease has been found (such reassurance, *by itself,* usually being useless in preventing continuing and worsening morbidity).[16, 19] Rather than treat the patients themselves, they should empathically refer the patient to a psychiatrist, the physician most knowledgeable about and experienced with antidepressant medication, "chemical imbalances" in the brain, drug-drug interactions, and psychotherapy. Even primary care physicians, who usually have more experience in prescribing antidepressants than cardiologists, have been consistently shown to treat about 50% of their patients with major depressive disorder ineffectively for various reasons (e.g., subtherapeutic dosages of antidepressants, too few visits, inadequate long-term monitoring, and inadequate medication instructions leading to premature medication discontinuation).[9]

Finally, it should be emphasized that major depressive disorder and panic disorder are treatable disorders with outcomes as good as those in almost any serious medical condition. In patients with "chest pain" related to a depressive and/or anxiety disorder, a biopsychosocial treatment strategy (reassurance about no heart disease *and* an explanation of what *is* causing the pain, psychotropic drugs *and* psychotherapy, all in the context of a truly caring and respectful doctor-patient relationship) has been shown to be effective.[16] In patients with coronary atherosclerotic heart disease-related angina or recent myocardial infarction and cormorbid major depressive disorder, such an approach may be lifesaving.[8]

References

1. Musselman DL, McDonald W, Nemeroff CB. Effects of mood and anxiety disorders on the cardiovascular system: Implications for treatment. In: Fuster V, Alexander RW, O'Rourke RA, et al. (eds): *Hurst's The Heart, 10th ed*, New York, McGraw, 2001;2227–2250.
2. Cormier LE, Katon W, Russo J, et al. Chest pain with negative cardiac dia nostic studies: Relationship to psychiatric illness. *J Nerv Ment Dis* 1988;176:351–357.
3. Barsky AJ, Palpitations, cardiac awareness, and panic disorder. *Am J Med* 1992;92 (Suppl 1A):31S–34S.
4. Wulsin LR, Yingling K. Psychiatric aspects of chest pain in the emergency department. *Med Clin N Amer* 1991;75:1175–1188.
5. Kroenke K, Spitzer RL, Williams JBW, et al. Physical symptoms in primary care: Predictors of psychiatric disorders and functional impairment. *Arch Fam Med* 1994;3:774–779.
6. American Psychiatric Association. *Diagnostic and Statistical Manual of Mental Disorders, 4th Ed*. Washington DC, American Psychiatric Association, 1994.
7. Katon W, Hall ML, Russo J, et al. Chest pain: Relationship of psychiatric illness to coronary angiographic results. *Am J Med* 1988;84:1–9.
8. Frasure-Smith N, Lesperance F, Talajic M. Depression following myocardial infarction: Impact on 6-month survival. *JAMA* 1993;270:1819–1825.
9. Wise MG, Rundell JR. *Concise Guide to Consultation Psychiatry, 2nd ed*. Washington, DC: American Psychiatric Press, Inc. 1994.
10. Bass C. Unexplained chest pain and breathlessness. *Med Clin N Amer* 1991;75:1157–1173.
11. Carter CS, Servan-Schreiber D, Perlstein WM. Anxiety disorders and the syndrome of chest pain with normal coronary arteries: Prevalence and pathophysiology. *J Clin Psychiat* 1997;58(suppl 3):70–75.
12. Hurst JW. Personal communication. July, 2000.
13. Mathew RJ, Weinman ML, Mirabi M. Physical symptoms of depression. *Br J Psychiat* 1981;139;293–296.
14. McDaniel JS, Brown FW, Cole SA. Assessment of depression and grief reactions in the medically ill. In: Stoudemire A, Fogel BS, Greenberg DB, eds. *Psychiatric Care of the Medical Patient. 2nd ed.*, New York; Oxford University Press, 2000, pp. 49–164.
15. Rouchell AM, Pounds R, Tierney JG, et al. Depression. In: Rundell JR, Wise

MG, eds. *Textbook of Consultation-Liaison Psychiatry*. Washington DC, American Psychiatric Press, 1996, pp. 312–345.

16. Mayou R. Patients' fears of illness: Chest pain and palpitations. In: Creed F, Mayou R, Hopkins A, (eds): *Medical Symptoms Not Explained by Organic Disease*. Washington DC, American Psychiatric Press, 1992, pp. 25–33.

17. Bradley LA, Richter JE, Scarinci IC, et al. Psychosocial and psychophysical assessments of patients with unexplained chest pain. *Am J Med* 1992;92(suppl 5A); 65S–73S.

18. Eifert GH. Cardiophobia: A paradigmatic behavioral model of heart-focused anxiety and non-anginal chest pain. *Behav Res Ther* 1992;30:329–345.

19. Ockene IS, Shay MJ, Albert JS, et al. Unexplained chest pain in patients with normal coronary angiograms. *N Engl J Med* 1980;303;1249–1252.

47

"Chest Pain" in Patients Who Are Malingering

James C. Hamilton, PhD and Marc D. Feldman, MD

General Considerations

Malingering in medical and surgical patients is defined by exaggerated, feigned, or self-induced physical signs and symptoms. The sick role is used to secure for the patient one or more material or social benefits. In some cases the patient may be motivated by financial incentives (e.g., legal settlements, worker's compensation). Non-financial incentives to malinger might include gaining access to narcotic medications, avoiding criminal prosecution, securing desirable work re-assignments, or access to a warm dry hospital bed on a cold wet night.[1] In other cases the rewards may be more subtle (e.g., the avoidance of interpersonal conflict or onerous household responsibilities, etc.) By definition, the false or exaggerated illness behavior is conscious and intentional.[2] In the most blatant cases, these patients are probably well aware of what they are doing and why they are doing it.[3,4] However, in other cases a mixture of self-deception and entitlement feelings may allow malingerers to regard their behavior as something less than blatantly fradulent.[5]

Clinical Setting

Of the chest pain conditions covered in this volume, the literature suggests that only two constitute settings in which malingering is often suspected, cervical pain and upper extremity pain. It is clear, however, that patients may feign the symptoms of myocardial ischemia in order to obtain a narcotic for "relief." There are no reliable data on demographic

From: Hurst JW, Morris DC (eds): *"Chest Pain"* →. © Futura Publishing Co., Inc., Armonk, NY, 2001.

characteristics that distinguish malingerers from patients who suffer from verifiable conditions known to produce chest pain.[6] The stereotypic medical malingerer is a patient of working age who is employed as a laborer, or as an unskilled clerical worker. The sterotypic malingerer will present with complaints of pain and disability that allegedly stem from an on-the-job injury (e.g., a fall or a lifting accident), or from the long-term effects of physically demanding job requirements (e.g., repetitive strain injuries) or an unhealthy work-place environment (e.g., "sick building syndrome").[7-9] These patients present to general practitioners, rheumatologists, neurologists, and orthopaedic and hand surgeons. The patients' stated or implied reason for the consultation will be to obtain medical certification of their putative pain or disability. However, there are few systematic empirical studies confirming this stereotype.

Patients of diverse demographic backgrounds may feign or exaggerate pain in order to secure prescriptions for narcotic-analgesic or hypnosedative medications, either for their own use or to re-sell. In addition to neck, shoulder, upper-back, and upper extremity pain, these patients may present with facial or dental pain. Drug-seekers are thought to "doctor shop" in order to find physicians who will accommodate their requests for prescriptions. The patients often present to emergency departments, urgent care centers, or to dentists on an emergency basis, complaining of acute pain. This includes patients who have known coronary disease who are seeking narcotics. The emergency provides a pretext for not visiting the patient's primary care physician. They may report an unusually large number of known drug allergies as a means of steering the physician toward prescribing their drug of choice, or simply insist on a specific product.[10,11]

Characteristics of the "Pain"

Patient's characterization of the "pain"

In malingering, reports of pain are used strategically to secure specific rewards or to avoid unpleasant responsibilities. The nature of the patient's complaints will fit the strategic purpose for which the report of illness or injury is intended. For example, a person who wishes to avoid an immediate predicament might feign an acute pain problem, like angina pectoris. A person wishing to secure a permanent disability judgement in a worker's compensation case will feign a medical problem that makes sense vis a vis the malingerer's job requirements.

The quality of the pain complaint will vary according to the medical sophistication of the patient; they may present with diffuse pain, or patterns of pain that are not consistent with known medical conditions or with the anatomy of the peripheral nervous system. More sophisticated malingerers may accurately feign signs and symptoms of a specific disease or injury. Therefore, they may feign the symptoms of myocardial ischemia. One unfortunate result of the wide availability of high quality medical information on the Internet is that malingerers now have plenty of guidance on how to accurately simulate pain and disability.

Common locations of the "chest pain"

Almost any chest pain syndrome described in this volume can be feigned by a malingering patient. Such patients might imitate angina pectoris or the symptoms of myocardial infarction (see Figure 47–1). However, there are some presentations that have received particular attention in the literature. Malingering is frequently suspected in unexplained hand, wrist or arm pain (see Figures 47–2 and 47–3). These cases may present as specific conditions (e.g. carpal tunnel syndrome, repetitive strain injury) or as more diffuse and varied limb pain (e.g., reflex sympathetic dystrophy, type I complex regional pain syndrome.)[12,13] Although the bulk of the literature on chronic pain syndromes and malingering has focused on low back pain, feigned or exaggerated pain related to the cervical and thoracic spine has also been suspected, especially in the context of whiplash injuries.[14–17] Diffuse or widely distributed pain locations, including chest pains, are described in patients with chronic fatigue syndrome and fi-

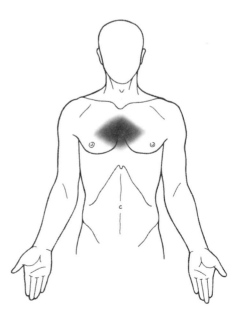

Figure 47–1. The malingerer can imitate the "chest pain" of angina pectoris or myocardial infarction due to coronary atherosclerotic heart disease (or any other condition for that matter).

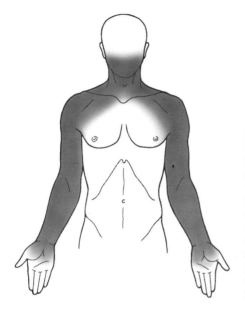

Figure 47–2. Frontal view. Malingering is often suspected when the pain is isolated to any part of the body shown in the shaded area above. The "pain" may be described as being in the hand, wrist, or arm. This location of pain also occurs in patients with angina pectoris or infarction due to coronary atherosclerotic heart disease and the malingerer 'wins his battle" because the physician "does not wish to miss a diagnosis of angina or infarction."

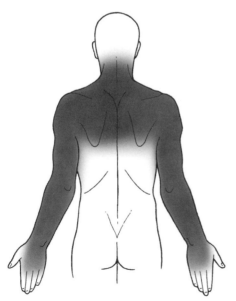

Figure 47–3. View of the back. The "pain" of angina pectoris is rarely located in the shaded area shown above. Malingerers who have not perfected their complaints may complain of pain located in the shaded areas shown above.

bromyalgia, with signs and symptoms that are sometimes referable to the chest. Because there are no definitive tests for diagnosing these syndromes they may produce a context that is conducive to malingering.[18,19]

Uncommon locations of the "chest pain"

The literature on malingering contains few reports of feigned or exaggerated pain suggestive of chest wall, cardiac, or pulmonary conditions.[3] Accordingly, the pain is only rarely located in a segment of the area illustrated in Figure 47–4. Nor are there any published reports of feigned peptic ulcer. However, it is important to understand that cases of malingered pain that are unrelated to the medicolegal context may simply go unrecognized or unreported. With the exception of pain in the upper back and upper extremities, the pain conditions described in this volume are not frequently linked to compensable injury.

Size of the painful "area"

The malingerer commonly knows the characteristics of the pain associated with the condition he or she is imitating. (See Chapter 29 for symptoms due to myocardial ischemia).

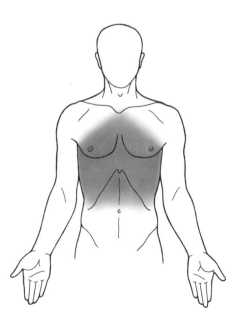

Figure 47–4. The "pain" feigned by the malingerer may, on rare occasion, be located in any segment of the shaded area shown above.

Duration of the "chest pain"

Here again, the malingerer can imitate any condition he or she wishes to present to the physician, including angina pectoris. We could find no unequivocal comparisons of the duration of malingered versus authentic pain complaints. Instead, there are a large number of studies comparing the recovery times of patients with and without a history of worker's compensation or civil litigation. The assumption made in these studies (it is often implicit) is that compensation serves as a powerful incentive to malinger, and so compensation status can serve as a proxy for direct evidence of malingering.[20] These studies are fairly consistent in showing that compensation is associated with longer recovery time,[21-23] but there are several exceptions.[15,16] Longer recovery times in compensation cases may reflect the fact that people in physically demanding occupations in which work related injuries might be sustained, might also require a more complete recovery before returning to work.[22,24,25]

Tenderness of the chest wall

Tenderness of the chest wall is not a part of the myocardial ischemic condition. Therefore, the drug-seeking malingerer does not complain of chest wall tenderness. The malingerer can, however, imitate those conditions in which tenderness to palpation is known to exist.

Precipitating causes of the "chest pain"

In patients seeking worker's compensation or those pursuing personal injury litigation, malingering may be unplanned. The patient may seize upon an industrial or motor vehicle accident as an opportunity for financial gain. In the most egregious cases accidents may be staged to create an opportunity for litigation. Several commentators have suggested that malingering behavior may be the result of modeling processes. This is supported by anecdotal accounts of increased frequency of disability claims in families in which someone has already been certified as disabled. Other commentators have observed a type of contagion effect for certain work-place injuries or illnesses.[7,8]

Relief of the "chest pain"

For patients who seek a disability claim, it is against their interests to acknowledge any improvement in their condition or even any palliative effects of medicine, corrective surgery, or physical therapy. The one exception to this may be in cases of sophisticated patients who admit to partial or temporary relief of pain in order to enhance their credibility. Patients who seek legal settlements may report some relief after their legal cases have been resolved. However, even in these cases the patient is subject to prosecution for fraud if evidence of the malingering is uncovered. This set of contingencies creates an ironic disincentive to recover.[5]

Patients who are fraudulently seeking prescription medications can either present with a chronic pain problem, such as angina pectoris, for which medications are constantly needed, or with a series of unrelated illnesses or injuries. In either case they may strategically report that addictive/abusable drugs are more effective than non-addictive ones. Or they may report only partial relief in response to narcotic medicines in the hope of convincing the physician to increase the strength or dosage.

The presence of non-organic signs has also been used to define groups of patients who may be malingering. Patients with non-organic signs appear to take longer to return to work than those who do not.[26] Findings of this sort do not necessarily represent malingered pain in people trying to avoid work. Both the non-organic signs and the hesitance to return to work could reflect a fear of pain and of reinjury.[27]

There has been some research done on self-report variables that might distinguish malingerers from non-malingerers, or ones that might at least distinguish organic from non-organic pain complaints. This research has focused primarily on information that can be derived from the patient's description of his or her symptoms, or from standardized self-report measures. There is some evidence that the pain reports of malingerers are exaggerated relative to patients with documented tissue damage.[28] Leavitt[28] found that a questionnaire measure of patients' responses to pain related words could discriminate pain patients from non-patients asked to simulate the responses of a pain patient. However, the same study found that the measure could not distinguish between pain patients who were instructed to exaggerate and those who were not. Several studies suggest that a combination of clinical and validity scales from the Minnesota Multi-Phasic Personality Inventory-2 (MMPI-2) can discriminate between patients with and without physical evidence of injury,[29,30] but the use of the MMPI-2 as a means of detecting malingered pain has not been very thoroughly studied. Fishbain, et al., in a comprehensive review of the literature on detecting feigned medical problems, found no consistent evidence to support the use of self-report measures to detect feigned pain.

Associated Signs

Physical examination

Expected signs of injury or disease will be absent or inadequate to account for the patient's reported degree of pain or disability. There may be non-organic signs, like Waddell's signs,[31] that would be unexpected in an uncomplicated case of authentic illness. However, it should be noted that the majority of research on the predictive validity of Waddell's signs is based on studies of low back pain suffers.[32] Furthermore, Waddell[33] himself has cautioned that the signs are not indicators of malingering per se, but rather they suggest that medicolegal or psychosocial variables may have an important effect on the way the patient interprets or responds to his or her injury.

An alternate approach to the direct detection of malingered musculoskeletal pain has been to test for malingered pain-related physical disability. For example, there is a large literature on patterns of submaximal performance and sincerity of effort on strength tests. Two careful reviews of the literature have independently concluded that the evidence concerning the diagnostic usefulness of non-organic signs and submaximal effort tests is inconclusive.[6,34] Both reviews caution against the uncritical use of these indicators, and against the assumption that their presence indicates malingering.

"Routine" laboratory tests

There are few tests that can be performed to definitively establish the inauthenticity of pain complaints. In rare instances of malingering in acute chest pain, negative finding in the electrocardiogram and isoenzyme tests assist in the exclusion of myocardial infarction but do not assist in the exclusion of angina. Otherwise, the best the physician can do is to take care to follow standard procedures for laboratory tests. In treating malingering patients, as with factitious disorder patients, clinical errors can result from placing too much trust in the patient's self-reported history, or on his or her outward appearance. A dishonest patient can easily use false claims and false appearances to cause the physician to assume that basic definitive diagnostic tests are unnecessary. For example, a new patient who falsely reports that she has advanced lung cancer might request help with pain control. A compassionate physician might make a crucial clinical error by deciding to forego the definitive chest x-ray and focus instead on pain management or discuss end of life issues with a patient.

Differential Diagnosis

There are five conditions from which malingering must be differentiated; undetected physical pathologies, three of the somatoform disorders, and factitious disorder.

Undiagnosed or Underestimated Physical Illness or Injury

Unfortunately, in many cases it is difficult to exclude the possibility of an occult physical pathology that is responsible for the patients' complaints.[35] Even more vexing is the fact that many patients malinger by exaggerating the severity or persistence of a verifiable medical problem.[1] *Patients with documented pain problems are particularly effective at simulating pain.*[36]

Pain Disorder and Somatization Disorder

Pain disorder is diagnosed in cases of persistent pain that is not accounted for by objective evidence of tissue damage. Unfortunately, many patients with myocardial ischemia have no objective signs of disease when they are first encountered. Somatization disorder is diagnosed in patients with chronic complaints of physical discomfort (including pain) or disability that cover multiple organ systems. Presumably, the patient truly experiences the pain as he or she reports it. The pain complaints may co-vary with psychological stresses or interpersonal conflicts. The pain reported in these disorders and malingered pain are distinguished by the fact that malingered pain complaints are conscious and voluntary, whereas those in pain disorder and somatization disorder are unconscious and not intentionally fraudulent. The differential diagnosis can sometimes be made with affirmative evidence of malingering (e.g., from video surveillance). We are not aware of any reliable method for affirmatively establishing that pain complaints are unconscious and involuntarily produced.

Hypochondriasis

Hypochondriasis is diagnosed in patients who engage in the perceptual amplification or catastrophic interpretation of physical sensations.[37] The patient presents with minor signs and symptoms (often minor pains) that he or she fears are indicators of some occult life-threatening illness. Presentations involving chest pain and fears of imminent cardiopulmonary failure are probably common among these patients.[38,39] The general demeanor of these patients is characterized by fear and anxiety. Unlike the malingerer, the patient with hypochondriasis is eager to undergo diagnostic evaluations of all sorts. They will often report at least a brief period of relief upon hearing that a test result was negative, though new fears and worries may soon return. In contrast, the malingerer is often uncooperative with the diagnostic process and is unlikely to show any positive affective reactions to negative test results. In some cases, persons with hypochondriasis lie about their past medical history or simulate or self-induce illness intentionally. However, in these cases the patient's deceptions reflect a desperate need to convince medical staff to perform further diagnostic tests.

Factitious Disorder with Physical Signs and Symptoms

In factitious disorder with physical signs or symptoms there is also exaggerated, feigned, or self-induced medical problems. By definition, in factitious disorder the fraudulent complaints cannot be adequately explained by external incentives. For factitious disorder patients the sick role is intrinsically rewarding, and so enactment of the sick role is their ultimate goal. Accordingly, the factitious disorder patient will seek out contacts with physicians, and welcome the chance to undergo medical and surgical procedures, even those that most people would regard as painful, embarrassing or otherwise aversive. Malingerers, on the other hand, are driven by the ultimate goal of gaining an external reward or dispensation. Sick role behavior is simply a means to that end, and so malingerers strive to attain medical certification of their disease or disability while minimizing medical contacts through which their deceptions might be uncovered.

Other Diagnostic Testing

Dozens of other methods for the detection of malingering have been proposed. The literature describes methods that can be used to definitely detect pathophysiological processes that can account for pain complaints that might be mistaken for malingering.[35,40,41] Several writers have discussed the use of covert videotaped surveillance[20] or extended observations as a means of collecting definite proof of malingering.[1] Extended observations of patients are feasible during inpatient hospital stays. Around the clock observation of the patients by members of a multidisciplinary treatment team can reveal inconsistencies in the patients' apparent level of disability across different activities, settings, and times of day.

Patients with "chest pain" who have symptoms simulating those due to myocardial ischemia seem to fall into one of two groups.

The patient who consciously feigns "chest pain" simulating a myocardial infarction may resist having additional studies performed to support the diagnosis. They may be seeking retirement benefits or some other useful financial or social gain.

Patients who have angiographically proven coronary atherosclerotic heart disease and angina pectoris may exaggerate their problem in an effort to avoid undesirable encounters or to gain access to narcotics because they "only obtain relief with narcotics." They may be willing to undergo coronary arteriography or other tests because they know coronary disease will be found and the doctor may have trouble deciding that minimal or no change in the test result explains the patient's increasing symptoms. The "chest pain" in these patients may be impossible to understand. A satisfactory solution to the problems is not always possible. The physician must rely on other information he or she collects from the patient to determine that the patient is exaggerating the symptoms of a proven disease. The constant request for narcotics and the failure to improve, and the identification of life situations that fit the malingering pattern are helpful but are not always sufficient to solve this problem satisfactorily.

Etiology and Basic Mechanisms Responsible for the "Pain"

Blatant malingering may arise from the same types of enduring personality traits that are observed in antisocial personality disorder, such as a lack of concern for the rights of others, a sense of entitlement, difficulty enduring steady employment, and a tendency to manipulate others for personal gain.[42] Antisocial personality disorder may also play a role in patients who use malingered pain as a means of obtaining prescription medicines. In both drug-seekers and less blatant cases of malingering, a number of other treatable psychological problems may contribute to the strategic use of illness behavior, including anxiety, depression, and personality disorders.[43–45] In assessing the role of psychological distress in pain patients it is important to remember that the distress could reflect a consequence of pain and disability,[46] or a consequence of the stresses associated with compensation claims or litigation.[44]

In more subtle cases of malingering, the sick role may be used to compensate for a variety of psychosocial deficits (e.g., assertiveness skills). Persons who feel powerless to escape an aversive situation may use the sick role to do so. For example, students who believe that they are destined to fail a college course may use illness as an excuse to withdraw from the class. A spouse who has lost interest in sexual relations with her partner may use illness as a legitimate excuse for rebuffing his sexual overtures. More chronic sick role behavior might serve as a way of protecting self-esteem.[47] In these cases, illness protects the malingerer from the negative personal implications of educational, occupational, and interpersonal failures.

Treatment

Malingering in its pure form is best described as a medicolegal designation, not a physical or mental disease. In the most blatant cases, the management of these patients amounts to detecting them and dismissing them from one's care. However, cases in which the patient's complaints are complete and total fabrications, strategically aimed at securing some obvious financial benefit, are probably rare. More commonly, malingerers are patients who have had real injuries and who may be experiencing real pain. If these patients coincidentally have jobs that they find aversive, or financial problems, or unfilfilling relationships, they may gradually convince themselves and others that their pain and disability merit special consideration or financial compensation. Cases like this may arise from psychological factors that are treatable, such as those just described. For cases like these many of the strategies developed for managing factitious disorder may be useful for managing malingerers.[48] Physicians who become angry and frustrated with a malingering patient may be tempted to confront the patient directly. However, the likely results of doing so will be to (a) pass the patient along to a colleague who also will become angry and frustrated with the patient, and (b) fuel the patient's rationalization of his or her malingering. Better results may be achieved with a non-confrontational approach that allows the patient to relinquish the sick role without admitting to having feigned or exaggerated his or her pain or disability. Multi-disciplinary pain clinics are well suited for this purpose.[1] A referral to such a clinic does not challenge the veracity of the patient's medical complaints, but at the same time brings the patient into contact with psychiatrists, psychologists, and social workers, who can begin to address some of the psychosocial deficits for which the patient compensates with illness behavior.

References

1. LoPiccolo CJ, Goodkin K, Baldewicz TT. Current issues in the diagnosis and management of malingering. *Ann Med* 1999;31:166–174.
2. American Psychiatric Association. Diagnostic and statistical manual of mental disorders: *DSM-IV. 4th ed.* Washington, DC: American Psychiatric Association, 1994.
3. Kissler F, Marsoner F, Stefenelli N, et al. [Self-inflicted injuries by injecting contaminated solutions through the chest wall (author's transl)]. *Medizinische Klinik* 1976;71:1200–1203.
4. Sousa JA, Cline DM, Stout RC, et al. Extortion in the emergency department [see comments]. *J Emerg Med* 1997;15:537–541.
5. Bellamy R. Compensation neurosis: Financial reward for illness as nocebo. *Clin Orthopaedics and Related Research* 1997;336:94–106.
6. Fishbain DA, Cutler R, Rosomoff HL, et al. Chronic pain disability exaggeration/malingering and submaximal effort research. *Clin J Pain* 1999;15:244–274.
7. Ford CV. Somatization and fashionable diagnoses: Illness as a way of life. *Scand J Work and Environ Health* 1997;23:7–16.
8. Rothman AL, Weintraub MI. The sick building syndrome and mass hysteria. *Neuro Clinics* 1995;13:405–412.

9. Ruhl RA, Chang CC, Halpern GM, et al. The sick building syndrome. II. Assessment and regulation of indoor air quality. *J Asthma* 1993;30:297–308.

10. Longo LP, Parran TJ, Johnson B, et al. Addiction: Part II. Identification and management of the drug-seeking patient. *Am Fam Physician* 2000;61:2401–2408.

11. Mitka M. Abuse of prescription drugs: Is a patient ailing or addicted? [news]. *JAMA* 2000;283:1126–1129.

12. Verdugo RJ, Ochoa JL. Abnormal movements in complex regional pain syndrome: Assessment of their nature. 2000;23:198–205.

13. Ochoa JL. Truths, errors, and lies around\"reflex sympathetic dystrophy and \"complex regional pain syndrome. *J Neurol* 1999;246:875–879.

14. Ferrari R, Kwan O, Russell AS, et al. The best approach to the problem of whiplash? One ticket to Lithuania, please. *Clin Experimental Rheumatol* 1999;17: 321–326.

15. Swartzman LC, Teasell RW, Shapiro AP, et al. The effect of litigation status on adjustment of whiplash injury. *Spine* 1996;21:53–58.

16. Kolbinson DA, Epstein JB, Burgess JA, et al. Temporomandibular disorders, headaches, and neck pain after motor vehicle accidents: A pilot investigation of persistence and litigation effects. *J Prosthetic Dentistry* 1997;77;46–53.

17. Freeman MD, Croft AC, Rossignol AM, et al. A review and methodologic critique of the literature refuting whiplash syndrome. *Spine* 1999;24:86–96.

18. Abbey SE. Psychiatric diagnostic overlap in chronic fatigue syndrome. In: Demitrack MA, Abbey SE (eds). *Chronic Fatigue Syndrome: An Integrative Approach to Evaluation and Treatment.* New York, The Guilford Press, 1996, pp. 48–71.

19. Bohr TW. Fibromyalgia syndrome and myofascial pain syndrome: Do they exist? *Neurol Clinics* 1995;13:365–384.

20. Kay NR, Morris-Jones H. Pain clinic management of medico-legal litigants. *Injury* 1998;29:305–308.

21. Coste J, Delecoeuillerie G, Cohen de lara A, et al. Clinical course and prognostic factors in acute low back pain: An inception cohort study in primary care practice. *Brit Med J* 1994;308:577–580.

22. Leavitt F. The physical exertion factor in compensable work injuries. A hidden flaw in previous research. *Spine* 1992;17:307–310.

23. Greenough CG, Fraser RD. The effects of compensation on recovery from low-back injury. *Spine* 1989;14:947–955.

24. Filan SL. The effect of workers' or third-party compensation on return to work after hand surgery (see comments). *Med J Australia* 1996;165:80–82.

25. Frieman BG, Fenlin JMJ. Anterior acromioplasty: Effect of litigation and workers' compensation. *J Shoulder and Elbow Surg* 1995;4:175–181.

26. Gaines WG, Jr., Hegmann KT. Effectiveness of Waddell's nonorganic signs in predicting a delayed return to regular work in patients experiencing acute occupational low back pain. *Spine* 1999;24:396–400; discussion 1.

27. Vlaeyen JW, Linton SJ. Fear-avoidance and its consequences in chronic musculoskeletal pain: A state of the art. *Pain* 2000;85:317–332.

28. Leavitt F. Predicting disability time using formal low back pain measurement: The Low Back Pain Simulation Scale. *J Psychosomatic Research* 1991;35:599–607.

29. Larrabee GJ. Somatic malingering on the MMPT and MMPI-2 in personal injury litigants. *Clin Neuropsychologist* 1998;12:179–188.

30. Lees-Haley PR, English LT, Glenn WJ. A Fake Bad Scale on the MMPI-2 for personal injury claimants. *Psychological Reports* 1991;68:203–210.

31. Kiester PD, Duke AD. Is it malingering, or is it 'real'? Eight signs that point to nonorganic back pain. *Postgrad Med* 1999;106:77–80,3–4.
32. Sobel JB, Sollenberger P, Robinson R, et al. Cervical nonorganic signs: A new clinical tool to assess abnormal illness behavior in neck pain patients: A pilot study. *Arch Phys Med Rehabil* 2000;81:170–175.
33. Main CJ, Waddell G. Behavioral responses to examination. A reappraisal of the interpretation of V'nonorganic signs. *Spine* 1998;23:2367–2371.
34. Lechner DE, Bradbury SF, Bradley LA. Detecting sincerity of effort: A summary of methods and approaches. *Physical Therapy* 1998;78:867–888.
35. Giles LG, Crawford CM. Shadows of the truth in patients with spinal pain: A review. *Canadian J Psychiatry. Revue Canadienne de Psychiatrie* 1997;42:44–48.
36. Leavitt F. Detection of simulation among persons instructed to exaggerate symptoms of low back pain. *J Occupational Med* 1987;29:229–233.
37. Barsky AJ, Klerman GL. Overview: Hypochondriasis, bodily complaints, and somatic styles. *Am J Psychiatry* 1983;140:273–283.
38. Barsky AJ. Somatoform disorders and personality traits. J Psychosomatic Res 1995;39:399–402.
39. Barsky AJ, Ahern DK, Bailey ED, et al. Predictors of persistent palpitations and continued medical utilization. *J Fam Pract* 1996;42:465–472.
40. Fishbain DA, Abdel-Moty E, Cutler RB, et al. Detection of a "faked strength task effort in volunteers using a computerized exercise testing system. *Am J Phy Med and Rehabil* 1999;78:222–227.
41. Thomas D, Aidinis S. Objective documentation of musculoskeletal pain syndrome by pressure algometry during thiopentone sodium (Pentothal) anesthesia. *Clin J Pain* 1989;5:343–350.
42. Clark CR. Sociopathy, malingering and defensiveness. In: Rogers R (ed). *Clinical Assessment of Malingerin and Deception, 2nd ed.* New York, The Guilford Press, 1997, pp. 68–84.
43. Melzack R, Katz J, Jeans ME. The role of compensation in chronic pain: Analysis using a new method of scoring the McGill Pain Questionnaire. *Pain* 1985;23:101–112.
44. Lee J, Giles K, Drummond PD. Psychological disturbances and an exaggerated response to pain in patients with whiplash injury. *J Psychosomatic Res* 1993;37:105–110.
45. Grillo J, Brown RS, Hilsabeck R, et al. Raising doubts about claims of malingering: Implications of relationships between MCMI-II and MMPI-2 performances. *J Clin Psychology* 1994;50–651–655.
46. Wallis BJ, Lord SM, Bogduk N. Resolution of psychological distress of whiplash patients following treatment by radiofrequency neurotomy: A randomised, double-blind, placebo-controlled trial (see comments). *Pain* 1997;73:15–22.
47. Hamilton JC, Janata JW. Dying to be ill. The role of self-enhancement motives in the spectrum of factitious disorders. *J Social and Clin Psychology* 1997;16:178–199.
48. Eisendrath SJ, Feder A. Management of factitious disorders. In: Feldman MD, Eisendrath SJ (eds): *The Spectrum of Factitious Disorders. Clin Prac, No. 40.* Washington, D.C.: American Psychiatric Press, Inc, 1996, pp. 195–213.

48

"Chest Pain" in Patients with Munchausen Syndrome

Marc D. Feldman, MD and James C. Hamilton, PhD

General Considerations

Factitious disorder, including the subtype known as *Munchausen syndrome*, is among the most daunting phenomena in clinical practice. This mental disorder involves the fabrication, simulation, exaggeration, aggravation, or induction of physical or, less commonly, psychological ailments.[1] The patient's principal goal is to garner gratifications intrinsic to the sick role, such as attention, care, and lenience. The best data indicate that, within large general hospitals, factitious disorder is diagnosed in approximately 1% of patients on whom psychiatrists consult.[2]

Around 10% of factitious disorder patients have Munchausen syndrome.[3] These individuals have a severe, chronic course characterized by *peregrination* (widespread travel in pursuit of additional medical treatment) and *pseudologia fantastica* (the creation of a captivating but specious personal history).[2]

Clinical Setting

Factitious disorder as a whole is more common in females than males. However, in Munchausen syndrome, men prevail.[4-6] The conditions usually develop during the third or fourth decade of life.[7] Factitious disorder patients often have families and hold responsible jobs, particularly as nurses or nurses' aides. In contrast, Munchausen syndrome is usually incompatible with the individual's maintaining steady employment and family ties.[7]

From: Hurst JW, Morris DC (eds): *"Chest Pain"* →. © Futura Publishing Co., Inc., Armonk, NY, 2001.

Characteristics of the "Chest Pain"

Patient's characterization of the "chest pain"

Pain is perhaps the most common and easily enacted manifestation of factitious disorder. Pain is inherently subjective and, since all individuals have experienced it, the features are well-known to those who choose to feign or exaggerate it. Accordingly, patients can imitate the "pain" of angina pectoris or myocardial infarction. Individuals can easily misrepresent themselves through facial expressions or answers on common pain assessment measures.[8,9] Their reports and, in many cases, the physical evidence they manufacture can be extremely persuasive. For instance, one patient underwent 16 bronchoscopies and three cardiac catheterizations—all with normal results—as physicians searched for the elusive cause of his signs and symptoms.[10]

Common location of the "chest pain"

The most common form of factitious chest pain is the simulation of myocardial infarction or another acute cardiac event. In this type of presentation, sometimes called *cardiopathia fantastica*, a patient reports crushing retrosternal pain that may radiate into the left arm or jaw and involve diaphoresis (see Figure 48–1). In a review of 204 patients presenting with acute precordial chest pain, Orchard, et al.[11] determined that 10 manifested Munchausen syndrome. Acute cardiac symptoms will inevitably receive immediate medical attention in the doctor's office, emergency department, or hospital, and thus they are particularly gratifying for factitious disorder patients. Other patients present with factitious unstable angina, with pain in the same distribution. One such case led to intra-aortic balloon counterpulsation,[12] and, as noted, repeated cardiac catheterizations are sometimes performed.

Other patients offer less specific complaints of chest discomfort that are associated with arrhythmias. In turn, the arrhythmias may be feigned or self-induced. Tizes[13] referred to a subset of these individuals as "professional cardioversion patients." In such cases, the frequent presence of a pacemaker lends credibility to the purported history, but the pacemaker itself has usually been inserted based on spurious signs.[14]

Another variation involves chest discomfort or tightness with associated dyspnea and hypoxemia. An effort to simulate asthma is sometimes at the root of these presentations.

Finally, some patients offer complaints of "pain" that are diffuse or nonspecific, yet severe. In doing so, they intend to force a comprehensive diagnostic battery of tests.

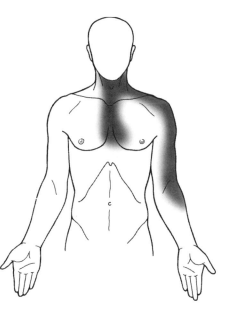

Figure 48–1. Patients with factitious "chest pain" may complain of symptoms that precisely imitate the chest discomfort of angina pectoris or myocardial infarction.

Factitious hemoptysis is present in association with all forms of factitious chest pain with surprising frequency. One patient claimed falsely that her hemoptysis stemmed from cystic fibrosis and that it had been severe enough to necessitate blood transfusions and bronchial artery embolization. This same patient later produced "blood" that proved to be a mixture of iodine and shampoo.[15] Another patient underwent serial bronchoscopies, bronchial arteriography, bronchography, and perfusion and ventilation lung scans before the bleeding was determined to be factitious.[16] In extreme cases, patients will go on to feign respiratory failure and even undergo prolonged ventilator support.[17] The ruse of hemoptysis often involves surreptitious laceration of the tongue or placement of blood (e.g., obtained through autophlebotomy) in the mouth. In one case, deliberate superwarfarin ingestion led to actual hemoptysis and respiratory failure.[18]

Uncommon locations of the "chest pain"

Some patients allege acute trauma to the chest, with pain centered around the site of ostensive damage. The site can be anywhere, but tends to be located where access is easy (e.g., the midline or left side in a right-handed person). If present, bruises, lacerations, and even penetrating injuries may have been self-inflicted through repeated battering, cutting, or piercing with knives, needles, or syringes. In one case, actual pericardial effusion and acute cardiac tamponade were self-induced in this fashion.[19]

Others have introduced bacteria (e.g., feces) into the wounds or even the pulmonary cavity, creating pneumonia and bacterial endocarditis as an example of the latter situation.[20]

Other variants are distinctly less common. One man presented with bilateral shoulder pain. Eventually, he was determined to have deliberately destroyed his glenohumeral joints to simulate neuropathic disease.[21] In a case of Munchausen syndrome presenting as a sexual assault, a young woman alleged pain from being bitten on both breasts during the attack. However, the nature of the lesions, combined with her history and ultimate confession, pointed to self-administered pinching.[22]

Size of the painful "area"

As indicated, reports of the size of the painful area are usually consistent with patients' understanding of the manifestations of myocardial infarction or angina. In general, they tailor their reports of size to the medical condition being represented. When self-harm has occurred, pain reports may be accurate but the cause of the injury is concealed.

Duration of the "chest pain"

The chest pain is often remarkably tenacious. Patients are loath to relinquish any symptoms, especially those that elicit the attention and care of the staff. Pain is often clearly disproportionate in both intensity and duration to any objective findings. Despite the presumptive pain, factitious patients rarely agree to or comply with behavioral pain management techniques.

Tenderness of the "chest pain"

Palpation is often met "with groans and exclamations of distress"[23] that appear overdramatized if not blatantly fabricated or exaggerated. However, this feature is imprecise because it requires the personal impression of the examiner. Discrepancies are more telling. For instance, a patient may be hypersensitive to light touch at one point during the examination but give no response when distracted.

Precipitating causes of the "chest pain"

Non-Munchausen factitious behavior is usually precipitated by heightened psychological and social conflicts. In Munchausen syndrome, the episodes are essentially continuous, interrupted only by impending or actual discovery of the truth.

The causes of chest-related signs and symptoms in factitious disorder are remarkably diverse. False reports (e.g., of hemoptysis) are most common. Other deceptions are more sophisticated and potentially more hazardous. A few examples will illustrate the range. Blood pressure peaks, hypotensive episodes, fluctuating heart rate, and dysrhythmias have all been induced by the Valsalva maneuver.[24] Recurrent Torsades de pointes resulting from hypokalemia has been caused by laxative abuse.[25] Bradycardia and recurrent cardiovascular collapse have been induced through the surreptitious intake of high doses of a calcium channel-[26] or beta-blocker.[27] Patients have tapped or otherwise manipulated electrodes to create abnormal tracings on the electrocardiogram. Factitious asthma and the associated chest symptoms have been caused by deliberate inhalation of baby powder or by ingestion or topical application of known allergens. Upper airway obstruction resulting in wheezing has also been induced by voluntary adduction of the vocal cords.[28]

Relief of the "chest pain"

In addition to those identified in the next section, a potential indicator of factitious disorder is the unresponsiveness of the patient's signs and symptoms to interventions that are consistently effective in other cases. Indeed, there may be a continual escalation regardless of the intensity of treatment, or an unwavering pattern of unexplained relapse following improvement.. Alternatively, a patient's presentation may become notably less acute upon his or her learning that hospital admission will occur. If the patient infers that physicians are doubting its authenticity or importance, the "chest pain" may resolve, only to be replaced by other manufactured symptoms. As in malingering, it is a paradox of factitious disorder that these individuals react with anger rather than pleasure when told that they do not have a serious medical affliction.

Associated Symptoms

Factitious disorder and malingering are unique in that the most important associated features often do not stem from the details of patients' symptom reports. Instead, these key elements include their behaviors during presentation and examination, and the degree of concordance between their reports and other sources of information, such as past medical records. Although none is diagnostic in isolation, potential indicators of factitious disorder include the following: (1) the magnitude of symptoms consistently exceeds objective pathology; (2) there has been a remarkable number of tests, consultations, and treatment efforts to little or no avail; (3) the patient is unusually willing to undergo medical/surgical procedures; (4) the patient disputes test results; (5) the patient predicts deteriorations, or there are exacerbations shortly before medical encounters are to end; (6) the patient emerges as an inconsistent, selective, or misleading informant; (7) the patient restricts access to outside information sources; (8) evidence from laboratory or other tests proves self-harm or disputes information provided by the patient; (9) signs and symptoms are present only when observation by others is evident to the patient; and (10) the patient engages in gratuitous lying.[29]

Associated Signs

Physical examination

When conditions are feigned or exaggerated, physicians will often find that expected physical findings are absent or that inconsistencies are evident. For example, despite his claim of pleuritic chest pain, a man who feigned lupus had no pericardial friction rub, pleural effusion, or other evidence of serositis.[23] There may be indications of self-harm or a startling number of surgical scars. One such patient had scars from venous cutdowns "over every named vein" that revealed the extensive medical/surgical history she had attempted to minimize.[30] In cases of a self-induced malady, physical findings will be consistent with the illness but needle marks and other signs may betray its origin.

"Routine" laboratory tests

Typically, tests such as the electrocardiogram, chest x-ray film, cardiac isoenzymes, and arterial blood gas and pH will be normal, though imaging studies may show evidence of prior surgery (e.g., surgical clips) not reported by the patient. However, manipulation of lab tests (e.g., adding blood to a urine specimen) can lead to spurious positive results, and some patients alter their charts to indicate abnormalities. Unexplained variations in test results from day to day should warrant suspicion, as should extreme abnormalities that are incompatible with the vitality of the patient. An individual's refusal to cooperate with studies, especially definitive tests, should also prompt suspicion. In cases of self-induced physical illness, there will be corresponding test results. For instance, a complete blood count will confirm a profound anemia caused by autophlebotomy.

Exceptions to The Usual Manifestations

The manifestations of factitious disorder including Munchausen syndrome are limited only by the patient's motivation and ingenuity. To illustrate, approximately 50 different factitious neurologic disorders have been reported in the medical literature. Although the variations of factitious disorder involving the chest are notably less abundant, additional inventive presentations will doubtless be described in the future. It is likely that there is no medical condition immune to a factitious representation.

Differential Diagnosis

Authentic Physical Illness

A true physical illness may account for the clinical presentation, as in the case of a patient who died of cancer after having been spurned by doctors as having feigned her lower thoracic pain. The diagnostic complexity is heightened by the fact that patients may self-induce conditions, such as profound bradycardia, that require vigorous medical intervention despite being manifestations of factitious disorder. There can also be iatrogenic complications, including "chest pain," from past procedures and medication trials.

Somatoform Disorders

In somatoform disorders such as hypochondriasis, the patient reports physical symptoms that suggest a medical problem. However, these symptoms cannot be accounted for by physical findings, by the use of legal or illegal drugs, or by another mental disorder. Unlike patients with factitious disorders, those with classical somatoform disorders do not intend to deceive others and do not intentionally produce their symptoms.

Mood or Anxiety Disorders

Patients with conditions such as major depression and panic disorder often describe chest symptoms such as pain, heaviness, and tightness. These symptoms generally respond to treatment of the underlying mental disorder and do not involve any effort to deceive others.

Malingering

In factitious disorders, the motivation is to assume the sick role. In malingering, external incentives are apparent, such as financial compensation, acquisition of opioids, avoidance of military duty, or evasion of criminal prosecution. Of course, when perceived incentives are used as a diagnostic criterion, imprecision in diagnosis is bound to arise at times. Clinicians should also be aware that an individual's goals, whether internal or external, can vary over time or co-exist.

Other Diagnostic Testing

When there are indications of factitious disorders, physicians should think carefully before ordering additional tests, especially if they have already been performed with negative results, are of potential risk to the patient, or are unlikely to provide important new information. The most common reason for delay in diagnosing factitious disorder is failure to include it in the differential diagnosis. Sometimes this step is overlooked in favor of less common possibilities. Physicians may need to resist the patient's demands for more testing and diagnostic procedures of increasing invasiveness. In one case, a patient presenting with factitious angina progressed to recurrent thromboembolism and limb amputations as a result of iatrogenic complications induced by angiographic and surgical procedures.[12]

Etiology and Basic Mechanisms Responsible for the "Pain"

By definition, the chest pain in factitious disorder including Munchausen syndrome is feigned, exaggerated, or self-induced. If any objective physical findings are present, there has been a determination that they are inconsistent with the presentation, are not explanatory, or have been deliberately created. Therefore, any discussion of etiology must focus not on medical, but on cognitive, social, and/or emotional factors.

Psychodynamic theories of factitious disorder have a long history. As early as 1934, Menninger[31] advanced the notion of "polysurgical addiction." He postulated that these patients experience intense aggression toward themselves and their physicians, the latter serving as surrogates for the "perceived sadistic parent." Later, Spiro[32] suggested that early deprivation and trauma, weak self-identity, and deficits in conscience and self-control were the causes. Overlapping hypotheses have involved gratification of patients' needs to be dependent on others; establishment of a well-defined role (that of "patient") to be played by individuals whose self-identity is weak; achievement of a sense of mastery to combat feelings of weakness and vulnerability; masochism, since such patients seek out situations that mix caring with pain; and enhancement of self-esteem.[33–35]

Behavioral theories view factitious disorder as the result of past social learning and current positive and negative reinforcement.[36,37] These patients may have experienced a critical illness as a child or had a relative who was seriously ill. This experience of assuming, or watching a model assume, the sick role may be positively reinforced when the child experiences or witnesses the sympathy and attention accorded occupants of this role. In addition, the sick role behavior may be negatively reinforced by an avoidance of responsibilities and duties.[38]

Biological theories have been less compelling. In small studies, a minority of factitious disorder or Munchausen patients have had some suggestion of brain dysfunction,[39] and there may be nonspecific findings on brain imaging[40,41] or neuropsychological testing.[42] No genetic pattern has been established.

Likely *predisposing factors* to factitious disorder include the presence of other mental disorders or general medical conditions during childhood or adolescence that led to extensive medical treatment; family disruption or abuse in childhood; a grudge against the medical profession; employment in a medically related position; and the presence of a severe personality disorder, most often borderline personality disorder.[2,43,44]

Treatment

Factitious disorder patients usually resist or decline psychiatric consultation or treatment because they wish to retain the role of medical/surgical patient. Refusals, along with threats, elopements, or discharges against medical advice, are especially likely in Munchausen syndrome. Face-saving or other non-confrontational approaches[45] may enhance the likelihood of success in presenting the diagnosis to the patient. Pharmacotherapy of factitious disorder is limited largely to treatment of any comorbid psychiatric diagnoses, such as mood or anxiety disorders. Medications should be carefully monitored because of these patients' propensity to misuse them. There is no "gold standard" for nonpharmacologic treatment, but psychotherapy and behavior therapy can sometimes facilitate the containment of symptoms.[46] Treating clinicians should have modest expectations, anticipating relapse and accepting periods of symptomatic relief rather than cure. The primary goal is to reduce the patient's medical/surgical over-utilization by helping the patient find alternate ways to gain the gratification provided by the sick role. Positive prognostic indicators include an ability to establish a therapeutic alliance; an underlying psychiatric diagnosis such as major depression; psychosocial supports, such as ongoing relationships with others; and an absence of borderline or antisocial personality traits.[47] Clinicians must be aware of and, as needed, attempt to modulate any angry reactions they experience toward these patients.[48]

Classic Descriptions

In 1843, Gavin[49] summarized the "feigned and factitious diseases of soldiers and seamen," observing that some engaged in medical deception simply "to excite compassion or interest." Sixty years later, Reiling reinforced the concept, describing individuals whose infirmities were "magnified, particularly when this creates interest from others. They take pleasure in becoming the centers of exacting attention, care, and sympathetic comment."[50] The term "Munchausen's syndrome" was coined by Asher in 1951.[51] He recounted the dilemma for physicians: "The doctor is confronted with a patient with apparently infinite inventiveness, who is turning into an adversary." He concluded that "the most remarkable feature of the syndrome is the apparent senselessness of it. Unlike the malingerer, who may gain a definite end, these patients often seem to gain nothing except the discomfiture of unnecessary investigations or operations."

References

1. Feldman MD, Ford CV. Factitious disorders. In: Sadock BJ, Sadock VA (eds). *Kaplan and Sadock's Comprehensive Textbook of Psychiatry*. Baltimore, Lippincott Williams & Wilkins, 1999.
2. American Psychiatric Association. *Diagnostic and Statistical Manual of Mental Disorders*. Washington, DC, American Psychiatric Association, 2000.
3. Reich P, Gottfried LA. Factitious disorders in a teaching hospital. *Ann Intern Med* 1983;99:240–247.
4. Ford CV. *The Somatizing Disorders: Illness as a Way of Life*. New York, Elsevier Biomedical, 1983.
5. Bock KD, Overkamp F. [Factitious disease. Observations on 44 cases at a medical clinic and recommendation for a subclassification]. *Klin Wochenschr* 1986; 64:149–164.
6. Freyberger H, Nordmeyer JP, Freyberger HJ, et al. Patients suffering from factitious disorders in the clinico-psychosomatic consultation liaison service: Psychodynamic processes, psychotherapeutic initial care and clinicointerdisciplinary cooperation. *Psychother Psychosom* 1994;62:108–122.
7. Eisendrath SJ. Current overview of factitious physical disorders. In: Feldman MD, Eisendrath SJ (eds). *The Spectrum of Factitious Disorders*. Washington, DC, American Psychiatric Press, 1996.
8. Robinson ME, Myers CD, Sadler IJ, et al. Bias effects in three common self-report pain assessment measures. *Clin J Pain* 1997;13:74–81.
9. Poole GD, Craig KD. Judgments of genuine, suppressed, and faked facial expressions of pain. *J Pers Soc Psychol* 1992;63:797–805.
10. Baktari JB, Tashkin DP, Small GW. Factitious hemoptysis. Adding to the differential diagnosis. *Chest* 1994;105:943–945.
11. Orchard RT, Yates DB, Taylor DJ. Acute precordial chest pain. *Practitioner* 1974;13:212–217.

12. Manolis AS, Sanjana VM. Cardiopathia fantastica and arteritis factitia as manifestations of Munchausen syndrome. *Crit Care Med* 1987;15:526–529.
13. Tizes R. The professional cardioversion patient: A new medical and psychiatric entity. *Chest* 1977;71:434–435.
14. Cavenar JO, Jr., Maltbie AA, Hillard JR, et al. Cardiac presentation of Munchausen's syndrome. *Psychosomatics* 1980;21:946–948.
15. Rusakow LS, Gershan WM, Bulto M, et al. Munchausen's syndrome presenting as cystic fibrosis with hemoptysis. *Pediatr Pulmonol* 1993;16:326–329.
16. Saed G, Potalivo S, Panzini L, et al. Munchausen's syndrome. A case of factitious hemoptysis. *Panminerva Med* 1999;41:62–67.
17. Roethe RA, Fuller PB, Byrd RB, et al. Munchausen syndrome with pulmonary manifestations. *Chest* 1981;79:487–488.
18. Barnett VT, Bergmann F, Humphrey H, et al. Diffuse alveolar hemorrhage secondary to superwarfarin ingestion. *Chest* 1992;102:1301–1302.
19. Dixon D, Abbey S. Cupid's arrow. An unusual presentation of factitious disorder. *Psychosomatics* 1995;36:502–504.
20. Halter U. [A case from practice (255). Munchausen syndrome in borderline personality. Bacterial right and left heart endocarditis following i.v. injection of feces. Abscessed pneumonia. Acute post-infection glornerulonephritis with reversible kidney failure. Multi-drug addiction with i.v. drug abuse (Temgesic and other opiates)]. *Schweiz Rundsch Med Prax* 1992;81:1290–1291.
21. Baran GA, Vas WG, Sundaram M, et al. Case report 544: Munchhausen syndrome with self-inflicted destruction of both shoulders simulating neuropathic disease. *Skeletal Radiol* 1989;18:459–461.
22. Gibbon KL. Munchausen's syndrome presenting as an acute sexual assault. *Med Sci Law* 1998;38:202–205.
23. Apfelbaum JD, Williams HJ. Factitious simulation of systemic lupus erythematosus. *West J Med* 1994;160:259–261.
24. Ludwigs U, Ruiz H, Isaksson H, et al. Factitious disorder presenting with acute cardiovascular symptoms. *J Intern Med* 1994;236:685–690.
25. Krahn LE, Lee J, Richardson JW, et al. Hypokalemia leading to torsades de pointes. Munchausen's disorder or bulimia nervosa? *Gen Hosp Psychiatry* 1997;19:370–377.
26. Eckert S, Mertens HM, Mannebach H, et al. [Bradycardia factitia]. *Dtsch Med Wochenschr* 1988;113:469–471.
27. Warwick GL, Boulton-Jones JM. Recurrent cardiovascular collapse due to surreptitious ingestion of propranolol. *BMJ* 1989;298:294–295.
28. Egan AJM, Tazelaar HD, Myers JL, et al. Munchausen syndrome presenting as pulmonary talcosis. *Archives of Pathology & Laboratory Medicine* 1999;123:736–738.
29. Eisendrath SJ, Rand DC, Feldman MD. Factitious disorders and litigation. In: Feldman MD, Eisendrath SJ (eds). *The Spectrum of Factitious Disorders.* Washington, DC, American Psychiatric Press, 1996.
30. Gadre AK, DeSautel MG, Senders CW. Otolaryngological manifestations of factitious disorders-a case and literature review. *J Laryngol Otol* 1996;110:981–983.
31. Menninger K. Polysurgery and polysurgical addiction. *Psychoanalytic Q* 1934;4: 173–199.
32. Spiro HR. Chronic factitious illness. Munchausen's syndrome. *Arch Gen Psychiatry* 1968;18:569–579.
33. Spivak H, Rodin G, Sutherland A. The psychology of factitious disorders. A reconsideration. *Psychosomatics* 1994;35:25–34.

34. Ford CV. *Lies! Lies!! Lies!!! The Psychology of Deceit.* Washington, DC, American Psychiatric Press, 1996.
35. Hamilton JC, Janata JW. Dying to be ill: The role of self-enhancement motives in the spectrum of factitious disorders. *J Soc Clin Psychol* 1997;16:178–199.
36. Barsky AJ, Wyshak G, Klerman GL. Psychiatric comorbidity in DSM-111-R hypochondriasis. *Arch Gen Psychiatry* 1992;49:101–108.
37. Schwartz SM, Gramling SE, Mancini T. The influence of life stress, personality, and learning history on illness behavior. *J Behav Ther Exp Psychiatry* 1994;25: 135–142.
38. Feldman MD, Hamilton JC, Deemer HN. A critical analysis of factitious disorders. In Phillips KA (ed). *Somatoform and Factitious Disorders.* Washington, DC, American Psychiatric Press, 2001.
39. King BH, Ford CV. Pseudologia fantastica. *Acta Psychiatr Scand* 1988;77:1–6.
40. Fenelon G, Mahieux F, Roullet E, et al. Munchausen's syndrome and abnormalities on magnetic resonance imaging of the brain. *BMJ* 1991;302:996–997.
41. Babe KS, Jr., Peterson AM, Loosen PT, et al. The pathogenesis of Munchausen syndrome. A review and case report. *Gen Hosp Psychiatry* 1992;14:273–276.
42. Pankratz L, Lezak MD. Cerebral dysfunction in the Munchausen syndrome. *Hillside J Clin Psychiatry* 1987;9:195–206.
43. Kapfbammer HP, Dobmeier P, Mayer C, et al. [Conversion syndromes in neurology. A psychopathological and psychodynamic differentiation of conversion disorder, somatization disorder and factitious disorder]. *Psychotherapie, Psychosomatik, Medizinische Psychologie* 1998;48:463–474.
44. Ford CV. The Munchausen syndrome: A report of four new cases and a review of psychodynamic considerations. *Int J Psychiatry Med* 1973;4:31–45.
45. Eisendrath SJ. Factitious physical disorders: Treatment without confrontation. *Psychosomatics* 1989;30:383–387.
46. Eisendrath SJ, Feder A. Management of factitious disorders. In Feldman MD, Eisendrath SJ (eds): *The Spectrum of Factitious Disorders.* Washington, DC, American Psychiatric Press, 1996.
47. Folks DG. Munchausen's syndrome and other factitious disorders. *Neurol Clin* 1995;13:267–281.
48. Feldman MD, Feldman JM. Tangled in the web: Countertransference in the therapy of factitious disorders. *Int J Psychiatry Med* 1995;25:389–399.
49. Gavin H. *On Feigned and Factitious Diseases, Chiefly of Soldiers and Seamen.* London, John Churchill, 1843.
50. Reiling J. Litigation symptoms and diseases. *JAMA* 1999;281:1.
51. Asher R. Munchausen's syndrome. *Lancet* 1951;1:339–341.

$$\boxed{49}$$

"Chest Pain" in Patients with Addiction

Karen Drexler, MD

General Considerations

Addictive disorders are common in patients presenting with chest pain. From the most commonly used addictive substances- alcohol and nicotine- to illicit drugs, addictive substances increase the risk of many medical problems presenting with chest pain. Alcohol dependence leads to dilated cardiomyopathy, peptic ulcer disease, gastritis, cardiac arrhythmias, and pancreatitis.[1] Inhalants and stimulants can also cause cardiac arrhythmias.[2] Intravenous drug use is associated with endocarditis. Cigarette, cocaine, and amphetamine smoking can lead to angina pectoris and acute myocardial infarction (MI).[3] Cocaine has also been associated with pneumonitis and acute aortic dissection.[4] The evaluation and treatment of these myriad medical complications of addiction are addressed elsewhere in this book.

Of the many medical complications of psychoactive substance use, one deserves particular attention. Cocaine dependence is less common than alcohol and nicotine dependence, yet it has dramatically changed the evaluation and treatment of chest pain in emergency settings. In the 1980s, cocaine-related emergency room visits increased 20-fold such that it became the leading cause of drug-related emergency room visits by 1987.[5] This chapter will concentrate on the unique aspects of cocaine-induced chest pain.

Some patients who are addicted to morphine may complain of pain in order to obtain the drug. Malingering such as this is described in Chapter

---

[1]This chapter, written by a psychiatrist, on "Chest Pain" in patients with Addiction is somewhat similar to Chapter 33 which was written by a cardiologist and his associate. Both chapters are included in an effort to characterize all aspects of a patient with chest pain who is an addict.

From: Hurst JW, Morris DC (eds): *"Chest Pain"* →. © Futura Publishing Co., Inc., Armonk, NY, 2001.

47. The addiction may have developed because the drug was originally given for a definite illness, but the continued use of the drug has led to addiction. Many times the malingerer complains of pain that can spontaneously subside. For example, kidney colic may disappear when the stone is passed. Therefore, a malingering patient is more likely to complain of kidney colic than "chest pain." This is true because with factitious chest pain, physicians may suggest that other procedures, such as a coronary arteriogram, should be performed to clarify the problem. On the other hand, the patient with kidney colic can claim that he or she passed the stone and no other procedures are needed. The point is, the malingering patient does not wish to have other procedures. This is unlike the behavior of patients with Munchausen syndrome (factitious disorder); they will gladly undergo any and all types of procedures.

The malingerer who complains of chest pain simulating myocardial ischemia is usually sophisticated and can put on a convincing performance, but at the same time knows how to avoid other procedures. In fact, the master malingerer is in control of the situation.

Clinical Setting

The cocaine epidemic has led to a dramatic rise in the number of younger patients presenting with the classic symptoms of myocardial ischemia, but with few of the traditional risk factors for heart disease except for tobacco use.[6] Compared to other chest pain patients, cocaine users tend to be younger (mean age 29–37 years), male (70%–85%), current tobacco smokers (80%–85%), and tend not to have diabetes mellitus, previous history of MI, or family history of coronary artery disease.[6,7] A disproportionately high number of cocaine-related emergency room visits occur from 11:00 PM to 7:00 AM.[8] Cocaine can cause acute MI, and among cocaine users with chest pain, neither cardiac risk factors, nor severity of cocaine use, distinguish those who develop acute MI from those who do not.[9]

Characteristics of the "Pain"

Patient's characterization of the "chest pain"

The quality of acute cocaine-induced "chest pain" is indistinguishable from that experienced in acute myocardial ischemia. Patients usually describe their pain as "pressure-like" or "crushing"(30%–50%).[2] One-fifth of patients describe "aching" or "dull" pain.[6] About 30%–40% of patients describe a sharp or stabbing pain which may not be due to myocardial ischemia (see Chapter 29).[6]

Common location of the "chest pain"

The location of the pain due to myocardial ischemia is illustrated in Figures 49–1 and 49–2.

Uncommon locations of the "chest pain"

Uncommon locations of the chest pain is shown in Figure 49–3.

Size of the painful "area"

See Figures 49–1 and 49–2.

Duration of the "chest pain"

The "pain" may last from several minutes to several hours.

Tenderness of the chest wall

There is no tenderness of the chest wall.

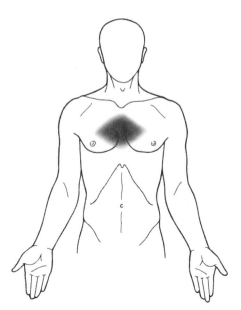

Figure 49–1. The usual location and size of the "chest pain" that is designated angina pectoris.

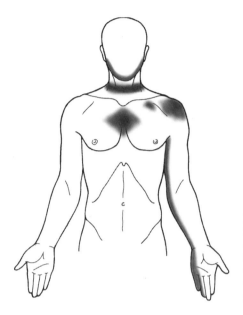

Figure 49–2. Common locations of the radiation of the "chest pain" that is designated angina pectoris. Note the radiation to the neck, jaw, left upper chest, left shoulder, inner surface of the left arm, left little finger, and left ring finger.

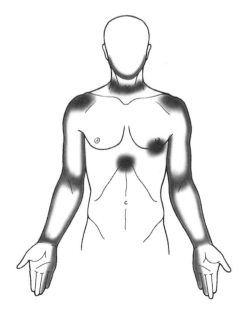

Figure 49–3. Unusual locations of the "pain" that is designated angina pectoris. The discomfort may be limited to the neck, jaw, right or left shoulder, left pectoral region, epigastrium, inner or outer surface of the right or left arms, elbows, wrists, or ring and little finger.

Precipitating causes of the "chest pain"

Cocaine-induced chest pain usually begins during or shortly after cocaine use. Risk of MI increases 24-fold within 1 hour of smoking crack and rapidly declines thereafter.[10] Cocaine-related chest pain usually occurs when patients are at rest, in contrast to non-cocaine related myocardial ischemia which is often triggered by exercise.

Relief of the "chest pain"

Cocaine-induced chest pain is relieved by stopping the use of cocaine; unless the patient has developed acute MI or a lethal ventricular arrhythmia. Most patients report that their pain began within 60 minutes of their last use of cocaine and persisted for about 120 minutes.[6]

The malingerer who craves morphine can imitate angina and infarction.

Associated Symptoms

Cardiac symptoms associated with cocaine-induced "chest pain" are typical of those associated with acute MI. Dyspnea and diaphoresis are common.[12] Other symptoms commonly associated with acute MI—nausea, vomiting, diaphoresis, palpitations and syncope do not distinguish cocaine users with acute MI from those patients who use no cocaine.[6]

Lethal ventricular arrhythmias can occur in 5% of patients with cocaine-induced chest pain.[11] Acute MI occurs in about 6% (range 0%–31% depending on the setting.)[6]

Symptoms of cocaine intoxication and withdrawal are often present and can help detect cocaine use in patients who are reluctant to report their drug use. Cocaine intoxication typically lasts 30 to 45 minutes after snorting, 10 to 20 minutes after injection and 8 to 10 minutes after smoking freebase or crack.[12] Cocaine withdrawal can begin 30 minutes to several hours after ingestion. Patients being evaluated for cocaine-induced "chest pain" may initially present with cocaine intoxication that evolves into cocaine withdrawal.

The "high" associated with crack smoking is described as intensely pleasurable- "like a whole body orgasm".[14] As the euphoria wanes, the intoxicated person, typically becomes more anxious and agitated, sometimes frankly paranoid and delusional. Other symptoms include affective blunting, hypervigilence, tension, confusion, or changes in interpersonal sensitivity.[15] Cocaine-induced psychosis (hallucinations and delusions) begins during intoxication, but can last 3 to 5 days.

Within several hours after cocaine ingestion, the person may experience withdrawal symptoms, lasting 12 hours to several days. He or she may describe depressed mood, regret, and guilt about drug use, often to the point of contemplating suicide. Marked fatigue, vivid unpleasant dreams, increased appetite, and insomnia or hypersomnia are also common.[16]

The symptoms of cocaine intoxication and withdrawal may be modified by the influence of alcohol, marijuana, or other drugs. The use of more than one addictive substance is common.

The malingerer can imitate the pain of angina or infarction (see General Considerations).

Associated Signs

Physical examination

Among cocaine users with "chest pain," neither vital signs, diaphoresis, vomiting, or syncope distinguish those who have acute MI from those who do not.

Physical signs of cocaine intoxication can help detect cocaine use when patients do not disclose their drug use. These signs include tachycardia or bradycardia, tachypnea, pupillary dilation, elevated or lowered blood pressure, perspiration or chills, nausea or vomiting, evidence of weight loss, psychomotor agitation or retardation, seizures, dyskinesias, dystonias, or coma.[8] Signs of cocaine withdrawal are less remarkable but can include psychomotor agitation or retardation. Pupils are typically of normal size and reactivity during withdrawal.

"Routine" laboratory tests

The *electrocardiogram* of patients with cocaine induced MI may show the telltale signs of MI. However, the electrocardiogram may be normal when the patient is first seen. Cardiac enzymes become elevated when there is an acute MI. These tests remain normal when the patient is malingering, but, because these tests may remain normal with acute coronary syndromes, the physician is left with a difficult diagnostic challenge.

Exceptions to the Usual Manifestations

Patients with cocaine-induced chest symptoms can also present with arrhythmias, cough, and/or cardiac arrest. Cocaine use has been associated with pneumonia, cardiomyopathy, arrhythmias, aortic dissection, pneumopericardium, and endocarditis.[8,11] An abrupt onset of severe pain often migrating and described as knifelike, tearing, or ripping may indicate aortic dissection.[16,17]

Differential Diagnosis

Cocaine causes chest pain that is indistinguishable from that associated with acute MI. Often the pain resolves without any detectable damage to the myocardium, but about 6% (0%–31%) develop acute MI.[6] This rate is similar to that in traditional patients in this age group (25–39 years) reporting chest pain (4.2%).[18] Every cocaine user presenting with anterior chest pain should be evaluated for possible acute MI.

Other Diagnostic Testing

Because patients can be reluctant to disclose drug use, laboratory tests for drug use are important. The presence of benzoylecgonine, a metabolite of cocaine, in the serum can detect cocaine use within the past few hours. Urine drug screens for benzoylecgonine can detect use from 1 hour to 3 days.[19]

In one study of cocaine-associated MIs, 38% of patients with cocaine-associated MI had a normal electrocardiogram on initial presentation.[6] In another report, 29% of patients with cocaine-associated chest pain and normal electrocardiograms had abnormal myocardial perfusion scans using Tecnetium-99m tetrofosmin.[20]

Creatinine kinase-MB isoform (CK-MB) is a protein marker used to diagnose acute MI. CK-MB levels rise to twice normal in about 6 hours after MI and peak within 24 hours. However, CK-MB is not completely cardiac specific. It is present in small quantities in skeletal muscle. Because cocaine use can damage skeletal muscle, patients with cocaine-induced chest pain can have elevated CK-MB without MI.[20]

Myoglobin is another protein marker used for early detection of acute MI. Because of its low molecular weight, myoglobin diffuses quickly from damaged muscle tissue. Its levels reach twice normal within 2 hours and peak within 4 hours of acute MI. In a general emergency department population, it has over 90% sensitivity and about 80% specificity for diagnosing acute MI within 2 hours of the onset of chest pain. However, in patients with recent cocaine use, the specificity drops to 50%.[20]

Troponin I is more specific than either myoglobin or CPK for determining myocardial damage in patients with cocaine-induced chest pain.[21] Troponin I levels become elevated within six hours of myocardial damage and peak in 12 hours. The level remains elevated for 6 to 10 days. It has been shown to have 94% specificity for diagnosing acute MI in patients with and without recent cocaine use.[20]

Etiology and Basic Mechanisms Responsible for the "Pain"

Cocaine blocks presynaptic reuptake of dopamine and norepinephrine. The resulting central adrenergic stimulation causes an increase in heart rate, blood pressure, and left ventricular contractility.[7] In addition, cocaine's local effects cause increased systemic blood pressure, decreased left ventricular ejection fraction, and coronary artery spasm.[22] Myocardial ischemia develops due to increased myocardial oxygen demand and decreased perfusion. Cocaine use also accelerates atherosclerosis and activates platelet aggregation. This can lead to acute MI through the formation of a thrombus that blocks coronary arteries. Cocaine also prolongs electrical conduction in the heart. In the setting of ischemia, this can lead to lethal ventricular arrhythmias.[11]

Treatment

For acute management, it is important to approach an acutely intoxicated stimulant user in a subdued manner. Speak softly and avoid touching the patient without warning. Benzodiazepines (lorazepam and others) can relieve agitation. Antipsychotic medication (such as haloperidol, risperidone, and others) can treat hallucinations and paranoia. Patients are often ashamed to admit even to themselves that their drug or alcohol use is a problem. Using a thorough search for clues from the history, physical examination, laboratory tests, and collateral history from friends and family members, the careful clinician will detect cocaine abuse, recommend abstinence, and, if indicated, refer the addicted patient to a rehabilitation program. A recent review describes motivational interviewing and brief intervention techniques for primary care physicians.[23] A high index of suspicion coupled with an open and understanding bedside manner will yield a much more satisfying treatment outcome when both the presenting medical condition and the underlying addiction are addressed.

As for the chest pain itself, emergency department chest pain centers can provide an efficient setting for evaluation and treatment of patients with chest pain who are at low to moderate risk for acute coronary syndromes.[24,25] Such settings may be ideal for assessment of stable patients with cocaine-associated chest pain, but without signs of acute MI or arrhythmia on initial presentation.[26] In one report of 197 patients admitted to a chest pain center, 171 (87%) were released to home after continuous 12-lead electrocardiogram S-T segment monitoring and serial CPK-MB for 9 hours or CPK-MB and troponin for 6 hours. None of the patients released to home had cardiac complications at 30-day follow-up (91% follow-up obtained).[27]

As stated in the section "General Considerations" the malingerer who is addicted is usually able to avoid further testing to determine the cause of the pain. Such patients need the care of a skilled psychiatrist who works with addicts.

References

1. Gordis E, (ed) et al. Eighth Special Report to the U.S. Congress on Alcohol and Health. US Department of Health and Human Services, 1993, pp. 165–201.
2. Zimmerman JL, Dellinger RP, Majid PA. Cocaine-associated chest pain. *Ann Emerg Med* 1991;20:611–615.
3. Moliterno DJ, Willard JE, Lange RA, et al. Coronary-artery vasoconstriction induced by cocaine, cigarette smoking, or both. *NEJM* 1994;330:454–459.
4. Chang RA, Rossi NF. Intermittent cocaine use associated with recurrent dissection of the thoracic and abdominal aorta. *Chest* 1995;108:1758–1762.
5. MacDonald DI. Cocaine heads ED drug visits. *JAMA.* 1987;258:2029.
6. Hollander JE, Hoffman RS, Gennis P, et al. Prospective multicenter evaluation of cocaine-associated chest pain. *Acad Emerg Med* 1994;1:330–339.
7. Mouhaffel AH, Madu EC, Satmary WA, et al. Cardiovascular complications of cocaine. *Chest* 1995;107:1426–1434.
8. Brody SL, Slovis CM, Wrenn KD. Cocaine-related medical problems: Consecutive series of 233 patients. *Am J Med* 1990;88:325–331.
9. Amin M, Gabelman G, Darpel J, et al. Acute myocardial infarction and chest pain syndromes after cocaine use. *Am J Cardiol* 1990;66:1434–1437.
10. Mittleman MA, Mintzer D, Maclure M, et al. Triggering of myocardial infarction by cocaine. *Circulation* 1999;99:2737–1741.
11. Gamouras GA, Monir G, Plunkitt K, et al. Cocaine abuse: Repolarization abnormalities and ventricular arrhythmias. *Am J Med Sci* 2000;320:9–12.
12. Gitter MJ, Goldsmith SR, Dunbar DN, et al. Cocaine and chest pain: Clinical features and outcome of patients hospitalized to rule out myocardial infarction. *Ann Intern Med* 1991;115:277–280.
13. Verbeny K, Gold MS. From cocaine leaves to crack: The effects of dose and routes of administration in abuse liability. *Psychiatr Ann* 1988;18:514.
14. Gold MS. Cocaine and crack: Clinical aspects. In Lowinson JH, Ruiz P, Millman RB. *Substance Abuse : A Comprehensive Textbook. Second Edition.* Baltimore: Williams & Wilkins 1992;205–221.
15. American Psychiatric Association. *Diagnostic and Statistical Manual of Mental Disorders, Fourth Edition.* Washington, DC, American Psychiatric Association, 1994.
16. Rashid J, Eisenberg M, Topol EJ. Cocaine-induced aortic dissection. *Am Heart J* 1996;132:1301–1304.
17. Fikar CR, Koch S. Etiologic factors of acute aortic dissection in children and young adults. *Clinical Pediatrics* 2000;39:71–80.

18. Lee TH, Cook EF, Weisberg M, et al. Acute chest pain in the emergency room: Identification and examination of low risk patients. *Arch Intern Med* 1985;145: 65–66.
19. Hollander JE, Levitt MA, Yound GP, et al. Effect of recent cocaine use on the specificity of cardiac markers for diagnosis of acute myocardial infarction. *Am Heart J* 1998;135:245–252.
20. Feldman JA, Bui LD, Mitchell PM, et al. The evaluation of cocaine-induced chest pain with acute myocardial perfusion imaging. *Acad Emerg Med* 1999;6:103–109.
21. Falahati A, Sharkey SW, Christensen D, et al. Implementation of serum cardiac troponin I as marker for detection of acute myocardial infarction. *Am Heart J* 1999;137:332–337.
22. Pitts WR, Vongpatanasin W, Cigarroa, JE, et al. Effects of the intracoronary infusion of cocaine on left ventricular systolic and diastolic function in humans. *Circulation* 1998;97:1270–1273.
23. Weaver MF, Jarvis MAE, Schnoll SH. Role of the primary care physician in problems of substance abuse. *Arch Intern Med* 1999;159:913–924.
24. Robinson B, Garcia TB, Walton JF, et al. Indigent patient's utilization of emergency department-based chest pain centers for nonmedical reasons. *Ann Emerg Med* 1999;34(supp):s48.
25. Zalenski RJ, Aurora M, McCarren M, et al. The comparative value of an emergency diagnostic and treatment unit protocol for acute cardiac ischemia (ACI) in patients with cocaine-associated chest pain. *Ann Emerg Med* 1999;34(supp): s22–s23.
26. Henderson SO, Ostrzega E, Genna T, et al. Coronary triage unit in an indigent county population. *Ann Emerg Med* 2000;35(supp):s51–s52.
27. Kushman SO, Storron AB, Liv T, et al. Cocaine-associated chest pain in a chest pain center. *Am J Cardiol* 2000;85:394–396.

Part XIII

"Chest Pain" of Controversial Origin

Although the definition of "chest pain"→ is discussed in Chapter 1, the definition is repeated here so that communication is clear.

The quotation marks around "chest" imply that different patients have different definitions of the word "chest." Here we use the word to indicate pain located above the waist. Then, too, *angina pectoris* is not always located in the pectoral region—it may be felt only in the jaw, neck, shoulder, elbow, or wrist. Therefore, the word "chest" implies that other parts of the upper body may also be involved with painful syndromes.

The quotation marks around "pain" imply that patients may assign other terms to their discomfort, such as indigestion, burning, ache, etc.

The arrow after "chest pain" implies that the physician initially may not know the cause of the symptom, so a differential diagnosis must be established that fits the available information.

50

"Chest Pain" in Patients with Syndrome X

Richard O. Cannon III, MD

General Considerations

Four decades after the recognition that patients with angina-like chest pain may have normal coronary angiograms,[1,2] consensus regarding the definition, pathophysiology, and management of this syndrome remains elusive. Even the definition of syndrome X is a matter of dispute, and often confused (or compared) with the metabolic syndrome X of insulin resistance. *Attempts have been made by many researchers and clinicians to restrict the use of the term cardiac syndrome X to those patients who have effort-provoked angina-like chest pain associated with ischemic-appearing ST segment depression on exercise electrocardiograms in the setting of normal coronary angiograms and absence of coronary spasm or cardiomyopathy.* However, other investigators (including this author) have not found the character of symptoms, response to therapy, or prognosis to differ in patients who fulfill this "restricted" definition of syndrome X compared with the much larger group of patients (approximately 10% of patients undergoing coronary angiography) with chest pain symptoms sufficiently angina-like to warrant cardiac catheterization, but who emerge from the lab with "clean coronaries".

Certain features of the symptom complex do set patients with syndrome X apart from patients with coronary atherosclerotic heart disease with regard to provoking circumstances, duration of pain, and response to therapy.

Clinical Setting

Syndrome X is more commonly seen in women than in men. The average age of those who suffer with this syndrome is about 50 years.

From: Hurst JW, Morris DC (eds): *"Chest Pain"* →. © Futura Publishing Co., Inc., Armonk, NY, 2001.

Characteristics of the "Pain"

Patient's characterization of the "chest pain"

Patients with syndrome X commonly describe the quality of their chest pain symptoms as being similar to the symptoms of patients with angina pectoris due to coronary atherosclerotic heart disease (see Chapter 29). That is, syndrome X patients commonly describe their "chest pain" as tightness, pressure, or burning.

Common location of the "chest pain"

The "chest pain" is usually located in the restrosternal area (see Figure 50–1). Further, the radiation patterns are similar to those of angina pectoris, including to the neck and lower jaw and to the medial aspect of one or both arms (see Figure 50–2).

Size of the "painful" area

The size of the "painful" area in patients with syndrome X is similar to the "painful area" that occurs in patients with myocardial ischemia caused

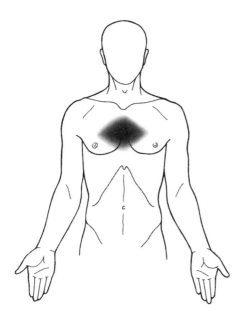

Figure 50–1. The usual location and size of the "chest pain" that occurs in patients with syndrome X. Note that the location of the pain is similar to that occurring in patients with angina pectoris.

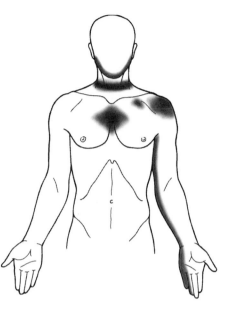

Figure 50–2. Common locations of the radiation of the "chest pain" that occurs in patients with syndrome X. Note the radiation to the neck, jaw, left upper chest, left shoulder, inner surface of the left arm, left little finger, and left ring finger.

by coronary atherosclerotic heart disease. The retrosternal "pain" is commonly the size of the fist or larger and the size of the referred "painful" area is limited to the size of the anatomic area (jaw, shoulder, elbow, etc).

Duration of the "chest pain"

In this author's experience, patients commonly report "chest pain" that can last over half an hour, and sometimes wax and wane for several hours. This differs from the duration of the "chest pain" in patients with angina pectoris. Remember, as discussed in Chapter 29 the chest pain of effort angina lasts 2 to 3 minutes and perhaps 20 minutes when the angina is provoked by emotional stimuli.

Tenderness of the "chest" wall

The chest wall is not tender.

Precipitating causes of "chest pain"

In the classic paper reporting the existence of patients with angina-like chest pain despite normal coronary angiograms, Kemp et al.[1] reported characteristics of patients' chest pain that are consistent with this author's experience. In their series of 50 patients (31 women, 19 men), the duration of pain from onset of symptoms to time of study ranged from 5 months to 25 years, indicative of the chronicity of pain in many patients. Fifteen of the 50 patient cohort reported chest pain only with effort, but in 6, effort-provoked pain was unpredictable. Twenty-two additional patients had chest pain that occurred with effort as well as protracted episodes of chest pain occurring at rest, commonly unpredictable in provocation or circumstance. In the remaining 13 patients, episodes of chest pain occurred only at rest and was often protracted. Further, "chest pain" that occurs at rest is not necessarily aggravated by superimposed activity. In 10 of the 50 patients, the pain was virtually disabling.

Relief of the "chest pain"

Although some patients report that sublingual nitroglycerin is of benefit, they often use several tablets in an attempt to relieve the pain, which commonly recurs after a brief period of respite. In general, response to anti-ischemic therapy (beta-blockers, calcium channel-blockers, long-acting nitrates) is often transient (raising the prospect of a placebo effect) and patients commonly present for additional evaluations on a multitude of medications.

Finally, the severity of pain is often pronounced, resulting in significant deleterious impact in the quality of life, and often refractory to reassurance of a benign prognosis.[3,4]

Associated Symptoms

In addition to "chest pain," breathlessness and fatigue are commonly reported by patients with chest pain despite normal coronary angiograms, including the more narrowly defined syndrome X cohort. Several researchers have reported a high prevalence of psychiatric morbidity on the basis of standardized testing, with significantly higher psychological scores on indices of anxiety and depression compared with age and gender-matched subjects.[4,5] In our study of 60 consecutive patients with chest pain despite normal coronary angiograms (one-third of whom had syndrome X on the basis of ischemic-appearing ST segment depression during exercise), 38 patients (63%) fulfilled DSM-III-R criteria for one or more psychiatric diagnoses at some time during their lives; panic disorder in 26 patients, history of major depression in 17, somatization in 11, current major depression in 3, hypochondriasis in 2, alcohol dependence in 2, other anxiety disorders in 5, and other non-anxiety disorders in 7.[6] Identification of psychiatric disorders during the patient interview may be of importance in patient management.

Associated Signs

Physical examination

The physical examination is usually normal.

"Routine" laboratory tests

There are no routine laboratory tests that separate patients with cardiac syndrome X from the population at large. By definition of the syndrome, the exercise electrocardiogram is positive and shows transient S-T segment displacement suggesting subendocardial injury.

Exceptions to the Usual Manifestations

The definition of syndrome X is sufficiently restrictive to almost eliminate exceptions to the description of the syndrome.

Differential Diagnosis

Patients with cardiomyopathies, including dilated or hypertrophic cardiomyopathy (familial or hypertensive) and amyloid heart disease, may present with chest pain, breathlessness and fatigue.

A history of dysphagia should prompt referral for esophageal manometry.

A trial of acid-inhibiting therapy may be sufficient to exclude gastroesophageal reflux. Chest wall tenderness that replicates the patient's "chest pain" complaint should lead to consideration of costochondritis or fibromyalgia.

Etiology and Basic Mechanisms Responsible for the "Pain"

Controversy has raged over the past four decades,[7] and continues to the present,[8–11] regarding the existence of inducible myocardial ischemia in syndrome X. We studied 70 patients with angina-like chest pain despite normal coronary angiograms (44 women, 26 men; average age 49 years), 22 of whom had syndrome X by virtue of ischemic-appearing ST segment depression during exercise.[12] All underwent dobutamine stress echocardiography, and the regional and transmural contractile responses were compared to those of 26 normal volunteer subjects (7 women and 19 men; average age 56 years). We used the transesophageal route for imaging in order to maximize the number of ventricular segments visualized and the quality of images for assessment of contractility. Dobutamine infused in step-wise increments up to 40 μg/kg/min induced chest pain in 59 patients (84%), but in none of the control subjects. Ischemic-appearing ST segment depression developed in 22 patients (19 with syndrome X) and in 2 control subjects. Wall motion abnormalities occurred in none of the patients or the control subjects. Importantly, no differences were observed in the transmural contractile response to dobutamine between patients and control subjects. Further, the quantitative myocardial response to dobutamine was similar in patients with and those without ischemic-appearing ST segment depression during the infusion. Thus, despite the frequent provocation of characteristic chest pain and, in the syndrome X subset, ischemic-appearing ST segment depression, patients with chest pain despite normal coronary angiograms do not demonstrate concomitant regional wall motion abnormalities and in fact show a quantitatively normal myocardial contractile response to dobutamine.

Patchy or diffuse microvascular constriction has been proposed as a mechanism to account for absence of evidence for ischemia by assessment of contractility, due to hyperfunctioning of adjacent normally perfused myocardium.[13] However, explanations for chest pain alternative to myocardial ischemia have been supported by several investigators. In this regard, chest pain is commonly provoked in patients with chest pain despite normal coronary angiograms by manipulation of catheters in the heart, during coronary angiography, and most commonly, during right ventricular pacing, suggesting that abnormal cardiac pain perception may be of fundamental importance in accounting for pain.[14-16] In this regard, we found that in 36 patients with chest pain despite normal coronary angiograms, that characteristic "chest pain" could be provoked in 56% of the patients during injection of contrast media into the left coronary artery and in 86% by electrical stimulation (right ventricular pacing) at a heart rate 5 beats faster than the resting heart rate, with the pain worsening by increasing the stimulus intensity.[15] In contrast, pain responses to the injection of contrast media or by right ventricular pacing were seen in only 2 of 42 patients with coronary atherosclerotic heart disease and in none of 10 patients with valvular heart disease.

It is unknown whether heightened intracardiac pain sensitivity demonstrated in patients with chest pain despite normal coronary angiograms represents one extreme of the normal bell curve of the distribution of visceral sensory function, or is indicative of a true abnormality in visceral sensory function. These patients may represent the opposite end of the cardiac pain spectrum from that subgroup of patients with coronary artery disease who have "silent ischemia", i.e., no chest pain despite myocardial ischemia. Similar observations of exaggerated visceral pain sensitivity have been made within the esophagus of patients with chest pain and normal or near normal coronary angiograms that may explain why high esophageal pressures or acid reflux, generally unrecognized by healthy subjects, causes "chest pain" in some patients.[17] Additionally, exaggerated visceral pain sensitivity has been demonstrated within the rectum, sigmoid colon, and small intestine of patients with irritable bowel syndrome.[18] Thus, patients with "sensitive hearts" may represent one manifestation of chronic pain associated with heightened visceral pain sensitivity. In addition, the mechanism of exaggerated visceral pain sensitivity may be neurophysiologically linked to whatever is responsible for anxiety and panic disorders commonly encountered in this patient population.

Treatment

The management recommendations that follow are predicated on determination of normal coronary pressures and angiograms during cardiac catheterization, a normal echocardiogram showing absence of myocardial or valvular disease, and no evidence of coronary spasm (absence of characteristic ST segment changes during spontaneous episodes of chest pain or negative ergonovine challenge in the cath lab). Given this constellation of findings, the patient should be reassured that he/she has a chest pain syndrome that poses no increased cardiovascular morbidity or mortality risk. For patients with luminal irregularities on coronary angiography, or with risk factors associated with endothelial dysfunction (hypercholesterolemia, hypertension, cigarette smoking, diabetes mellitus), the risk of subsequent coronary events is higher than patients with entirely smooth coronary arteries and who have no risk factors for endothelial dysfunction. Accordingly, these patients should undergo aggressive risk factor management and begin daily aspirin therapy. All patients should be started on a regular exercise program in order to improve their stamina (many patients are severely deconditioned) and to encourage a positive attitude regarding their state of health. This effort is assisted by discontinuing all unnecessary medications. In some, this approach will sufficiently alleviate symptoms, and no further evaluation is necessary. Should symptoms persist despite reassurance, performance of exercise or dobutamine echocardiography can provide evidence for or against myocardial ischemia. Should a wall motion abnormality or diminished transmural contractility be induced, a trial of anti-ischemic therapy may be considered, if this approach has not already been tried. If dobutamine infusion is associated with "chest pain" despite a uniform increase in contractility, myocardial ischemia *alone* is unlikely to account for symptoms, and a trial of tricyclic antidepressant therapy coupled with beta-blockers (to block anticholinergic effects of this therapy) may be of symptom benefit by reducing visceral pain sensitivity.[6] If chest pain persists despite these therapeutic trials, gastroesophageal evaluation may be necessary with endoscopy to rule out chronic inflammation. Should these evaluations and therapeutic trials fail to control chest pain symptoms, referral to a pain clinic may be necessary for a multi-disciplinary approach to pain management.

Regardless of the path taken, sympathetic appreciation by the physician of the deleterious impact of "chest pain" on the patient's quality of life can go a long way towards reassuring the patient that an earnest attempt is being made to help alleviate symptoms.

References

1. Kemp HG, Elliott WC, Gorlin R. The anginal syndrome with normal coronary arteriography. *Trans Assoc Am Phys* 1967;80:59–70.
2. Likoff W, Segal BL, Kasparin H. Paradox of normal selective coronary arteriograms in patients considered to have unmistakable coronary heart disease. *N Engl J Med* 1967;276:1063–1066.
3. Ockene IS, Shay MJ, Alpert JS, et al. Unexplained chest pain in patients with normal coronary arteriogram. *N Engl J Med* 1980;303:1249–1252.
4. Bass C, Wade C, Hand D, et al. Patients with angina with normal and near normal coronary arteries: Clinical and psychosocial state 12 months after angiography. *Br Med J* 1983;287:1505–1508.
5. Beitman BD, Mukerji V, Lamberti JW, et al. Panic disorder in patients with chest pain and angiographically normal coronary arteries. *Am J Cardiol* 1989;63: 1399–1403.
6. Cannon RO III, Quyyumi AA, Mincemoyer R, et al. Imipramine in patients with chest pain despite normal coronary angiograms. *N Engl J Med* 1994;330: 1411–1417.
7. Cannon RO III, Camici PG, Epstein SE. Pathophysiological dilemma of syndrome X. *Circulation* 1992;85:883–892.
8. Zeiher AM, Krause T, Shachinger V, et al. Impaired endothelium-dependent vasodilation of coronary resistance vessels is associated with exercise-induced myocardial ischemia. *Circulation* 1995;91:2345–2352.
9. Hasdai D, Gibbons RJ, Holmes DR Jr, et al. Coronary endothelial dysfunction in humans is associated with myocardial perfusion defects. *Circulation* 1997;96: 3390.
10. Buchthal SD, Den Hollander JA, Bairey Merz CN, et al. Abnormal myocardial phosphorus-31 nuclear magnetic resonance spectroscopy in women with chest pain but normal coronary angiograms. *N Engl J Med* 2000;342:829–835.
11. Cannon RO III, Balaban RS. Chest pain in women with normal coronary angiograms. *N Engl J Med* 2000;342:885–886.

12. Panza JA, Laurienzo JM, Curiel RV, et al. Investigation of the mechanism of chest pain in patients with angiographically normal coronary arteries using transesophageal dobutamine stress echocardiography. *J Am Coll Cardiol* 1997; 29:293–301.

13. Masseri A, Crea F, Kaski JC, et al. Mechanisms of angina pectoris in syndrome X. *J Am Coll Cardiol* 1991;17:499–506.

14. Shapiro LM, Crake T, Poole-Wilson PA. Is altered cardiac sensation responsible for chest pain in patients with normal coronary arteries? Clinical observation during cardiac catheterization. *BMJ* 1988;296:170–171.

15. Cannon RO III, Quyyumi AA, Schenke WH, et al. Abnormal cardiac sensitivity in patients with chest pain and normal coronary arteries. *J Am Coll Cardiol* 1990;16:1359–1366.

16. Pasceri V, Lanza GA, Buffon A, et al. Role of abnormal pain sensitivity and behavioral factors in determining chest pain in syndrome X. *J Am Coll Cardiol* 1998;31:62–66.

17. Richter JE, Barish CF, Castell DO. Abnormal sensory perception in patients with esophageal chest pain. *Gastroenterology* 1986;91:845–852.

18. Lynn RB, Friedman LS: Irritable bowel syndrome. *N Engl J Med* 1993;329: 1940–1945.

51

"Chest Pain" in Patients with Mitral Valve Prolapse

J. Willis Hurst,MD

General Considerations

Discussions of the midsystolic click, with or without a late systolic murmur, heard on auscultation at the cardiac apex have filled the medical literature for several decades. The systolic click was formerly believed to be extracardiac in origin. Reid, in 1961, reported his belief that the systolic clicks originated in the mitral valve.[1] Barlow et al., using left ventricular angiography, proved that systolic clicks and late systolic murmurs were caused by prolapse of the mitral valve leaflets into the left atrium.[2,3] Their observations were followed by numerous clinical observations, not only describing the auscultatory findings, but enumerating the symptoms, electrocardiographic findings, and complications associated with the condition.[4,5] Later, echocardiography proved to be the superior method of identifying the condition. Each step of the way different authors offered different criteria for diagnosis and, because of this, the results of various studies differed considerably. The important study by Freed et al. of 1845 women and 1646 men was reported in 1999.[6] She and her colleagues used new criteria for the diagnosis and studied ambulatory outpatients in order to gain more insight into the prevalence and seriousness of the condition.

Clinical Setting

Previous reports of the prevalence of mitral valve prolapse (MVP) have suggested the condition occurred in about five% of the adult population.[7] The condition was believed to occur about twice as commonly in

From: Hurst JW, Morris DC (eds): *"Chest Pain"* →. © Futura Publishing Co., Inc., Armonk, NY, 2001.

females as males. Using Freed's criteria for diagnosis in a Framington survey cohort, the condition was found in only 2% to 3% of the population and was almost as common in males as females.[6]

Characteristics of the "Pain"

Most subjects with MVP do not have chest pain. Freed, et al. reported that the prevalence of chest pain in subjects with MVP was 21.9% and the prevalence of chest pain in patients without MVP was 17.5% ($P=0.12$).[6] The prevalence of chest pain found by Freed et al. in the population of subjects at large is, as expected, much less than it is in patients who see physicians because of symptoms. Even when chest pain is present in patients with MVP it is usually due to another cause such as anxiety (see Chapter 45). Still, experts are unwilling to state that MVP alone does not produce chest pain in an occasional patient. Barlow writes:

> "Most of my patients complaining of chest pain were anxious.
> However, there was a minority of somewhat placid young
> women who originally knew nothing of their mitral valve anomaly
> and did complain bitterly about the intermittent chest pain.
> I am uncertain whether the pain is causally related to the valve
> anomaly but favor that it sometimes is."[8]

> John Michael Criley writes:
> "I honestly don't know what causes the chest pain in most of patients with mitral valve prolapse, but I was compelled to believe in the papillary muscle stretch theory when I saw a patient who developed intense chest pain every time I brought out an intermittent click by having her roll on her left side or perform a Valsalva strain. It was the loudest click I ever heard, and every time I provoked it, she grabbed my wrist (the one holding the stethoscope) and dug in her fingernails to let me know how much it hurt!"[9]

"Chest pain," and associated symptoms due to anxiety are so common in patients with MVP that a physician must not casually attribute the symptoms to the prolapse.

Patients characterization of the "chest pain"

Patients may complain of "sharp stabs" of pain or a "prolonged ache." This is also characteristic of the "pain" associated with anxiety or depression.

Common location of the "chest pain"

The "pain" is located at or near the cardiac apex (see Figures 51–1 and 51–2). This is similar to the location of the "pain" associated with anxiety

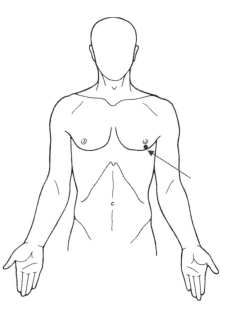

Figure 51–1. The "chest pain" of many patients with mitral valve prolapse is located near the cardiac apex and may be no larger than the tip of the finger; this is similar to the "chest pain" described by patients with anxiety or depression and many observers do not believe it is caused by prolapse of the mitral valve.

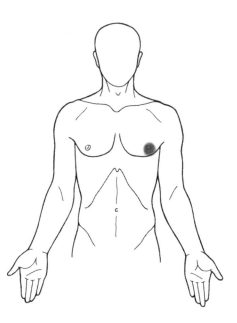

Figure 51–2. The "chest pain" of many patients with mitral valve prolapse is located near the cardiac apex and may be about the size of half of a hand; this is similar to the "chest pain" described by patients with anxiety or depression and many observers do not believe it is caused by prolapse of the mitral valve.

or depression. The location of the chest pain in Criley's patient as described above is shown in Figure 51–3.

Uncommon locations of the "chest pain"

The "pain" is rarely located in other regions of the "chest" other than the areas mentioned above.

Size of the "painful" area

The area of pain may be no larger than the tip of the finger, but may be as large as the hand. This does not differ from the size of pain the painful area observed in patients with anxiety or depression (see Figures 51–1 and 51–2).

Duration of the chest pain

The "sharp stabs" of discomfort may last no longer than it takes to "snap the fingers" or the dull ache may last for hours and days. The duration of the "pain" is similar to the duration of "pain" observed in patients with anxiety or depression.

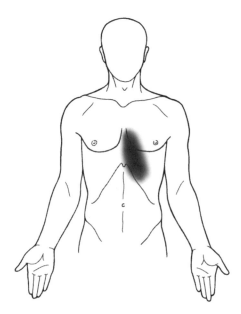

Figure 51–3. The figure shows the location of the chest pain in Criley's patient with mitral valve prolapse. Each time Criley had the patient roll on her left side or perform a Valsalva strain he brought out a loud intermittent systolic click and severe chest pain.[9]

Tenderness of the chest wall

The painful area may be tender but this also occurs in patients with anxiety.

Precipitating causes of the chest pain

The "pain" is rarely related to effort. When the discomfort is definitely related to effort one is forced to consider the possibility of angina pectoris.

The "sharp pain" of brief duration may be caused by premature cardiac contractions. Perhaps the powerful systolic ejection due to enhanced cardiac contraction following the longer than usual diastolic pause that follows a premature contraction causes more tension on the mitral valve apparatus than occurs with normal contractions.

Dr. Criley described the patient (see description earlier in this chapter) who had intense pain when she performed a Valsalva maneuver, or rolled to her left side, at which time the systolic click became louder. The chest pain occurring under these circumstances is usually brief in duration.

Patients with MVP are more likely to have atrial and ventricular arrhythmias than patients who do not have the condition. It is likely, but unproven, that patients with MVP have more "chest pain" during cardiac arrhythmias than subjects with palpitation who do not have MVP.

Relief of chest pain

The chest pain occurring in patients with MVP may be helped with beta-blockers, especially when premature atrial or ventricular contractions are controlled.

Associated Symptoms

Patients with MVP may complain of fatigue but this symptom was not mentioned in Freed's report. In most instances, fatigue is associated with anxiety or depression.

Dyspnea was reported by Freed et al. in 26.4% of their patients with MVP and in 21.1% of subjects without MVP ($P=0.13$).[6]

Syncope occurred in 3.6% of Freed's subjects with MVP, but occurred in 3% of patients without the condition.[6] None of Freed's patients died, but it is accepted that sudden death does occur rarely.

Freed did not comment on palpitation as a common symptom.[6] Others have previously reported that episodes of palpitation are more common in patients with MVP than in patients without the condition, but few investigators studied as many subjects in the general population as Freed and her group.

Associated Signs

Physical examination

Freed, et al. found that the body habitus of their patients supported the view of past observers; the patients with MVP were "leaner on the basis of body-mass index and waist-to-hip ratio than subjects without prolapse."[6] Because MVP is associated with other diseases it is prudent to remember to search for the clues to the diagnosis of Marfan syndrome, Ehlers-Danlos disease, and other collagen diseases.

Auscultation should be carried out by placing the diaphragm of the stethoscope at the cardiac apex, or left mid precordium, and listen while the patient squats and then stands. The systolic murmur of mitral valve regurgitation will decrease in intensity and move toward the second heart sound when the patient or subject squats and increase in intensity and move toward the first heart sound when the patient or subject stands. The systolic click also moves toward the second heart sound when the patient squats and toward the first heart sound when the patient stands but the intensity of the click changes very little with the change in posture. The click itself increases in intensity during handgrip, by turning the patient or subject to the left lateral decubitus, and after breathing amyl nitrite. The papillary muscles, chordae tendineae, and mitral valve leaflets are less slack when the left ventricle enlarges, as it does when the patient squats, compared to tenseness of these structures when the heart is smaller, as it is when the patient stands. Therefore, there is less mitral valve regurgitation when the subject squats than there is when the subject stands. There, of course, may be no audible mitral valve regurgitation or it may be mild to severe.

Signs of heart failure may develop in patients with severe mitral valve regurgitation but Freed and her group observed no patients with heart failure in the general population of subjects with MVP. Accordingly, patients who are hospitalized for heart failure represent exceptions to the rule.

"Routine" laboratory tests

Electrocardiograms may reveal left atrial abnormalities and left ventricular hypertrophy in patients with mitral regurgitation.[6]

The mean T vector may be directed away from the cardiac apex in some patients. The T wave may return to normal after mitral valve valvuloplasty.[10]

Freed et al. observed atrial fibrillation in only 1.2% of patients with MVP whereas the prevalence was 1.7% in patients without MVP. Obviously, hospitalized patients due to a complication of MVP would exhibit atrial fibrillation more often than patients with no prolapse.

The chest x-ray film is usually normal except when there is severe mitral regurgitation causing left atrial enlargement and left ventricular enlargement.

The "routine" blood work and chemical studies are within normal limits.

Exceptions to the Usual Manifestations

The following statements are included to emphasize that the "chest pain" observed in patients with MVP is usually due to anxiety or depression. The "chest pain" may, at times, be iatrogenetically created by the words and action of the physician. Still, as described above, a small percentage of patients have chest pain due to the prolapse.

The unusual manifestation of MVP are actually complications of the condition. *Rupture of one or more chordae tendineae* may produce abrupt mitral regurgitation. The systolic murmur may radiate up and down the spine, to the sacrum and top of the head. Acute pulmonary edema may develop, but the heart size may be only minimally enlarged.

Patients may develop *chronic heart failure* due to severe mitral regurgitation with intermittent episodes of increasing severity suggesting more prolapse, perhaps due to the breakage of secondary chords. In such patients the heart is usually enlarged.

A small number of patients with MVP will develop *infective endocarditis.* Some patients with MVP and normal rhythm have *cerebral emboli* thought to be due to fibrin deposits in the valve leaflets. Freed, however, observed strokes in 1.2% of their patients with MVP and in 1.5% of their control group.[6] Gilon, et al. have recently reported on the lack of evidence of an association between MVP and strokes in young women.[11]

Ventricular tachycardia may develop and sudden death may occur. Although these events are rare they leave a lasting impression on the physician and contribute to the erroneous view that MVP is always serious.

These complications serve to emphasize that the study of hospitalized patients gives an erroneous view of the prevalence of the disease and its complications.

Differential Diagnosis

The differential diagnosis of the "chest pain" related to MVP is discussed above.

The diagnosis of MVP is made by auscultation of the cardiac apex. The systolic click and late systolic murmur are diagnostic of the condition. Auscultating the area of the cardiac apex and left mid precordium in patients or subjects in whom the condition is suspected in the squat-stand positions and during a Valsalva maneuver usually confirms the diagnosis. See discussion under Physical Examination.

Other Diagnostic Testing

A two-dimensional echocardiogram should be performed at least once on patients believed to have MVP. It is needed for baseline purposes and to study the root of the aorta for possible forme fruste Marfan disease. Additional echocardiograms are not indicated after the initial echocardiogram in patients with isolated MVP unless the auscultatory findings change or endocarditis is suspected. Performing echocardiograms every 6 months on patients such as those described by Freed is probably harmful because it suggests to the patient that they have a serious disease, whereas most of them do not.

Freed et al., using two-dimensional echocardiography on a large number of community-based subjects, used the following echocardiographic criteria for the diagnosis of MVP.[6] *Classic mitral valve prolapse* was diagnosed when, in the parasternal long axis view, the mitral valve leaflets were displaced at least 2 millimeters above a line connecting the annular-hinge points and showing mitral valve thickness of ≥ 5 millimeters during diastole.[6] *Nonclassic prolapse* was diagnosed when the valve leaflets were displaced 2 millimeters above a line connecting the annular-hinge points but measured < 5 millimeters in thickness during diastole.[6] The degree of mitral regurgitation was graded as a trace, mild, moderate, or severe determined by relating the area of regurgitant jet to the size of the left atrium.[6]

Etiology and Basic Mechanisms Responsible for the "Pain"

Barlow states the most common cause of MVP in South Africa is rheumatic heart disease.[10] Mitral valve prolapse in the United States is sometimes due to *myxomatous degeneration* of the mitral valve leaflets and chordae tendineae. The aortic and tricuspid valve may be affected with the condition, but this is much less common than MVP. Mitral valve prolapse usually occurs as an isolated condition, but is commonly observed in patients with Marfan disease, Ehlers-Danlos disease, and other collagen diseases. Mitral valve prolapse also occurs as an *anatomic misfit* when the mitral valve leaflets and chords are not intrinsically diseased, at least early in life, but are simply larger and longer than they need to be to function in a harmonious manner. This anatomic misfit may be referred to *as a normal variant, or non-classic prolapse* as described by Freed.[6] Mitral valve prolapse may occur in several family members and a genetically determined predisposition is likely. The details of the genetic aspect of this condition, however, must wait until diagnostic criteria are agreed upon by all those investigating the problem.

The "chest pain" in most patients with MVP is not due to the prolapse. The mechanism responsible for the "chest pain" that *is* due to the prolapse is not actually known but the following hypothesis seems reasonable. When one views an echocardiogram or left ventricular angiogram of a patient with severe MVP and observes a portion of the left ventricular wall being pulled toward the mitral valve, one wonders why pain does not occur each time the left ventricle contracts. During the day the heart responds to normal activity by varying its size. For example, the heart is smaller when a patient stands than when he or she squats. Accordingly, as discussed earlier, there would be more vigorous pull on the chords and papillary muscles and the wall of the left ventricle, when the heart is small and the mitral valve apparatus is more relaxed. Many observers have wondered if this sequence of events could produce ischemia of the papillary muscles and left ventricle but this has not been proven.

It is more likely that simply stretching the papillary muscles plus the abnormal pull on the myocardium causes the "pain" as the heart changes in size in response to the usual maneuvers that occur during the day.

Treatment

Iatrogenic heart disease can be produced when physicians alarm patients with mild MVP by over-testing with too many echocardiograms and when they offer poor explanations for the cardiac findings. If the "chest pain," which is often due to anxiety or depression, is erroneously attributed to MVP by the physician, the patient may not improve. The anxiety or depression itself must be dealt with (see Chapters 45 and 46).

The reader is referred to the article by Carabello and Crawford[12] and the book *Hurst's The Heart* for the details of treatment for MVP.[13] Mitral valve surgery, including valvuloplasty or replacement, is indicated in a small percentage of patients. Antiarrhythmic treatment is commonly prescribed in patients with atrial and ventricular arrhythmias and endocarditis prophylaxis, as recommended by the American Heart Association, should be implemented.

References

1. Reid JV. Mid-systolic clicks. *S Afr Med J* 1961;35:353–355.
2. Barlow JB, Pocock WA, Marchand P, et al. The significance of late systolic murmurs. *Am Heart J* 1963;66:443–452.
3. Barlow JB, Bosman CK. Aneurysmal protrusion of the posterior leaflet of the mitral valve. *Am Heart J* 1966;71:166–178.
4. Devereux RB, Perloff JK, Reichek N, et al. Mitral valve prolapse. *Circulation* 1976;54:3–14.
5. Chesler E, Gornick CC. Maladies attributed to myxomatous mitral valve. *Circulation* 1991;82:328–332.
6. Freed LA, Levy D, Levine RA, et al. Prevalence and clinical outcome of mitral-valve prolapse. *N Engl J Med* 1999;341:1–7.
7. Levy D, Savage D. Prevalence and clinical features of mitral valve prolapse. *Am Heart J* 1987;113:1281–1290.
8. Barlow JB. Personal communication. March 23, 2000.
9. Criley JM. Personal communication. April 3, 2000.
10. Barlow JB. Idiopathic (degenerative) and rheumatic mitral valve prolapse: Historical aspects and an overview. *J Heart Valve Disease* 1992;1:163–174.
11. Gilon D, Buonanno FS, Joffe MLM, et al. Lack of evidence of an association between mitral-valve prolapse and stroke in young patients. *N Engl J Med* 1999;341:8–13.
12. Carabello BA, Crawford FA. Valvular heart disease. *N Engl J Med* 1997;337:32–41.
13. O'Rourke RA. Mitral valve prolapse syndrome. In: Alexander RW, Schlant RC, Fuster V (eds): *Hurst's The Heart, 9th Ed.* New York, McGraw-Hill Book Co, 1998, pp.1829–1830.

Part XIV

Final Comments

52

The Evolution of Our Knowledge and Remaining Problems

J. Willis Hurst, MD

The competence of a physician is tested when he or she attempts to establish the etiology of "chest pain." There are many causes of chest pain, and the physician who attempts to establish the cause must have a large knowledge base that includes all of the causes of "chest pain." The physician must also be highly skilled at extracting accurate information from patients, of whom they must ask carefully constructed questions. This skill is not learned in lectures. It is only learned by observing patients and correlating their symptoms with other data, including that obtained by high-tech procedures, and by follow-up observations.

At present the most skilled physicians are not always correct in their assessment of a patient's "chest pain." Experts are still humbled when their diagnoses are proven to be wrong. Knowing this we hope this little book will be helpful, although we recognize that it is far from complete. On the other hand, we believe we can do better than state that a patient has *noncardiac chest pain* after the coronary arteriogram shows no permanently obstructive coronary disease, or stating that a patient has *atypical chest pain*.

It is interesting to note how some of the "chest pain" syndromes of the past have "disappeared." The explanation lies in the fact that the conditions have not disappeared—only the *names* of the syndromes have disappeared.

Perhaps the most notable example of the disappearing act described above is the abandonment of the term *"neurocirculatory asthenia."* Before that term, the terms Decosta syndrome, soldier's heart, and effort syndrome were all used. One of the last articles written by Mandel Cohen and Paul

From: Hurst JW, Morris DC (eds): *"Chest Pain"* →. © Futura Publishing Co., Inc., Armonk, NY, 2001.

White in 1972 discusses the disorder under *anxiety* or *depression* and by doing so passes the syndrome to the psychiatrists or a combination of both conditions.[1]

The term pre-infarction angina has given way to the term *unstable angina pectoris.*

The term shoulder-hand syndrome, which has almost vanished, has been replaced by the term *complex regional pain syndrome.*

The term *pseudo-angina* was used in Osler's day. The term is no longer used. I suppose it has been replaced by "atypical angina" which is equally nondescript and confusing.

It is apparent at this point in the evolution of our knowledge that many patients have more than one cause for "chest pain." For example, the patient with stable angina pectoris may also be depressed. This creates a serious problem because depression alone can be associated with chest pain and, in the setting of proven stable angina, may alter the patient and physician's perception of what is actually happening.

Because anxiety and depression are so common, it is of paramount importance for the physician to recognize these conditions because they may be the sole cause of the patient's "chest pain" or the symptoms associated with these conditions may be superimposed on the "chest pain" due to angina pectoris. The anxiety and depression must be treated as serious conditions along with the angina pectoris.

High-tech procedures have enabled physicians to arrive at more correct diagnoses than they were able to make a few decades ago. In fact, coronary arteriography and echocardiography commonly clarify confusing clinical situations. No one can doubt the contribution these procedures have made. Still, it is the wise physician who chooses which of his patients with "chest pain" should have such procedures. Does the patient with end-stage Alzheimer's disease who seems to have "chest pain" really need to have a coronary arteriogram? I use that extreme question to highlight the fact that the impact of co-morbid diseases should have considerable influence on the decision to perform high-tech procedures on patients with "chest pain." Then, too, when a coronary arteriogram shows a 30%–40% narrowing of a coronary artery, the physician must then decide if the symptom complex could actually be caused by what was found. By all means the arteriographer and referring physicians should not tell the patient, "You have no significant coronary disease." They should say, "We found no lesions that are obstructing coronary blood flow at this time, but we did identify some non-obstructing lesions." The patient should be treated vigorously using all preventive measures that are known. Any lesion is significant whether or not it is obstructing. Under these circumstances the cause of the patient's chest pain has not been solved, but must not be ignored. The physician should, under these circumstances, look for one of the other causes of the chest pain that are discussed in this book.

Reference

1. Cohen ME, White PD. Neurocirculatory Asthenia: 1972 Concept. *Military Medicine* 1972;173(4):142–144.

Index

Page numbers followed by "t" indicate tables.